D1519796

EXERCISE
and
IMMUNE FUNCTION

NUTRITION in EXERCISE and SPORT

Editors, Ira Wolinsky and James F. Hickson, Jr.

Published Titles

Nutrients as Ergogenic Aids for Sports and Exercise
Luke Bucci

Nutrition in Exercise and Sport, 2nd Edition
Ira Wolinsky and James F. Hickson, Jr.

Exercise and Disease
Ronald R. Watson and Marianne Eisinger

Nutrition Applied to Injury Rehabilitation and Sports Medicine
Luke Bucci

Nutrition for the Recreational Athlete
Catherine G.R. Jackson

NUTRITION in EXERCISE and SPORT

Editor, Ira Wolinsky

Published Titles

Nutrition, Physical Activity, and Health in Early Life
Jana Pařízková

Exercise and Immune Function
Laurie Hoffman-Goetz

Sports Nutrition: Minerals and Electrolytes
Constance Kies and Judy Driskell

Forthcoming Titles

Nutrition and the Female Athlete
Jaime S. Rudd

Body Fluid Balance: Exercise and Sport
E.R. Buskirk and S. Puhl

Biochemical Methods for Exercise Assessment
Jon Karl Linderman

Handbook of Sports Nutrition: Vitamins and Trace Minerals
Ira Wolinsky and Judy Driskell

EXERCISE
and
IMMUNE
FUNCTION

Edited by
Laurie Hoffman-Goetz

CRC Press
Boca Raton   New York   London   Tokyo

Library of Congress Cataloging-in-Publication Data

Exercise and immune function / edited by Laurie Hoffman-Goetz
    p.   cm.— (Nutrition in exercise and sport)
    Includes bibliographical references and index.
    ISBN 0-8493-8190-8
    1. Exercise—Immunological aspects. I. Hoffman-Goetz, Laurie
II. Series.
QP301.E935   1996
616.07'9—dc20   95-46107
                                                                      CIP

© 1996 by CRC Press, Inc.

No claim to original U.S. Government works
International Standard Book Number 0-8493-8190-8
Library of Congress Card Number 95-46107
Printed in the United States of America 1 2 3 4 5 6 7 8 9 0
Printed on acid-free paper

SERIES PREFACE

The CRC series on *Nutrition in Exercise and Sport* provides a setting for in-depth exploration of the many and varied aspects of nutrition and exercise, including sports. The topic of exercise and sports nutrition has been a focus of research among scientists since the 1960s, and the healthful benefits of good nutrition and exercise have been appreciated. As our knowledge expands, it will be necessary to remember that there must be a range of diets and exercise regimes that will support excellent physical condition and performance. There is not a single diet-exercise treatment that can be the common denominator, or the single formula for health, or panacea for performance.

This series is dedicated to providing a stage to explore these issues. Each volume provides a detailed and scholarly examination of some aspect of the topic.

Contributors from any bona fide area of nutrition and physical activity, including sports and the controversial, are welcome.

We welcome to the series the invaluable contribution *Exercise and Immune Function* by L. Hoffman-Goetz.

Ira Wolinsky, Ph.D.
Series Editor

Over the past few years, numerous experimental and clinical studies have been published on the effect of exercise on various facets of specific and innate immunity. This work has led to the formation of a new field of exercise immunology within the larger parent disciplines of immunology and of exercise physiology. What has accounted for the rapid development of this new interdisciplinary subdiscipline? First, there has been increased interest by coaches and athletes to find ways to reduce the perceived risk of respiratory tract infections associated with competition and overtraining. This approach is grounded in a strategy of illness prevention that involves high-risk individuals. Exercise immunology could theoretically contribute to preventive action by helping to identify the critical exposure window when an athlete is most susceptible. The second factor leading to the development of exercise immunology as a field of scientific inquiry is rooted in the population health perspective. This approach focuses on identifying relevant risk factors and shifting the whole risk distribution of a population for any given disease (such as colon cancer or rheumatoid arthritis). In this strategy, even though individual health benefits may be quite small, the total benefit to the health of the population may be substantial. Here, exercise-associated changes in immune functions could have applications in risk reduction of certain cancers by enhancing innate immune surveillance or by slowing the progression of tumors which are responsive to immunotherapeutic modalities. The third factor which has contributed to the growth of exercise immunology as a field is the parallel development of psychoneuroimmunology. Exercise can be viewed as a repeatable and quantifiable stressor which can be easily manipulated experimentally. This allows the controlled testing of hypotheses on the roles of neuroendocrine and cytokine signals in the feedback between the central nervous and the immune systems in response to physical stress.

This volume brings together experts in the area of exercise immunology to critically review the evidence for exercise-induced changes in immunity, and to evaluate this evidence within a framework for human health. The two opening chapters consider the hormonal consequences of exercise and stress, and how neuroendocrine factors influence the immune system. Chapters 3 and 4 focus on cytokine and acute-phase responses during exercise: cytokines will likely prove to be key players in the exercise-immune response link involved in local regulation of immune responses and providing coordinated information to the brain about systemic immunological changes occurring with exercise. Current reviews on the specific immunological responses, primarily in humans, to acute exercise, training, and overtraining are included in Chapters 5, 6, and 7. Chapters 8 through 11 deal specifically with the health implications of exercise-induced changes in immune function for infectious disease, autoimmunity, colon cancer, and aging. Chapters 12 and 13 address contemporary health behavioral concerns of addiction and substance abuse, and the increasingly prevalent phenomenon of dieting in the context of exercise and exercise-associated changes in immunity.

The work presented in this book provides strong evidence that exercise is an important human behavior which influences the immune response. While some of the effects observed are quite transient, others appear to have more long-lasting consequences for immune regulation. The question of whether such changes can contribute to the developent of individual and population-based health promotion strategies to reduce the development of certain pathological states will need to be addressed in the future.

Laurie Hoffman-Goetz, Ph.D.

THE EDITOR

Laurie Hoffman-Goetz, Ph.D., is Professor of Health Studies and Gerontology and of Kinesiology, in the Faculty of Applied Health Sciences at the University of Waterloo, Ontario, Canada.

Dr. Hoffman-Goetz obtained her B.A. degree from the State University of New York at Binghamton in 1974, and her M.A. and Ph.D. degrees in 1976 and 1979 from the University of Michigan. she was appointed an Assistant Professor of Health Studies at the University of Waterloo in 1980, an Associate Professor in 1986 and a Full Professor in 1992. She has also worked as a Fellow in the Division of Cancer Prevention and Control, National Cancer Institute, National Institutes of Health, Bethesda, Maryland.

Dr. Hoffman-Goetz is a member of the American Physiological Society, American Society for Cancer Research, American College of Sports Medicine, Canadian Society for Immunology, Canadian Society for Nutritional Sciences, and International Society of Exercise and Immunology. She has served on the editorial boards of the *Journal of Sports Medicine* and *Physical Fitness.* She has been the recipient of many research grants and contracts from the National Sciences and Engineering Research Council of Canada, the Canadian Lifestyle and Fitness Research Institute, and the Department of Defence (Canada).

Dr. Hoffman-Goetz is the author of more than 50 papers and 10 book chapters. Her current major research interests relate to the modulation of innate immunity by physical activity and stress and population-based studies on exercise and cancer.

CONTRIBUTORS

Gregory J. Bagby, Ph.D.
Department of Physiology, Louisiana State University Medical Center, New Orleans, Louisiana

Sally E. Blank, Ph.D.
Department of Kinesiology and Leisure Studies, Washington State University, Pullman, Washington

Joseph G. Cannon, Ph.D.
Noll Physiological Research Center, Pennsylvania State University, University Park, Pennsylvania

Carole A. Conn, Ph.D.
The Lovelace Institutes, IBAMR, Albuquerque, New Mexico

Larry D. Crouch, Ph.D.
Department of Physiology, Louisiana State University Medical Center, New Orleans, Louisiana

Flemming Dela, Ph.D.
Department of Medical Physiology, The Panum Institute and Department of Orthopedic Surgery, Gentofte Hospital, Copenhagen, Denmark

Arnaud Ferry, Ph.D.
Laboratoire de Physiologie des Adaptations, University of René Descartes, Paris, France

Laurie Hoffman-Goetz, Ph.D.
Department of Health Sciences and Gerontology, Faculty of Applied Health Sciences, University of Waterloo, Ontario, Canada

Janice Husted, Ph.D.
Department of Health Sciences and Gerontology, Faculty of Applied Health Sciences, University of Waterloo, Ontario, Canada

David Keast, Ph.D.
Department of Microbiology, The University of Western Australia, Nedlands, Australia

Michael Kjaer, M.D., D.M.Sci.
Copenhagen Muscle Research Center, National University Hospital and Department of Rheumatology, Bispeberg Hospital, Copenhagen, Denmark

Alex Kusnecov, Ph.D.
Department of Pathology, University of Pittsburgh School of Medicine, Pittsburgh, Pennsylvania

Robert S. Mazzeo, Ph.D.
Department of Kinesiology, University of Colorado, Boulder, Colorado

Gary G. Meadows, Ph.D.
Department of Pharmaceutical Sciences, Washington State University, Pullman, Washington

Niall M. Moyna, Ph.D.
Department of Pathology, University of Pittsburgh School of Medicine, Pittsburgh, Pennsylvania

David C. Nieman, Dr. PH.
Department of Health and Exercise Science, Appalachian State University, Boone, North Carolina

Bente Klarlund Pedersen, M.D., D.M. Sci.
Copenhagen Muscle Research Center and Department of Infectious Diseases, National University Hospital, Copenhagen, Denmark

Bruce S. Rabin, M.D., Ph.D.
Division of Clinical Immunology, Department of Pathology, University of Pittsburgh School of Medicine, Pittsburgh, Pennsylvania

Pang N. Shek, Ph.D.
Department of Clinical Immunology, University of Toronto and Defence and Civil Institute of Environmental Medicine, North York, Ontario, Canada

Roy J. Shephard, M.D., Ph.D., D.P.E.
School of Physical and Health Education, University of Toronto and Health Sciences Programme, Brock University, St. Catharines, Ontario, Canada

Raymond E. Shepherd, Ph.D.
Department of Physiology, Louisiana State University Medical Center, New Orleans, Louisiana

Michael R. Shurin, Ph.D.
Department of Pathology, University of Pittsburgh School of Medicine, Pittsburgh, Pennsylvania

Daohong Zhou, M.D.
Department of Pathology, University of Pittsburgh School of Medicine, Pittsburgh, Pennsylvania

CONTENTS

Chapter **1**

ENDOCRINE RESPONSES TO EXERCISE

Michael Kjaer
Flemming Dela

CONTENTS

0-8493-8190-8/96/$0.00+$.50
© 1996 by CRC Press, Inc.

1

I. INTRODUCTION

Exercise causes a 20- to 25-fold increase in whole body energy metabolism, and oxygen uptake can increase from resting levels of approximately 0.3 l/min and up to 6–7 l/min in highly trained endurance athletes. This results in an increased glycolysis and glycogenolysis in muscle tissue, an increased glycogenolysis and gluconeogenesis in the liver, an increased lipolytic activity in adipose tissue as well as in intramuscular fat depots, and to a minor extent an increased protein breakdown in muscle tissue. These dramatic changes in fuel requirements, together with cardiovascular adjustments needed to accomplish the increased demand for muscle tissue oxygen supply, require a strong regulation in order to maintain internal homeostasis during exercise. Changes in autonomic nervous activity and in hormone secretion are central in this respect; and the present chapter will review the hormonal responses to acute exercise as well as the adaptation to training, in order to provide basis for understanding of a possible coupling of changes in the hormonal system and the immune system during physical activity[47] (see Chapter 5).

II. HORMONAL RESPONSES TO ACUTE EXERCISE REGULATION

A. CATECHOLAMINES (NOREPINEPHRINE, EPINEPHRINE)

Arterial plasma concentrations of norepinephrine and epinephrine increase almost linearly with duration of dynamic exercise (Figure 1), and exponentially with intensity (Figure 1) when this is expressed relative to the individual's maximal oxygen uptake (% $\dot{V}O_2$max).[12,24,51,56,66,126] The fact that the catecholamine response is related to the relative (% $\dot{V}O_2$max) rather than to the absolute work load (watts) is derived from experiments comparing exercise performed with small and large muscle groups at similar $\dot{V}O_2$,[71] and by manipulating the relative work load comparing exercise responses at normoxia and hypoxia.[27,63] The catecholamine response to exercise is detectable in arterial blood within 30 to 60 s from start of muscle contraction, and stimulation of this release starts immediately after onset of exercise. This is supported by experiments in which high intensity exercise of only 6-s duration resulted in marked increases in plasma levels of norepinephrine and epinephrine.[67]

Epinephrine is released from the adrenal medulla, and increases in plasma levels during exercise are likely to reflect true changes in hormonal release, inasmuch as clearance only changes slightly with duration and intensity of exercise both in humans and in dogs.[5,64,83] The half-life of epinephrine is approximately 2 min, which stresses the point that blood sampling of this hormone (and others) should be done during, rather than after, exercise.[54]

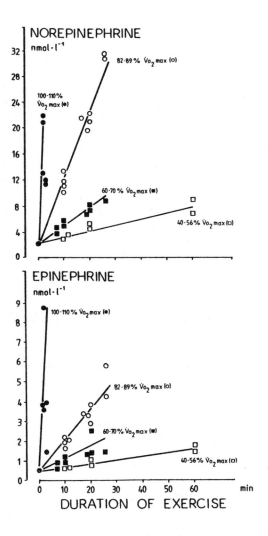

FIGURE 1 Arterial plasma concentrations of plasma norepinephrine and epinephrine in healthy subjects at rest (circle with cross) and during treadmill or cycle exercise at various intensities expressed as percent of individual maximal oxygen uptake. Data are given for mild (40 to 56%), moderate (60 to 70%), hard (82 to 89%), or intense (100 to 110%) exercise. Rest values are means of 63 subjects of different training status, and exercise values represent a mean value of 6 to 10 subjects. (Modified from *Int. J. Sports Med.*, 10, 2–15, 1989. With permission.)

Norepinephrine is released from sympathetic nerve terminals, and turnover studies have shown that skeletal muscle is a major source for the rise in plasma norepinephrine during exercise in both humans and other species.[83,91,97,98] In addition, probably a release from adrenergic neurons in the central nervous system (CNS) takes place during intense exercise,[89] a release that may contribute to adrenergic acceleration of brain metabolism, and is responsible for the increase in peripheral sympathoadrenergic activity during exercise.[99]

Several factors influence the catecholamine response. From experiments using tubocurarine to produce partial neuromuscular paralysis, whereby muscle strength was markedly reduced and motor center activity therefore increased in order to produce a certain work output, it was shown that catecholamine responses were exaggerated compared to experiments without blockade.[60] This indicates, together with findings in paralyzed and decorticated cats undergoing electrical stimulation of subthalamic motor centers, that motor center activity in the brain can directly stimulate sympathoadrenergic activity during exercise — independent of feedback from the contracting muscle.[60,116] However, it is also evident that motor center activity cannot explain the full catecholamine response to exercise,[60] and feedback mechanisms are equally important — either mediated as blood-borne metabolic or nonmetabolic error signals or through afferent nerves from exercising muscles. In evidence of an importance of neural reflex mechanisms for catecholamine responses during exercise, the response was diminished during static exercise in man when afferent nerve fibers from the contracting muscles were blocked by epidural anesthesia.[61] Furthermore, evidence has been provided from cat studies in which electrical stimulation of the muscle afferents in anesthetized animals increased catecholamines, and electrically induced isometric muscle contractions reflexly increased sympathetic nerve activity to adrenomedullary chromaffin cells.[115,117] What the exact signal from the muscle is due to is at present not fully explained, but it is suggested that both mechanoreceptors and metaboreceptors are involved and that factors such as pH — and maybe potassium and adenosine — may play a role for sympathoadrenergic response to exercise.[26,114] Temperature influences the catecholamine responses, and during hyperthermia the norepinephrine response is exaggerated.[96] Epinephrine is in contrast to norepinephrine largely influenced by the plasma glucose concentration,[33] emphasizing that the preexercise state of feeding (fasted vs. fed, high carbohydrate vs. carbohydrate poor) can markedly influence the epinephrine response to exercise; the lower the plasma glucose, the higher the epinephrine response will be. Especially during prolonged exercise, a decrease in plasma glucose results in dramatic changes in plasma epinephrine.[33] Finally, it is noteworthy that in women the catecholamine response to exercise changes with the menstrual cycle, and is more pronounced in the follicular phase compared with the luteal phase.[106]

Norepinephrine not only has major cardiovascular effects, regulating cardiac output as well as redistribution of blood flow to exercising muscles during exercise, but also exerts metabolic effects. It has been demonstrated that norepinephrine is a strong stimulator of lipolysis in adipose tissue, whereas the stimulation of muscle lipolysis is moderate.[11,120,130] Norepinephrine is only a very weak stimulator of muscle glycogenolysis and is unlikely to play any important role in hepatic glycogenolysis and gluconeogenesis during exercise.[123]

The primary effect of epinephrine during exercise is to increase glycogenolysis in muscle and to some extent in liver,[41,52,80,92-94,103] as well as to increase lipolysis in both adipose tissue and muscle.[4,120]

B. PANCREATIC HORMONES (INSULIN, GLUCAGON)

Insulin is secreted from the pancreatic beta cells and exerts three important effects: (1) facilitation of glucose uptake in muscle and adipose tissue by translocation of glucose transporting proteins (so-called GLUT4) to the sarcolemma, (2) inhibition of glucose output from the liver, and (3) inhibition of lipolysis by reducing activity of hormone-sensitive lipases. During exercise, however, insulin is not needed for the glucose uptake in skeletal muscle, and the effects of insulin and muscle contraction are additive.[87] A presence of high insulin plasma levels will therefore result in exercise-induced hypoglycemia due to accelerated glucose uptake in peripheral tissue (e.g., contracting muscle). Therefore it seems appropriate that insulin concentrations in contrast to most other hormones decrease with exercise in an intensity-dependent (Table 1) fashion if this is above 40 to 50% $\dot{V}O_2$max.[32,54,56,88,119] This decrease is due to alpha-adrenergic inhibition of insulin secretion,[32,42,48] and the decreased insulin during exercise facilitates fuel supply for the contracting muscle (Figure 2).

During mild exercise plasma glucagon increases almost linearly with duration in several nonhuman species,[8,121,122] whereas only a moderate increase in glucagon in humans is found approximately 1 h into prolonged exercise[31] (Table 1). This rise is mainly regulated by the plasma concentration of glucose, a decrease in plasma glucose being a potent stimulator for glucagon release.[33] Although adrenergic inhibition of insulin release is evident, adrenergic mechanisms are likely to play only a minor role for glucagon responses. However,

TABLE 1   Typical Changes in Arterial Plasma Levels of Hormones During Intense Exercise (90–100% VO₂max) and Moderate Exercise (60–70% VO₂max) to Exhaustion in Sedentary or Moderately Trained Postabsorptive Individuals

Hormone	Intense Exercise (5–10 min)	Moderate Exercise (60–90 min)
Norepinephrine	1200–1800%	800–1200%
Epinephrine	1200–1800%	500–800%
Insulin	60–70%	40–75%
Glucagon	70–75%	100–150%
Growth hormone	700–900%	300–500%
Adrenocorticotropin	150–200%	150–200%
Cortisol	—	—
Beta endorphin	300–500%	150–200%

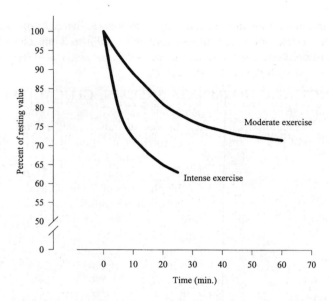

FIGURE 2 Typical changes in arterial plasma concentration of insulin during moderate (60 to 70% VO_2max) or intense exercise (90-100% VO_2max).

because during intense exercise glucagon levels decrease for the first 15 to 20 min (Table 1), it is likely that neural mechanisms inhibit glucagon release during early stages of intense exercise.[54]

The most important metabolic effect of an increased plasma concentration of glucagon probably is the rise in hepatic glucose production which has been demonstrated in running dogs.[94] In humans, no rise is found in glucagon until late during prolonged exercise, and in humans glucagon might therefore be important for regulation of hepatic glycogenolysis and gluconeogenesis only in the latter phase of exercise where blood glucose is likely to decrease.[33,52,128]

C. PITUITARY AND ADRENOCORTICOTROPIC HORMONES (GH, ACTH, ENDORPHINS, CORTISOL)

Plasma levels of pituitary hormones increase in response to exercise both with duration and with intensity of exercise[31,63] (Table 1). Growth hormone (GH), adrenocorticotropin (ACTH), and beta endorphin are all released from the anterior pituitary gland in a pulsatile manner. Irregular time courses for changes in plasma GH have therefore been found; and if exercise duration is short, peak GH values are not obtained until after termination of exercise.[54,107,113] Taken together, GH response is more related to the peak exercise intensity rather than to duration of exercise or total work output.[113] This fits well with the concept that growth hormone responses are closely linked to the degree of perceived exertion and probably motor center activity.[60] This is supported by findings in spinal cord injured individuals in whom GH did not rise during involuntary electrically induced exercise with paralyzed muscle where no motor center activity was present, whereas GH rose when voluntary exercise was conducted with the arms[59] (Figure 3).

Concentration of ACTH increases with duration of exercise if intensity is above 25% $\dot{V}O_2$max, and with a delay of approximately 10 min plasma cortisol also increases during exercise[31,54,107] (Figure 4). Regulation of ACTH response to exercise is influenced by both motor center activity,[60] by activity in muscle afferent nerves,[62,115] and by a drop in blood glucose levels.[109] The metabolic importance of cortisol during exercise is not clear. Lack of glucocorticoids in rats inhibits their endurance capacity, suggesting a role for cortisol in activating gluconeogenesis during mild prolonged exercise.[102]

Beta-endorphin concentrations rise in plasma during prolonged exercise if intensity is above 50% $\dot{V}O_2$max, and during maximal exercise if this is performed for a minimum of 3 min.[29,54,68,76] At low work loads no rise in beta-endorphin levels was found despite extremely long exposure time (1000 km running over 7 d).[85] In animals, not only plasma changes, but also increases in beta-endorphin content in the cerebrospinal fluid have been found in running rats.[40] Feedback mechanisms mediated via afferent muscle nerves are probably important for beta-endorphin responses to exercise in man. This is true since blockade of afferent muscle nerves abolishes the beta-endorphin responses to submaximal exercise,[62] and furthermore since beta-endorphin levels increased as a result of electrical stimulation of the muscle afferents in paralyzed cats.[115]

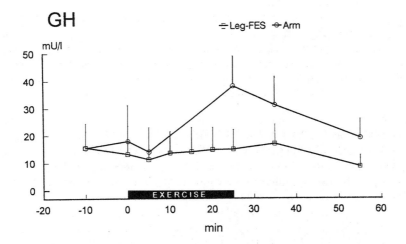

FIGURE 3 Plasma concentrations of growth hormone (GH) before, during, and after involuntary electrically induced bicycling with paralyzed legs (Leg-FES) on an ergometer equipment in six spinal cord injured tetraplegic males. Control experiments consisted of voluntary arm cranking in the tetraplegics (Arm). Although GH rose in response to voluntary arm cranking, no rise was found during involuntary exercise with the paralyzed legs.

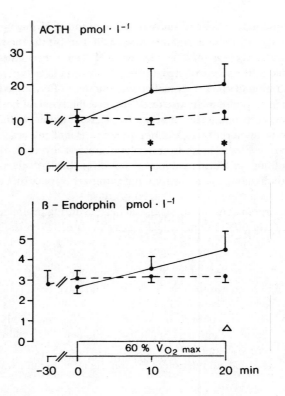

FIGURE 4 Plasma concentrations of adrenocorticotropin (ACTH) and beta endorphin at rest and during exercise at 65 to 70% VO₂max with and without afferent neural feedback from working muscles due to epidural blockade at vertebrae L3–L4 in six healthy males. Concentrations of ACTH and beta endorphin only increased in experiments without blockade. (●—●) Control; (●- - -●) epidural blockade; n = 6. (Adapted from *Am. J. Physiol.,* 257, E95–101, 1989. With permission.)

The role of beta endorphin in exercise metabolism and especially in relation to exercise euphoria (so-called runners high) is unclear. Changes in mood during and after exercise in humans have not been influenced by administration of naloxone, an opioid receptor blocker; and despite an increased pain threshold in response to exercise, this was not altered by opioid receptor blockade.[25,75]

D. FLUID-REGULATING HORMONES (RENIN, ALDOSTERONE, ANGIOTENSIN, VASOPRESSIN, ANF, ERYTHROPOIETIN)

Acute exercise results in increased levels of renin, aldosterone, angiotensin, and vasopressin.[34] This is following the exercise-induced reduction in plasma volume,[34] and is to a large extent mediated via sympathetic activation.[53,72,131] In addition to this, high levels of potassium that are found during intense exercise may influence aldosterone responses.[77] Futhermore, in women the concentration of these hormones varies with time of the menstrual cycle.[45] Atrial natriuretic peptide (ANP) or factor (ANF) increases during acute exercise, and this is probably related to the exercise-induced increase in atrial filling pressure[35] and due to sympathetic activation.[110] Erythropoietin levels do not increase in response to acute exercise of less than several hours,[27,100,101] but after a period of training the increase in plasma volume is followed by an increased erythropoietin level and in turn a rise in red cell mass.[118] However, during everyday life conditions serum erythropoietin levels are identical in sedentary and highly trained subjects,[65] but large diurnal variations in serum erythropoietin levels exist irrespective of the level of physical activity.[65]

E. REPRODUCTIVE HORMONES (FSH, LH, ESTRADIOL, PROGESTERONE, TESTOSTERONE)

In general, there are no changes in gonadotropic hormones FSH and LH during exercise either in females or in males.[31] Independent of this, the plasma levels of gonadal hormones, estradiol, progesterone, and testosterone increase during exercise dependent on the work load.[7,45,105] The main reason for this increase in plasma hormonal levels is a decrease in metabolic clearance of the hormones rather than an increased secretion during exercise.[49] With prolonged physical training, resting levels of both gonadotropic and gonadal hormones are diminished. This results in hypothalamic hypogonadism in both sexes.[15,74] Endurance-trained women experience a reversible amenorrhea; and endurance-trained male athletes have lower testosterone levels compared to sedentary counterparts,[36,124] but maintain their pulsatile release of LH. The functional significance of this latter finding is, however, unclear.

F. VASOACTIVE PEPTIDES (NPY, VIP, ENDOTHELIN, CGRP)

Neuropeptide Y (NPY) is cosecreted with norepinephrine from sympathetic nerve endings and is released in response to intense exercise.[62,82] The peptide is not known to have metabolic effects during exercise, but is probably involved in the sympathetic control of vascular tone both in skeletal muscle and in the splanchnic and the renal region during exercise.[2]

Vasoactive intestinal polypeptide (VIP) increases in plasma during prolonged exercise, but not during short-term intense exercise;[31] and the increase can be blunted by ingestion of glucose.[81]

Endothelin is known to be released from endothelial cells and acts as a vasoconstrictor.[129] During exercise, levels initially decrease, followed by an increase after more than 1 h of exercise at submaximal levels.[90]

Calcitonin gene related peptide (CGRP) is a potent vasodilator. Recently a rise was found during intense exercise in healthy subjects only if this was of a certain duration[9,112] (M. Kjaer, T. Mohr, and F. Dela, unpublished observation). The release of CGRP did not originate from the contracting muscle and occurred too slow to be important for the increased blood flow in exercising muscle. Furthermore, in spinal cord injured individuals, the rise in CGRP was marked during involuntary electrically induced exercise with paralyzed muscle; and it is possible that CGRP release in these subjects is involved in regulation of cardiac function and vascular tone, e.g., regulation of subcutaneous blood flow during exercise.[39,50]

III. ADAPTATION OF HORMONAL SECRETION TO TRAINING

A. RESTING HORMONAL LEVELS

Plasma norepinephrine levels are, in general, found to be unrelated to training status;[51,84,108] and the same goes for muscle sympathetic nerve activity to leg muscle,[108] indicating that training does not influence sympathetic nervous activity. However, a few studies have shown conflicting results, suggesting a decrease in norepinephrine levels after a period of training[38,43] Several studies indicate that epinephrine concentrations are not altered by short periods of training [43,70,108,126] whereas studies on athletes who have been training for years have shown elevated levels of epinephrine, indicating that long-term adaptations to training may result in increased adrenal medullary secretion capacity.[51] In the fasting state, plasma levels of insulin are found to be lower in athletes compared to sedentary subjects;[54,127] and during everday life conditions, plasma insulin concentrations are also lower in athletes compared to sedentary people.[21] This is probably due to an increased hepatic clearance of insulin in athletes, as plasma concentrations of C peptide (which is not metabolized in the liver) do not differ between trained and untrained subjects.[21] Some authors have found an increased level of ACTH and cortisol in highly trained subjects.[73] This was, however, not a uniform finding;[36,54] and the difference between results obtained from different experiments could be related to lack of sufficient recovery between training sessions. In accordance with this, it has been suggested that the ratio between cortisol and testosterone — where cortisol increases and testosterone decreases — is an indicator of periods with so-called overtraining.[3] Although the overall correlation between this ratio and overtraining (expressed as a reduction in performance) might be acceptable, the day-to-day variation in these measurements makes it unlikely for it to be of any practical value for the individual athletes in monitoring training intensity and duration.[37]

B. HORMONAL CHANGES DURING EXERCISE

The magnitude of hormonal responses to a given absolute work load decreases after just a short a period of physical training.[126] In addition to this, highly trained athletes (who have trained for several years) also have a lower hormonal response to a given absolute work load as compared to untrained subjects.[63] This supports that the hormonal response to exercise is dependent on the relative ($\dot{V}O_2$max) rather than on the absolute work load, and is supported by findings in man manipulating the relative work load with the use of hypoxia.[63] Interestingly, however, the adaptation of the hormonal response to training occurs very rapidly and is even faster than the adaptation of $\dot{V}O_2$max.[126] This indicates that factors other than the relative work load influence the response. In highly long-term trained endurance athletes, the hormonal response to a given relative work load and to maximal exercise has been found to be higher compared to responses for untrained subjects.[51] This holds true for both catecholamines and pituitary hormones.[10,29,54] For epinephrine, clearance is identical for trained and untrained subjects, indicating that the higher epinephrine response in trained subjects may be due to increased adrenal medullary secretion capacity.[64] This increased secretion capacity in long-term trained athletes has also been found in response to nonexercise stimuli such as hypoglycemia, hypoxia, hypercapnia, glucagon, and caffeine.[55,57,63,69] In addition to this, 10 weeks of endurance training in rats resulted in a higher content of epinephrine in adrenal medullary tissue as well as in a larger adrenal medullary volume as compared to rats that were weight-matched sedentary controls, sham trained, or cold stressed.[104] The development of such a sports adrenal medulla probably requires a long-term adaptation to training, since short-term changes in the level of physical training, such as 5 weeks of detraining in athletes, did not result in any major alteration in the epinephrine response to hypoglycemia.[58] Trained subjects probably stimulate their adrenal medullary release of epinephrine more than untrained subjects because the 24-h release of epinephrine, defined as the total elevation above baseline values (during everyday activity including training sessions), is more pronounced in well-trained endurance athletes compared to sedentary controls.[22] An increased capacity to secrete epinephrine might be important for exercise performance, taking into account the variety of effects this hormone has on cardiovacular and muscle function, and the fact that adrenergic blockade reduces the exercise performance.[28,44,46,111]

IV. ADAPTATION OF TARGET TISSUE HORMONE SENSITIVITY TO TRAINING

A. CATECHOLAMINES

In addition to an increased epinephrine secretion capacity in trained subjects, the peripheral effects of catecholamines are also enhanced, which explains why trained individuals at submaximal work loads require a smaller rise in plasma catecholamines than sedentary subjects. As an example, the sensitivity of beta-receptor-mediated lipolysis in adipose tissue to catecholamines is increased after training without increasing the numbers of receptors.[13,14,30,125] Training has been shown to decrease alpha-adrenergic and to increase beta-adrenergic pathway efficiency, favoring utilization of fatty acids relative to carbohydrate as fuel in the trained organism.[4,95]

B. INSULIN

Insulin-stimulated glucose uptake in skeletal muscle increases with physical training. The mechanism behind the increased insulin action is partly due to a training-induced increase in insulin-mediated blood flow (increasing glucose delivery to the trained muscles), and partly due to an increase in the ability to extract glucose from the blood.[17,18] The latter is the consequence of a training-induced increase in the content of GLUT4 in the muscles, an increase in capillary density (resulting in longer mean transit time), and an increase in enzyme activities in the glycogenic and glycolytic pathway.[1,16,17,23,78,86] The increased tissue-insulin sensitivity in trained subjects should allow for a reduction in insulin release in response to a certain stimulus, and interestingly it seems that the pancreatic beta cells adapt to training by lowering the response to hyperglycemia. Thus, in healthy endurance-trained humans the glucose- and arginine-stimulated insulin secretion is decreased in the resting state.[19,20,79] The mechanism behind this adaptation is not fully understood. It is not due to a lower average daily plasma glucose concentration in the athletes.[21] Rather it is possibly due to frequent high sympathoadrenal activity elicited during the necessary exercise bouts.[22]

The decreased insulin level in trained subjects both during rest and during stimulation could be considered beneficial in relation to health because high plasma insulin concentrations has been associated with the risk of developing atherosclerosis. However, during daily life, the sparing of insulin secretion in response to a given stimulus is outweighed by a higher food intake in athletes compared with sedentary people.[20,21]

V. CONCLUSIONS

During exercise the metabolic processes are regulated by increases in autonomic nervous activity as well as by increased secretion of hormones from endocrine glands. The most important neuroendocrine response is an increased sympathoadrenal activity with a resultant suppression of insulin secretion from the pancreas. Signals involved in these exercise-induced responses are both related to motor center activity in the brain (feed-forward) and to metabolic and neural feedback from contracting muscle. Physical training alters both resting concentrations and exercise responses of most hormones. These changes are accompanied by changes in target tissue sensitivity/responsiveness to both catecholamines and insulin.

ACKNOWLEDGMENTS

The study was supported by grants from The Danish National Research Foundation (J.nr. 504-14), The Danish Medical Association Research Foundation, and The Danish Sports Research Council.

REFERENCES

1. Abernethy, P. J., Thayer, R., and Taylor, A. W., Acute and chronic responses of skeletal muscle to endurance and sprint exercise, *Sports Med.*, 6, 365, 1990.
2. Ahlborg, G., Weitzberg, E., and Lundberg, J. M., Neuropeptide Y modifies the splanchnic glycogenolytic response to epinephrine, *Proc. 8th Int. Biochem. Exerc. Conf.*, 134 (Abst.), 1992.
3. Alen, M., Pakarinen, A., Häkkinen, K., and Komi, P. V., Responses of serum androgenic-anabolic and catabolic hormones to prolonged strength training, *Int. J. Sports Med.*, 9, 229, 1988.
4. Arner, P., Kriegholm, E., Engfeldt, P., and Bolinder, J., Adrenergic regulation of lipolysis in situ at rest and during exercise, *J. Clin. Invest.*, 85, 893, 1990.
5. Beliveau, L., Peronnet, F., Trudeau, F., Brisson, G., and Nadeau, R., Plasma catecholamines in the aorta and the phrenicoabdominal vein in exercising dogs, *J. Appl. Physiol.*, 69, 604, 1990.
6. Bloom, S. R., Johnson, R. H., Park, D. M., Rennie, M. J., and Sulaiman, W. R., Differences in the metabolic and hormonal response to exercise between racing cyclists and untrained individuals, *J. Physiol.*, 258, 1, 1976.
7. Bonen, A., Ling, W. Y., MacIntyre, K. P., Neil, R., McGrail, J. C., and Belcastro, A. N., Effects of exercise on the serum concetrations of FSH, LH, progesterone and estradiol, *Eur. J. Appl. Physiol. Occup. Physiol.*, 42: 15, 1979.
8. Brockman, R. P., Effect of somatostatin on plasma glucagon and insulin, and glucose turnover in exercising sheep, *J. Appl. Physiol.*, 47, 273, 1979.
9. Brooks, S., Nevill, M. E., Meleagros, L., Lakomy, H. K. A., Hall, G. M., Bloom, S. R., and Williams, C., The hormonal response to brief maximal exercise in humans, *Eur. J. Appl. Physiol. Occup. Physiol.*, 60, 144, 1990.
10. Bunt, J. C., Boileau, R. A., Bahr, J. M., and Nelson, R. A., Sex and training differences in human growth hormone levels during prolonged exercise, *J. Appl. Physiol.*, 61, 1796, 1986.
11. Cleroux, J., van Nguyen, P., Taylor, A., and Leenen, F. H., Effects of ß1 vs ß1+ß2 blockade on exercise endurance and muscle metabolism in humans, *J. Appl. Physiol.*, 66, 548, 1989.
12. Cosineau, D., Ferguson, R. J., de Champlain, J., Gauthier, P., Cote, P., and Bourassa, M., Catecholamines in coronary sinus during exercise in man before and after training, *J. Appl. Physiol.*, 43, 80, 1978.
13. Crampes, F., Beauville, M., Riviere, D., and Garrigues, M., Effect of indurance training and chronic isoproterenol treatment on skeletal muscle sensivity to norepinephrine, *Life Sci.*, 37, 695, 1968.
14. Crampes, F., Beauville, M., Riviere, D., and Garrigues, M. Effect of physical training in humans on the response of isolated fat cells to epinephrine, *J. Appl. Physiol.*, 61, 25, 1986.
15. Cumming, D. C., Vickovic, M. M., Wall, S. R., and Fluker, M. R., Defects in pulsatile LH release in normally menstruating runners, *J. Clin. Endocrinol. Metab.*, 60, 810, 1985.
16. Dela, F., Handberg, A., Mikines, K. J., Vinten, J., and Galbo, H., GLUT 4 and insulin receptor binding and kinase activity in trained human muscle, *J. Physiol. (London)*, 469, 615, 1993.

17. Dela, F., Mikines, K. J., Larsen, J. J., Ploug, T., Petersen, L. N., and Galbo, H., Insulin stimulated muscle glucose clearance in patients with type 2 diabetes mellitus. Effects of one-legged physical training, *Diabetes*, 44, 1010, 1995.

18. Dela, F., Mikines, K. J., Von Linstow, M., Secher, N. H., and Galbo, H. Effect of training on insulin mediated glucose uptake in human skeletal muscle, *Am. J. Physiol.*, 26, E1134, 1992.

19. Dela, F., Mikines, K. J., Tronier, B., and Galbo, H., Diminished arginine-stimulated insulin secretion in trained men, *J. Appl. Physiol.*, 69, 261, 1990.

20. Dela, F., Mikines, K. J., Von Linstow, M., and Galbo, H., Effect of training on response to a glucose load adjusted for daily carbohydrate intake, *Am. J. Physiol.*, 260, E14, 1991.

21. Dela, F., Mikines, K. J., Von Linstow, M., and Galbo, H., Twenty-four-hour profile of plasma glucose and glucoregulatory hormones during normal living conditions in trained and untrained men, *J. Clin. Endocrinol. Metab.*, 73, 982, 1991.

22. Dela, F., Mikines, K. J., Von Linstow, M., and Galbo, H., Heart rate and plasma catecholamines during 24 h of everyday life in trained and untrained men, *J. Appl. Physiol.*, 73, 2389, 1992.

23. Dela, F., Ploug, T., Handberg, A., Petersen, L. N., Larsen, J. J., Mikines, K. J., and Galbo, H., Physical training increases muscle GLUT4 protein and mRNA in patients with NIDDM, *Diabetes*, 43, 862, 1994.

24. Deuster, P. A., Chouros, G. P., Luger, A., DeBolt, J. E., Bernier, L. L., Trostmann, U. H., Kyle, S. B., Montgomery, L. C., and Loriaux, D. L., Hormonal and metabolic responses of untrained, moderately trained, and highly trained men to three exercise intensities, *Metabolism*, 38, 214, 1989.

25. Droste, C., Greenlee, M. W., Schreck, M., and Roskamm, H., Experimental pain thresholds and plasma beta-endorphin levels during exercise, *Med. Sci. Sports Exerc.*, 23, 334, 1991.

26. Ehrsam, R. E., Heigenhauser, G. J. F., and Jones, N. L., Effect of respiratory acidosis on metabolism in exercise, *J. Appl. Physiol.*, 53, 63, 1982.

27. Engfred, K., Kjaer, M., Secher, N. H., Friedman, D. B., Hanel, B., Nielsen, O. J., Bach, F. W., Galbo, H., and Levine, B. D., Hypoxia and training-induced adaptation of hormonal responses to exercise in humans, *Eur. J. Appl. Physiol. Occup. Physiol.*, 68, 303, 1994.

28. Epstein, S. E., Robinson, B. F., Kahler, R. L., and Braunwald, E., Effect of beta-adrenergic blockade on the cardiac response to maximal and sub-maximal exercise in man, *J. Clin. Invest.*, 44, 1745, 1965.

29. Farrell, P. A., Kjaer, M., Bach, F. W., and Galbo, H., Beta-endorphin and adrenocorticotropin response to supramaximal treadmill exercise in trained and untrained males, *Acta Physiol. Scand.*, 130, 619, 1987.

30. Fell, R. D., Lizzo, F. H., Cervoni, P., and Crandall, D. L., Effect of contractile activity on rat skeletal muscle beta-adrenoceptor properties, *Proc. Soc. Exp. Biol. Med.*, 180, 527, 1985.

31. Galbo, H., *Hormonal and Metabolic Adaptation to Exercise*, Thieme Verlag, New York, 1983.

32. Galbo, H., Christensen, N. J., and Holst, J. J., Catecholamines and pancreatic hormones during autonomic blockade in exercising man. *Acta Physiol. Scand.*, 101, 428, 1977.

33. Galbo, H., Christensen, N. J., and Holst, J. J., Glucose-induced decrease in glucagon and epinephrine responses to exercise in man, *J. Appl. Physiol. Respir. Environ. Exerc. Physiol.*, 42, 525, 1977.

34. Geyssant, A., Geelen, G., Denis, C., Allevard, A., and Vincent, M., Plasma vasopressin, renin activity and aldosterone: effect of exercise and training, *Eur. J. Appl. Physiol. Occup. Physiol.*, 46, 21, 1981.

35. Goetz, K., Physiology and pathophysiology of atrial peptides, *Am. J. Physiol.*, 254, E1, 1988.

36. Hackney, A., Sinning, W., and Bruot, B., Reproductive hormonal profiles of endurance-trained and untrained males, *Med. Sci. Sports Exerc.*, 20, 60, 1988.

37. Häkkinen, K., Pakarinen, A., Alen, M., Kauhanen, H., and Komi, P. V., Relationship between training volume, physical performance capacity and serum hormone concentrations during prolonged training in elite weightlifters., *Int. J. Sports Med.*, 8(*Suppl.*), 6, 1987.
38. Hespel, P., Lijnen, P., VanHoof, R., Fagard, R., Goossens, W., Lissens, W., Moerman, E., and Amery, A., Effects of physical endurance training on the plasma renin-angiotensin-aldosterone system in normal man, *J. Endocrinol.*, 116, 443, 1988.
39. Hjeltnes, N. and Vokac, Z., Circulatory strain in everyday life of paraplegics, *Scand. J. Rehabil. Med.*, 11, 67, 1979.
40. Hoffmann, P., Terenius, L., and Thoren, P., Cerebrospinal fluid immunoreactive beta-endorphin concentration is increased by voluntary exercise in the spontaneously hypertensive rat, *Regul. Pept.*, 28, 233, 1990.
41. Jansson, E., Hjemdahl, P., and Kaijser, L., Epinephrine-induced changes in muscle carbohydrate metabolism during exercise in male subjects, *J. Appl. Physiol.*, 60, 1466, 1986.
42. Jarhult, J. and Holst, J., The role of the adrenergic innervation to the pancreatic islets in the control of insulin release during exercise in man, *Pflugers Archi. Eur. J. Physiol.*, 383, 41, 1979.
43. Jennings, G., Nelson, L., Nestel, P., Esler, M., and Korner, P., The effects of changes in physical activity on major cardiovascular risk factors, hemodynamics, sympathetic function and glucose utilization in man: a controlled study of four levels of activity, *Circulation*, 73, 3040, 1986.
44. Joyner, M. J., Freund, B. J., Jilka, S. M., Hetrick, G. A., Martinez, E., Ewy, G. A., and Wilmore, J. H., Effects of beta-blockade on exercise capacity of trained and untrained men: a hemodynamic comparison, *J. Appl. Physiol.*, 60, 1429, 1986.
45. Jurkowski, J. E., Sutton, J. R., Keane, P. M., and Viol, G. W., Plasma renin activity and plasma aldosterone during exercise in relation to the menstrual cycle, *Med. Sci. Sports Exerc.*, 10, 41, 1978.
46. Kaiser, P., Tesch, P. A., Frisk-Holmberg, M., Juhlin-Dannfelt, A., and Kaijser, L., Effect of beta 1-selective and non-selective beta-blockade on work capacity and muscle metabolism, *Clin. Physiol.*, 6, 197, 1986.
47. Kappel, M., Tvede, N., Galbo, H., Haahr, P. M., Kjaer, M., Von Linstow, M., Klarlund, K., and Pedersen, B. K., Evidence that the effect of physical exercise on NK cell activity is mediated by epinephrine, *J. Appl. Physiol.*, 70, 2141, 1991.
48. Karlsson, S. and Ahren, B., Insulin and glucagon secretion in swimming mice: effects of autonomic receptor antagonism, *Metab. Clin. Exp.*, 39, 724, 1990.
49. Keizer, H. A., Poortmans, J., and Bunniks, J., Influence of physical exercise on sex hormone metabolism, *J. Appl. Physiol.*, 50, 545, 1981.
50. Kessler, K. M., Pina, I., Green, B., Burnett, B., Laighold, M., Bilsker, M., Palomo, A. R., and Myerburg, R. J., Cardiovascular findings in quadriplegic and paraplegic patients and in normal subjects. *Am. J. Cardiol.*, 58: 525, 1986.
51. Kjaer, M., Epinephrine and some other hormonal responses to exercise in man: with special reference to physical training, *Int. J. Sports Med.*, 10, 2, 1989.
52. Kjaer, M., Engfred, K., Fernandes, A., Secher, N. H., and Galbo, H., Regulation of hepatic glucose production during exercise in man — influence of sympathoadrenergic activity, *Am. J Physiol.*, 265, E275, 1993.
53. Kjaer, M., Engfred, K., Sonne, B., Rasmussen, K., Galbo, H., and Keiding, S., Glucose homeostasis during exercise in humans with a liver or kidney transplant, *Am. J. Physiol. (Endocrinol. Metab.)*, 268, in press.
54. Kjaer, M., Farrell, P. A., Christensen, N. J., and Galbo, H., Increased epinephrine response and inaccurate glucoregulation in exercising athletes, *J. Appl. Physiol.*, 61, 1693, 1986.
55. Kjaer, M. and Galbo, H., Effect of physical training on the capacity to secrete epinephrine, *J. Appl. Physiol.*, 64, 11, 1988.

56. Kjaer, M., Kiens, B., Hargreaves, M., and Richter, E. A., Influence of active muscle mass on glucose homeostasis during exercise in humans, *J. Appl. Physiol.*, 71, 552, 1991.

57. Kjaer, M., Mikines, K. J., Christensen, N. J., Tronier, B., Vinten, J., Sonne, B., Richter, E. A., and Galbo, H., Glucose turnover and hormonal changes during insulin-induced hypoglycemia in trained humans, *J. Appl. Physiol. Resp. Environ. Exerc. Physiol.*, 51, 21, 1984.

58. Kjaer, M., Mikines, K. J., Linstow, M. V., Nicolaisen, T., and Galbo, H., Effect of 5 weeks detraining on epinephrine response to insulin induced hypoglycemia in athletes, *J. Appl. Physiol.*, 72, 1201, 1992

59. Kjaer, M., Pollack, S. F., Weiss, H., Galbo, H., Gleim, G., and Ragnarsson, K. T., Glucose turnover during electrically induced exercise in spinal cord injured individuals, *Am. J. Physiol. (Regul.)*, in press.

60. Kjaer, M., Secher, N. H., Bach, F. W., and Galbo, H., Role of motor center activity for hormonal changes and substrate mobilization in humans, *Am. J. Physiol.*, 253, R687, 1987.

61. Kjaer, M., Secher, N. H., Bach, F. W., Galbo, H., Reeves, Jr., D. R., and Mitchell, J. H., Hormonal, metabolic, and cardiovascular responses to static exercise in humans: influence of epidural anesthesia, *Am. J. Physiol.*, 261, E214, 1991.

62. Kjaer, M., Secher, N. H., Bach, F. W., Sheikh, S., and Galbo, H., Hormonal and metabolic responses to exercise in humans: effect of sensory nervous blockade, *Am. J. Physiol.*, 257, E95, 1989.

63. Kjaer, M., Bangsbo, J., Lortie, G., and Galbo, H., Horomonal responses to exercise in humans: influence of hypoxia and physical training, *Am. J. Physiol.*, 254, R197, 1988.

64. Kjaer, M., Christensen, N. J., Sonne, B., Richter, E. A., and Galbo, H., Effect of exercise on epinephrine turnover in trained and untrained male subjects, *J. Appl. Physiol.*, 59, 1061, 1985.

65. Klausen, T., Dela, F., Hippe, E., and Galbo, H., Diurnal variations of serum erythropoietin in trained and untrained subjects. *Eur. J. Appl. Physiol. Occup. Physiol.*, 67, 545, 1993.

66. Kraemer, W. J., Endocrine responses to resistance exercise, *Med. Sci. Sports Exerc.*, 20, S152, 1988.

67. Kraemer, W. J., Patton, J. F., Knuttgen, H. G., Hannan, C. J., Kettler, T., Gordon, S. E., Dziados, J. E., Fry, A. C., Frykman, P. N., and Harman, E. A., Effects of high-intensity cycle exercise on sympathoadrenal-medullary response patterns, *J. Appl. Physiol.*, 70, 8, 1991.

68. Kraemer, W. J., Patton, J. F., Knuttgen, H. G., Marchitelli, L. J., Cruthirds, C., Damokosh, A., Harman, E., Frykman, P., and Dziados, J. E., Hypothalamicpituitary-adrenal responses to short-duration high-intensity cycle exercise, *J. Appl. Physiol.*, 66, 161, 1989.

69. LeBlanc, J., Jobin, M., Cote, J., Samson, P., and Labrie, A., Enhanced metabolic response to caffeine in exercise-trained human subjects, *J. Appl. Physiol.*, 59, 832, 1985.

70. Lehmann, M., Dickhuth, H. H., Schmid, P., Pozig, H., and Keul, J., Plasma catecholamines, beta-adrenergic receptors, and isoproterenol sensitivity in endurance trained and non-endurance trained volunteers, *Eur. J. App. Physiol. Occup. Physiol.*, 52, 362, 1984.

71. Lewis, S. F., Snell, P. G., Taylor, W. F., Hamra, M., Graham, R. M., Pettinger, W. A., and Blomqvist, C. G., Role of muscle mass and mode of contraction in circulatory responses to exercise, *J. Appl. Physiol.*, 58, 146, 1985.

72. Lijnen, P. J., Amery, A. K., Fagard, R. H., Reybrouck, T. M., Moerman, E. J., and DeSchaepdryver, A. F., The effects of ß-adrenergic receptor blockade on renin, angiotensin, aldosterone and catecholamines at rest and during exercise, *Br. J. Clin. Pharmacol.*, 7, 175, 1979.

73. Luger, A., Deuster, P., Kyle, S., Gallucci, W., Montgomery, L., Gold, P. W., Loriaux, D. L., and Chrousos, G. P., Acute hypothalamic-pituitary-adrenal responses to the stress of treadmill exercise, *N. Engl. J. Med.*, 316, 1309, 1987.

74. MacConnie, S. E., Barkan, A., Lampman, R. M., Schork, M. A., and Beitins, I. Z., Decreased hypothalamic gonadotropin releasing hormone secretion in male marathon runners, *N. Engl. J. Med.* 315, 411, 1986.

75. Markoff, R. A., Ryan, P., and Young, T., Endorphins and mood changes in long-distance running, *Med. Sci. Sports Exerc.*, 14, 11, 1982.

76. McMurray, R. G., Forsythe, W. A., Mar, M. H., and Hardy, C. J., Exercise intensity-related responses of beta-endorphin and catecholamines, *Med. Sci. Sports Exerc.*, 19, 570, 1987.

77. Medbø, J. and Sejersted, O., Plasma potassium changes with high intensoty exercise, *J. Physiol.*, 421, 105, 1990.

78. Mikines, K. J., Sonne, B., Farrell, P. A., Tronier, B., and Galbo, H., Effect of training on the dose-response relationship for insulin action in men, *J. Appl. Physiol.*, 66, 695, 1989.

79. Mikines, K. J., Sonne, B., Tronier, B., and Galbo, H., Effects of training and detraining on dose-response relationship between glucose and insulin secretion, *Am. J. Physiol.*, 256, E588, 1989.

80. Moates, J. M., Lacy, D. B., Goldstein, R. E., Cherrington, A. D., and Wasserman, D. H., Metabolic role of the exercise-induced increment in epinephrine in the dog, *Am. J. Physiol.*, 255, E428, 1988.

81. Oktedalen, O., Opstad, P. K., Fahrenkrug, J., and Fonnum, F., Plasma concentrations of vasoactive intestinal polypeptide during prolonged physical exercise, calorie supply deficiency, and sleep deprivation, *Scand. J. Gastroenterol.*, 18, 1057, 1983.

82. Pernow, J., Lundberg, J. M., Kaijser, L., Hjelmdahl, P., Theodorsson-Nordhein, E., Martinsson, A., and Pernow, B., Plasma neuropeptide Y-like immunoreactivity and catecholamines during various degrees of sympathetic activation in man, *Clin. Physiol.*, 6, 56, 1986.

83. Peronnet, F., Beliveau, L., Boudreau, G., Trudeau, F., Brisson, G., and Nadeau, R., Regional plasma catecholamine removal and release at rest and exercise in dogs, *Am. J. Physiol.*, 254, R663, 1988.

84. Peronnet, F., Cleroux, J., Perrault, H., Cosineau, D., de Champlain, J., and Nadeau, R., Plasma norepinephrine response to exercise before and after training in humans, *J. Appl. Physiol.*, 51, 812, 1992.

85. Pestell, R. G., Hurley, D. M., and Vandongen, R., Biochemical and hormonal changes during a 1000 km ultramarathon, *Clin. Exp. Pharmacol. Physiol.*, 16, 353, 1989.

86. Piehl, K., Adolfsson, S., and Nazar, K., Glycogen storage and glycogen synthetase activity in trained and untrained muscle of man, *Acta Physiol. Scand.*, 90, 779, 1974.

87. Ploug, T., Galbo, H., Vinten, J., Jorgensen, M., and Richter, E. A., Kinetics of glucose transport in rat muscle: effects of insulin and contractions, *Am. J. Physiol.*, 253, E12, 1987.

88. Pruett, E.D.R. Plasma insulin concentrations during prolonged work at near maximal oxygen uptake, *J. Appl. Physiol.*, 2, 155, 1970.

89. Radosevich, P. M., Nash, J. A., Lacy, D. B., O'Donovan, C., Williams, P. E., and Abumrad, N. N., Effects of low- and high-intensity exercise on plasma and cerebrospinal fluid levels of ir-beta-endorphin, ACTH, cortisol, norepinephrine and glucose in the conscious dog, *Brain Res.*, 498, 89, 1989.

90. Richter, E. A., Emmeluth, C., Bie, P., Helge, J., and Kiens, B., Biphasic response of plasma endothelin-1 concentration to exhausting submaximal exercise in man, *Clin. Physiol.*, 14, 379, 1994.

91. Richter, E. A., Kiens, B., Hargreaves, M., and Kjaer, M., Effect of arm-cranking on leg blood flow and noradrenaline spillover during leg exercise in man, *Acta Phys. Scand.*, 144, 9, 1992.

92. Richter, E. A., Ruderman, N. B., and Galbo, H., Alpha and beta adrenergic effects on metabolism in contracting, perfused muscle, *Acta Physiol. Scand.*, 116, 215, 1982.

93. Richter, E. A., Ruderman, N. B., Gavras, H., Belur, E. R., and Galbo, H., Muscle glycogenolysis during exercise: dual control by epinephrine and contractions, *Am. J. Physiol.*, 242, E25, 1982.

94. Richter, E. A., Sonne, B., Christensen, N. J., and Galbo, H. ,Role of epinephrine for muscular glycogenolysis and pancreatic hormonal secretion in running rats, *Am. J. Physiol.*, 240, E526, 1981.

95. Riviere, D., Crampes, F., Beauville, M., and Garrigues, M., Lipolytic response of fat cells to catecholamines in sedentary and exercise-trained women, *J. Appl. Physiol.*, 66, 330, 1989.

96. Rowell, L. B., Brengelmann, G. L., and Freund, P. R., Unaltered norepinephrine-heart rate relationship in exercise with exogenous heat, *J. Appl. Physiol.*, 62, 646, 1987.

97. Savard, G., Strange, S., Kiens, B., Richter, E. A., Christensen, N. J., and Saltin, B., Noradrenaline spillover during exercise in active versus resting skeletal muscle in man, *Acta Physiol. Scand.*, 131, 507, 1987.

98. Savard, G. K., Richter, E. A., Strange, S., Kiens, B., Christensen, N. J., and Saltin, B., Norepinephrine spillover from skeletal muscle during exercise in humans: role of muscle mass, *Am. J. Physiol.*, 257, H1812, 1989.

99. Scheurink, A. J., Steffens, A. B., and Gaykema, R. P., Hypothalamic adrenoceptors mediate sympathoadrenal activity in exercising rats, *Am. J. Physiol.*, 259, R470, 1990.

100. Schmidt, W., Eckardt, K. U., Hilgendorf, A., Strauch, S., and Bauer, C., Effects of maximal and submaximal exercise under normoxic and hypoxic conditions on serum erythropoietin level, *Int. J. Sports Med.*, 12, 457, 1991.

101. Schwandt, H. J., Heyduck, B., Gunga, H. C., and Röcker, L., Influence of prolonged physical exercise on the erythropoietin concentration in blood, *Eur. J. Appl. Physiol. Occup. Physiol.*, 63, 463, 1991.

102. Sellers, T. L., Jaussi, A. W., Yang, H. T., Heninger, R. W., and Winder, W. W., Effect of the exercise-induced increase in glucocorticoids on endurance in the rat, *J. Appl. Physiol.*, 65, 173, 1988.

103. Spriet, L. L., Ren, J. M., and Hultman, E., Epinephrine infusion enhances muscle glycogenolysis during prolonged electrical stimulation, *J. Appl. Physiol.*, 64, 1439, 1988.

104. Stallknecht, B., Kjaer, M., Mikines, K. J., Maroun, L., Ploug, T., Ohkuwa, T., Vinten, J., and Galbo, H., Diminished epinephrine response to hypoglycemia despite enlarged adrenal medulla in trained rats, *Am. J. Physiol.*, 259, R998, 1990.

105. Sutton, J. R., Coleman, M. J., Casey, J., and Lazarus, L., Androgen responses during physical exercise, *Br. Med. J.*, 1, 520, 1973.

106. Sutton, J. R., Jurkowski, J. E., Keane, P., Walker, W. H. C., Jones, N. L., and Toews, C. J., Plasma catecholamine, insulin, glucose and lactate responses to exercise in relation to menstrual cycle, *Med. Sci. Sports Exerc.*, 12, 83, 1980.

107. Sutton, J. R., Young, J. D., Lazarus, L., Hickie, J. B., and Maksvytis, J., The hormonal response to physical exercise, *Aust. Ann. Med.*, 18, 84, 1969.

108. Svedenhag, J., The sympatho-adrenal system in physical conditioning, *Acta Physiol. Scand.*, 125, 1, 1985.

109. Tabata, I., Atomi, Y., and Miyashita, M., Blood glucose concentration dependent ACTH and cortisol responses to prolonged exercise, *Clin. Physiol.*, 4, 299, 1984.

110. Thamsborg, G., Sykulski, R., Larsen, J., Storm, T., and Keller, N., Effect of beta 1-adrenoreceptor blockade on plasma levels of atrial natriuretic peptide during exercise in normal man, *Clin. Physiol.*, 7, 313, 1987.

111. Trudeau, F., Peronnet, F., Beliveau, L., and Brisson, G., Metabolic and endocrine responses to prolonged exercise in rats under beta 2-adrenergic blockade, *Can. J. Physiol. Pharmacol.*, 67, 192, 1989.

112. Valdemarsson, S., Andersson, D., Bengtsson, A., Bogren, M., Edvinsson, L., and Ekman, R., y2-MSH increases during graded exercise in healthy subjects: comparison with plasma catecholamines, neuropeptides, aldosterone and renin activity, *Clin. Physiol.*, 10, 321, 1990.

113. Vanhelder, W. P., Radomski, M. W., and Goode, R. C., Growth hormone responses during intermittent weight lifting exercise in men, *Eur. J. Appl. Physiol. Occup. Physiol.*, 53, 31, 1984.

114. Victor, R. G., Bertocci, L. A., Pryor, S. L., and Nunnally, R. L., Sympathetic nerve discharge is coupled to muscle cell pH during exercise in man, *J. Clin. Invest.*, 82, 1301, 1988.

115. Vissing, J., Iwamoto, G. A., Fuchs, I. E., Galbo, H., and Mitchell, J. H., Reflex control of glucoregulatory exercise responses by group III and IV muscle afferents, *Am. J. Physiol.*, 266, R824, 1994.

116. Vissing, J., Iwamoto, G. A., Rybicki, K. J., Galbo, H., and Mitchell, J. H., Mobilization of glucoregulatory hormones and glucose by hypothalamic locomotor centers, *Am. J. Physiol.*, 257, E722, 1989.

117. Vissing, J., Wilson, L. B., Mitchell, J. H., and Victor, R. G., Static muscle contraction reflexly increases adrenal sympathetic nerve activity in rats, *Am. J. Physiol.*, 261, R1307, 1991.

118. Vitali, E. D. P., Guegliemini, C., Casoni, I., Vedovato, M., Gilli, P., Fainelli, A., Salvatorelli, G., and Conconi, F., Serum erythropoietin in cross country skiers, *Int. J. Sports Med.*, 9, 99, 1988.

119. Wahren, J., Felig, P., Ahlborg, G., and Jorfeldt, L., Glucose metabolism during leg exercise in man, *J. Clin. Invest.*, 50, 2715, 1971.

120. Wahrenberg, H., Engfeldt, P., Bolinder, J., and Arner, P., Acute adaptation in adrenergic control of lipolysis during physical exercise in humans, *Am. J. Physiol.*, 253, E383, 1987.

121. Wasserman, D. H., Lickley, H. L., and Vranic, M., Interactions between glucagon and other counterregulatory hormones during normoglycemic and hypoglycemic exercise in dogs, *J. Clin. Invest.*, 74, 1404, 1984.

122. Wasserman, D. H., Spalding, J. A., Lacy, D. B., Colburn, C. A., Goldstein, R. E., and Cherrington, A. D., Glucagon is a primary controller of hepatic glycogenolysis and gluconeogenesis during muscular work, *Am. J. Physiol.*, 257, E108, 1989.

123. Wasserman, D. H., Williams, P. E., Lacy, D. B., Bracy, D., and Cherrington, A. D., Hepatic nerves are not essential to the increase in hepatic glucose production during muscular work, *Am. J. Physiol.*, 259, E195, 1990.

124. Wheeler, G. D., Simgh, M., Pierce, W. D., Epling, W. F., and Cumming, D. C., Endurance training decreases serum testoterone levels in men without change in luteinizing hormone pulsatile release, *J. Clin. Endocrinol. Metab.*, 72, 422, 1991.

125. Williams, R., Caron, M., and Daniel, K., Skeletal muscle beta-adrenergic receptors: variations due to fiber type and training, *Am. J. Physiol.*, 246, E160, 1984.

126. Winder, W. W., Hagberg, J. M., Hickson, R. C., Ehsani, A. A., and McLane, J. A., Time course of sympathoadrenal adaptation to endurance exercise training in man, *J. Appl. Physiol.*, 45, 370, 1978.

127. Wirth, A., Diehm, C., Mayer, H., Mörl, H., Vogel, I., Björntorp, P., and Schlierf, G., Plasma C-peptide and insulin in trained and untrained subjects. *J. Appl. Physiol.*, 50, 71, 1981.

128. Wolfe, R. R., Nadel, E. R., Shaw, J. H., Stephenson, L. A., and Wolfe, M. H., Role of changes in insulin and glucagon in glucose homeostasis in exercise, *J. Clin. Invest.*, 77, 900, 1986.

129. Yanagisawa, M., Kurihara, H., Kimura, S., Tomboe, Y., Kobayshi, M., Mitsui, Y., Yazaki, Y., Goto, K., and Masaki, T., A novel potent vasocontrictor peptide produced by vascular endothelial cells, *Nature (London)*, 332, 411, 1988.

130. Yeaman, S., Hormone-sensitive lipase-a multipurpose enzyme in lipid metabolism, *Biochem. Biophys. Acta*, 1052, 128, 1990.

131. Zambraski, E. J., Tucker, M. S., Lakas, C. S., Grassl, S. M., and Scanes, C. G., Mechanism of renin release in exercising dog, *Am. J. Physiol.*, 246, E71, 1984.

Chapter **2**

NEUROENDOCRINE EFFECTS ON IMMUNITY

Bruce S. Rabin
Niall M. Moyna
Alex Kusnecov
Daohong Zhou
Michael R. Shurin

CONTENTS

0-8493-8190-8/96/$0.00+$.50
© 1996 by CRC Press, Inc.

I. INTRODUCTION

Communication occurs between organs and tissues of the body so that alterations of metabolic function can be detected. Subsequent to the presence of alterations of metabolic function, a biochemical response to restore baseline metabolism is initiated as a means of maintaining homeostasis in the body. For example, communication between plasma glucose concentrations and the beta-islet cells of the pancreas results in an adjustment in the concentration of insulin released with a restoration of glucose to physiological levels. Hormones released from endocrine tissue bind to specific receptors either on a cell membrane or within the cytoplasm of a cell, and modify an intracellular chemical process, often leading to an alteration of cell function. Just as cells within organs and tissues of the body have receptors for hormones, so too do the cells of the lymphoid system. Thus, the means for interactions between the endocrine and immune systems are present, as will be discussed below.

Immune function involves an extensive array of interactions between lymphocytes and mononuclear phagocytes. For example, the cytokine interleukin-1 (IL-1) produced by mononuclear phagocytes (monocytes and macrophages) binds to receptors on T lymphocytes. The mononuclear phagocyte and the lymphocyte adhere to each other through membranous adhesion molecules. This type of interaction is reminiscent of the type of anatomic interaction which occurs across a synapse between two neurons.

In addition to having receptors for products of the immune system, lymphocytes are known to have receptors for hormones produced by the nervous system and to have receptors for endocrine hormones.[37] In addition, neurons are known to synapse with lymphocytes.[1] The presence of hormone receptors on lymphocytes and the anatomic contact between the nervous and immune systems reveal the existence of pathways of communication between the immune system, the nervous system, and the endocrine system. If bidirectional pathways of communication between the immune and endocrine, immune and nervous, and endocrine and nervous systems can be functionally identified, regulation of one or two of these systems by the other may occur as part of the body's mechanism of maintaining homeostasis.

Stress is known to produce alterations in the function of the immune, endocrine, and nervous systems.[35,51] Stressors can take many forms such as fear, pain, or physical activity. Even the activation of an immune response to an infectious agent may be a stressor to the body as the immune system works to rid the body of the invading microorganism. If there is activation of a neuroendocrine response to fear or pain, there will be the necessity of perception of the stressor by the brain. If there is an immune response to a foreign microorganism, the brain must be made aware of the ongoing immune response occurring in the periphery. Thus, this chapter will review (1) the areas of the brain which are activated by stress, stressor-induced activation of the sympathetic nervous system; (2) the stressor-induced activation of the hypothalamic-pituitary-adrenal (H-P-A) axis; and (3) the effect of hormones on modifying immunological function. Finally, communication from the immune system to the brain will be discussed.

II. PERCEPTION OF STRESS BY THE BRAIN

The use of markers which indicate that a cell has been functionally activated provides a means of identifying neurons in the brain which become activated subsequent to a stressor. Recently, studies have identified the presence of a marker which appears in the nuclei of cells which are functionally activated. The marker commonly used is the protein product of the c-Fos protooncogene, to which an antibody can be produced.[28,52] The protein product has a size of approximately 62 kDa. There are epitopes on the c-Fos protein which are shared by other molecules, but there are also epitopes which are specific for c-Fos. Thus, production of antibody to the Fos-specific epitopes can be used to identify cells which have been activated. We have found this technique extremely useful and have identified those areas of the rat forebrain and brainstem which become c-Fos reactive following either an unconditioned aversive stimulus or a conditioned aversive stimulus.[48,50]

The presence of the c-Fos protein will identify neurons which are activated and allow a differentiation to be made between quiescence and activated areas of the brain. For example, a resting animal that is in a room with the lights on will show c-Fos staining, using immunohistochemistry, in neurons of the visual and auditory areas of the brain. Areas associated with autonomic function are negative for the presence of c-Fos. Obviously, the areas of the brain involved with autonomic function are not inactive. However, c-Fos is present in very low concentrations in cells which are constantly being activated; and only when an acute event takes place is there a marked increase in the concentration of the c-Fos marker. Therefore, this allows this procedure to be used to identify areas of the brain that are acutely activated by a stressor.

To separate the psychological effects of a stressor from other stimuli which may activate neurons we have used a conditioned stressor to identify areas of the brain activated by stress. Stimuli such as electrical shock, swimming, or restraint may, in addition to producing stress, produce pain or rage, which may activate neurons in the brain that would then produce c-Fos. A conditioned stressor produces fear or anxiety without pain or physical activity.

In our studies rats were conditioned by an electrical footshock which was preceded by a clicking sound.[36] After 2 weeks of remaining undisturbed the animals are then reexposed to the clicking sound without footshock. The areas of the brain which are activated when the rats are reexposed to the conditioned stressor include

Forebrain nuclei activated by a conditioned aversive stimulus:
  Corticotropin-releasing hormone (CRH)-containing neurons of the
    paraventricular nucleus of the hypothalamus
  Ventral lateral septal nuclei
  Medial amygdaloid nuclei
  Sensorimotor cortex
  Basal ganglia
  Thalamic nuclei
Brainstem nuclei activated by a conditioned aversive stimulus:
  Locus coeruleus
  Nucleus of the solitary tract
  Ventral lateral medulla
  A5
  A7
  Dorsal and ventral subdivisions of the periaqueductal gray area
  Serotonergic neurons of the dorsal raphe nuclei

Thus, areas of the brain which are associated with H-P-A axis activation and sympathetic nervous system activation, and areas which project neurons to the intermediolateral cell column of the spinal cord are activated.

To confirm that areas of the brain which are induced to synthesize c-Fos are involved in the alteration of immune function subsequent to a stressor, lesioning of these areas and determination of whether there is an effect on immune function are required. When lesioning is done, areas of the brain which may prevent stressors from suppressing immune function as well as areas of the brain which are associated with the suppression of immune function by stress can be identified.

For example, lesioning of the paraventricular nucleus of the hypothalamus prior to reexposing an animal to a conditioned stressor results in greater suppression of spleen lymphocyte responsiveness to nonspecific mitogenic stimulation than is found in animals experiencing a sham lesion.[49] Lesions of the anterior hypothalamus, amygdala, or hippocampus produce changes in the response of lymphocytes of rats in their responsiveness to nonspecific mitogen.[10,17] Experimentally induced lesions of the lateral septal area of the rat brain prior to immunization with specific antigen is associated with decreased antibody production of immunoglobulin G (IgG), IgA, and IgM; however, a lesion of the hippocampus is associated with an elevation of IgG and IgM antibody to ovalbumin.[45] Thus, as stated by Blalock,[8] "…the immune and neuroendocrine systems exert profound and biologically relevant effects on one another *in vivo* and such crosstalk is undoubtedly important to homeostasis."

It is likely that the interaction between several brain areas which are activated by a stressor results in stressor-induced immune alteration. How the brain areas interact to activate the H-P-A axis and release of neuropeptides from nerve terminals in the spleen remains to be determined. However, it is unlikely that stress functions as an on or off switch to modulate immune function. For example, the characteristics of neuropeptides released in the spleen vary depending on the intensity of the stressor.[47]

It has been reported in human subjects experiencing an acute laboratory stressor that not all individuals react to the stressor.[40] However, if the same stressor, the Stroop color word test, is made more difficult, it will elicit a reaction from all subjects (S. Manuck, B. Rabin, and S. Cohen, unpublished observations). Therefore, it is likely either that areas of the brain in different individuals will be activated by different intensities of stressor or that regulatory pathways will be activated by different stress intensities. Whether these differences are associated with coping capabilities, habituation to stress, or other mechanisms associated with activation of the brain, remains to be determined.

Following the experience of a stressor, an individual may or may not respond with an alteration of immune function. If there is a response that alters immune function, it may be assumed that the stressor is activating the areas of the brain which produce the various neurotransmitters, neuropeptides, or hormones which modify immune function. If they do not respond with an alteration of immune function, it may be interpreted that the individual is not perceiving the stressor to be aversive or the pathways within the brain responsible for inducing immunological alterations are not functionally active. However, it is also possible that individuals who do not alter immune function following a stressor are vigorously activating those areas of the brain which suppress the areas of the brain whose activation is associated with immune alteration.

It is apparent that the central mechanisms of stressor-induced immune alteration are highly complex. Similar to the functioning of the immune system, which requires interactions between various subpopulations of lymphocytes, there are complex regulatory interactions between areas of the brain which are part of the mechanism of stressor-induced immune alteration.

III. SYMPATHETIC NERVOUS SYSTEM ACTIVATION AND STRESSOR-INDUCED IMMUNE ALTERATION

The sympathetic nervous system participates in stressor-induced immune alteration in both rodents and humans. However, the lymphoid compartments that are functionally altered by the sympathetic nervous system differ in these two species. In rats, spleen lymphocyte function is altered by the sympathetic nervous system while in humans, the function of peripheral blood lymphocytes is modified by the sympathetic nervous system.[3,40,53]

In rats, severing of the splenic nerve prior to stress[63] or injection of an adrenergic antagonist[19] prevents stress from modifying lymphocyte function. Although catecholamines are essential in the process by which stress suppresses the function of rodent spleen lymphocytes, it is uncertain whether the catecholamines activate second messenger pathways in lymphocytes or induce other mediators to alter lymphocyte function. For example, following a stressor, if spleen lymphocytes and macrophages are separated and the lymphocytes are stimulated with nonspecific mitogens, lymphocytes from stressed and non-stressed animals respond in an identical manner. This suggests that catecholamines may activate mononuclear phagocytic cells to mediate stressor-induced immune suppression. Indeed, suppression of the production of nitric oxide in cultures of spleen mononuclear cells obtained from rats exposed to a stressor prevents suppression of spleen lymphocyte mitogenic function.[15]

In humans, epinephrine will cause both quantitative and qualitative alterations of peripheral blood lymphocytes. There is an increase in numbers of natural killer (NK) cells and lymphocytes bearing the CD8 surface receptor.[16,38] In addition, the responsiveness of peripheral blood lymphocytes to nonspecific mitogens decreases. In humans who experience an acute laboratory stressor, the same changes caused by the injection of epinephrine are found in the peripheral blood.[2,40,44]

To confirm that catecholamines are responsible for the alterations of the peripheral blood lymphocyte populations following a stressor, subjects were pretreated with an adrenergic antagonist prior to being exposed to a psychological stressor.[3] Lymphocyte subsets, NK cell function, and responsiveness of T lymphocytes to stimulation with nonspecific mitogens were compared in specimens obtained prior to and after the mental stressor in subjects who received an injection of saline or the adrenergic antagonist. Both quantitative and qualitative alterations of the immune system occurred in those subjects who were exposed to the stressor and were injected with saline. However, in those subjects who received the adrenergic antagonist, the psychological stressor failed to produce alterations of immune function. This confirms that in humans, the immunological response to acute psychological stress is mediated by activation of the sympathetic nervous system.

If sympathetic nervous system activation is associated with a suppression of lymphocyte activity, a predisposition to immunologically mediated disease may be associated with activation of the sympathetic nervous system. Thus, if the activity of the sympathetic nervous system is low, the immune system may have an elevated level of activity and a predisposition to the development of an autoimmune disease may exist.[9] Similarly, increased activity of the sympathetic nervous system with a resultant suppression of immunological function may predispose to the development of infectious disease.[14,22] As indicated, both of these sequelae of altered activity of the sympathetic nervous system have been reported. This suggests that a cause and effect relationship may exist between sympathetic nervous system function, immune function, and health.

In addition to catecholamines, neuropeptide Y elevation, rather than an elevation of catecholamines, has been reported to be the mediator of altered NK cell function in humans experiencing a chronic stress.[29] As neuropeptide Y is released from the terminus of sympathetic neurons, studies need to be performed to determine whether receptors for neuropeptide Y, when activated by a specific ligand, result in an alteration of lymphocyte or NK cell activity.

Following the infusion of catecholamines into humans,[16] the immunological alterations persist for approximately 2 h. In subjects who experience laboratory stressors, lymphocyte function returns to baseline within 2 h of cessation of the stressor. Therefore, the effects of catecholamines on alteration of immune function are transient. This suggests that if catecholamines are to have an effect on immune function which then predisposes to an immunologically mediated disease, catecholamine levels must be chronically elevated. Thus, the association of stress with an altered predisposition to disease in humans is likely to result from chronic sympathetic nervous system activation rather than effects of acute stressors which have a short-lived effect on immune function. It is also important to determine possible differences between the effects of acute and chronic stress in regard to the alterations of immune function which are induced by each. For example, acute stress increases the number of circulating CD8 lymphocytes while chronic stress decreases their numbers.[27]

Chronic stress is difficult to produce experimentally in humans. Therefore, situations in which life events are creating chronic stress are more appropriate for study. In this regard, family members of individuals with Alzheimer's disease and subjects involved in marital difficulties have been studied. In such individuals, chronic activation of the sympathetic system is found to occur with a decreased functional activity of the immune system and an increase susceptibility to upper respiratory viral infections.[32,33]

IV. LYMPHOCYTE ADRENERGIC RECEPTORS

Receptors for catecholamines are present on lymphocyte membranes. However, different subpopulations of human lymphocytes have different numbers of adrenergic receptors.[30,39,60] NK cells contain the highest number of adrenergic receptors with CD4 lymphocytes having the lowest number. B lymphocytes and CD8 lymphocytes are intermediate between NK cells and CD4 lymphocytes. Macrophages have a greater number of adrenergic receptors then do lymphocytes; however, macrophages are much larger than lymphocytes and the greater number of adrenergic receptors may reflect their size rather than receptor density.

Recently, the CD4 population of lymphocytes (defined as the helper/inducer population) has been subdivided into two subpopulations with different funtional activities.[46] The Th1 population promotes cellular immune reactions involved with eliminating pathogens which are located within tissue cells. The Th2 population of lymphocytes is involved with promoting antibody production by B lymphocytes, and as such is involved with resistance to infection with bacteria which are located outside of tissue cells (extracellularly). In addition, the two populations of CD4 lymphocytes regulate each other's function. For example, an increase of the functional activity of the Th1 population results in a suppression of the Th2 function and vice versa. Therefore, it is possible that dysregulation of the function of one of the CD4 subpopulations will produce an alteration of function of the other population. This would be expressed *in vivo* as a decrease in cellular immune function and an increase of antibody production, a frequently reported effect of stress on the immune system. For example, it is known from the studies of Glaser et al.[22] and Kiecolt-Glaser et al.[31] that stress in medical students suppresses cellular immune function and is associated with an increase in production of antibody to the Epstein–Barr virus. This suggests a decrease in the activity of the Th1 population which may lead to increased activity of the Th2 population. Studies regarding how stress affects the Th1 and Th2 lymphoycte populations are urgently needed.

A relationship exists between adrenergic receptor numbers and a stress-induced quantitative increase in the number of NK lymphocytes in the peripheral blood. NK cells have the highest number of adrenergic receptors and is the cell population which has the largest quantitative increase in the peripheral blood subsequent to a stressor.[30,39] However, the lymphocyte population with the second highest number of adrenergic receptors, the B lymphocyte, shows very little quantitative change in the peripheral blood subsequent to a stressor.[40,44] A possible explanation is that B lymphocytes show little increase in cyclic adenosine 5′-monophosphate (cAMP) when incubated with a beta-adrenergic agonist, in comparison to other lymphocyte populations which have large increases in cAMP.[39] Thus, it is possible that the second messenger system is important in determining whether catecholamine release into the peripheral blood subsequent to a stressor will modify immune function. T lymphocytes have an increase in the content of cAMP when incubated with catecholamines.[11]

V. DO CATECHOLAMINES ALTER IMMUNE FUNCTION?

Evidence has been presented above that (1) the areas of the brain which are involved with activation of the sympathetic nervous system are activated by stress; (2) stress causes an increase in catecholamine production; (3) lymphocytes have receptors for catecholamines; and (4) in humans, blocking of catecholamine binding to adrenergic receptors prevents stress from modifying immune system function. What is missing, however, is an indication that catecholamines have a direct effect on modifying lymphocyte function. It is of course possible that there is a direct relationship between catecholamine production and alteration of immune function. However, in rodents, modification of immune function by stress is dependent on nitric oxide production by spleen macrophages.

After a rat has been exposed to a stressor there is a decreased ability of spleen lymphocytes to be induced into mitotic division by nonspecific mitogen.[53] However, if the spleen lymphocytes are separated from the spleen macrophages, the spleen lymphocytes from stressed animals will respond identically as do spleen lymphocytes from nonstressed animals when incubated with nonspecific mitogen. Therefore, the macrophages appear to be essential for stressor-induced suppression of spleen lymphocyte function.

Macrophages produce mediators such as prostaglandin, transforming growth factor beta, and nitric oxide. Preventing production or neutralization of prostaglandin and transforming growth factor beta production by macrophages from stressed animals does not prevent the suppression of spleen lymphocyte mitogenic activity by stress. However, spleen lymphocytes from stressed animals respond identically to spleen lymphocytes from control animals when nitric oxide production is inhibited. Therefore, this suggests that nitric oxide may be an important mediator of stressor-induced alteration of spleen lymphocyte function. We have found that nitric oxide production by spleen macrophages is dependent on catecholamine binding to adrenergic receptors.

Further, different concentrations of catecholamines may produce different effects on lymphocytes. Catecholamines can produce either suppression or enhancement of lymphoid cell function depending on the concentration of catecholamines that the lymphocytes are exposed to.[25,34] It is possible that the number of adrenergic receptors occupied by catecholamines can exert either a positive or a negative effect on a lymphocyte. Another consideration is that low concentrations of catecholamines may modify the function of one type of lymphoid cell and higher concentrations may modify the function of another type of lymphoid cell. Until studies can be done with isolated populations of different types of lymphocytes, it will be difficult to determine the mechanism of different concentrations of catecholamines either enhancing or suppressing lymphocyte function.

VI. STRESSOR-INDUCED ACTIVATION OF THE HYPOTHALAMIC-PITUITARY-ADRENAL AXIS

Subsequent to a stressor sympathetic nervous system activation occurs extremely rapidly (within seconds). Activation of the H-P-A axis is slower and may not produce an increase in plasma levels of glucocorticoids until several minutes after stressor exposure, possibly as long as 20 to 30 min. As an example, when subjects were exposed to a psychological stressor, the Stroop color word test for 20 min, there was no elevation of plasma corticosterone although plasma catecholamines were markedly elevated.[40] As both quantitative and qualitative aspects of immune function become altered within 5 min of stressor exposure[26] and at a time preceding the elevation of plasma gluco-corticoid, it is apparent that catecholamines are responsible for stressor-in-duced immune alteration in humans, subsequent to exposure to an acute stressor. However, lymphocytes possess glucocorticoid receptors[42] and a com-plex interrelationship exists between free plasma glucocorticoids and gluco-corticoid receptors.

It is likely that when glucocorticoid receptors become occupied in the cytoplasm of the lymphocyte that the receptors move into the nucleus and bind to glucocorticoid regulatory sites on DNA. Regulation of processes associated with lymphocyte function or lymphocyte trafficking through tissue may then occur if the glucocorticoids modify the amount of cytokines being produced by the lymphocyte or alter the concentration of surface adhesion molecules. If the concentration of glucocorticoids increases in plasma at a time when all recep-tors for glucocorticoids are occupied in lymphoid cells, the increase in gluco-corticoids will not have an effect on altering lymphocyte function. Thus, at times when glucocorticoid concentrations are high, such as at the beginning of the dark cycle (for rodents), it is likely that all glucocorticoid receptors may be occupied and a further increase in plasma glucocorticoids would not alter lymphocyte function. The ability of glucocorticoid receptors in rat spleen lymphocytes to bind a glucocorticoid tracer is reduced following stressor exposure in the daylight, indicating that the glucocorticoid receptors were unoccupied.[57] However, when the rats are stressed during the dark cycle, the amount of a glucocorticoid tracer bound by spleen lymphocytes does not differ between control and stressed rats. This indicates that all glucocorticoid recep-tors were occupied in the dark cycle.

In plasma, the concentration of free, but not bound, glucocorticoid is available to enter the cytoplasm of cells and bind to glucocorticoid receptors. Plasma glucocorticoids are transported by plasma proteins, and the concentra-tion of the carrier protein determines the concentration of free glucocorticoid. Thus, an increase in total plasma glucocorticoids with a concomitant increase in the glucocorticoid carrier protein may not increase the concentration of free glucocorticoid. Therefore, in assessing the influence of glucocorticoids on lymphocyte function it is important to know the baseline concentration of glucocorticoid, the baseline degree of occupancy of glucocorticoid receptors in lymphocytes, and the stressor-induced alteration of free plasma glucocorticoids.

Regardless of the complexities of understanding glucocorticoid interac-tion with lymphocytes, it is likely that glucocorticoids binding to DNA can produce changes which modulate lymphocyte viability and function. Apoptosis may be mediated by glucocorticoid binding. Glucocorticoids may alter the concentration or characteristics of adhesion molecules on lymphocyte surfaces causing them either to adhere to or to disassociate from sites of attachment such as endothelial cells or possibly reticulin fibers. However, as indicated above, it is likely that different responses will occur at different times of the day.

Glucocorticoids are released from the adrenal gland in response to ACTH release from the pituitary subsequent to CRH release from the hypothalamus. Lymphocytes have receptors for both ACTH and CRH,[12] and lymphocyte function may be modulated by both of these hormones. Thus, it is apparent that in assessing how the H-P-A axis modulates lymphocyte function a summation effect of numerous hormones acting simultaneously will have to be considered.

VII. OPIOID INFLUENCE ON THE IMMUNE SYSTEM

There is considerable evidence that the various opioid peptides which include endorphins, enkephalins, and dynorphins can alter the function of lymphocytes and macrophages.[55,56] Receptors for opioids are found on lymphoid cells, and the plasma concentration of opoids increases with stress. Whether all lymphocyte populations have their function modulated by opioids has not yet been determined.

In studies which we have performed we have found that suppression of spleen NK cell function in rodents exposed to a stressor is modulated by opoids.[18] However, lymphocyte function in the spleen of the same animals is modulated by catecholamines.

VIII. CYTOKINE INFLUENCE IN THE BRAIN

Besedovsky et al.[5-7] reported that an injection of sheep erythrocytes into experimental animals produced an increase of plasma corticosterone and an increase in the firing rate of neurons in the ventromedial hypothalamus at the peak of the antibody response. This suggests that products of the activated immune system may be responsible for the increased CNS electrical activity and that the immune system may be involved in its own regulation through interactions with the CNS.

Cytokines, released from lymphocytes, are known to have autocrine, paracrine, and endocrine activities. Cytokines which find a means of crossing the the blood–brain barrier and bind to receptors in the brain have characteristics of part of the endocrine system. If the immune system communicates to the CNS (likely through the production of cytokines derived from immunologically active cells), it can be hypothesized that the functional disruption of those areas of the brain which are activated during an immune response would lead to an alteration of immune system activity.

Injecting IL-1 into the ventricle of a rodent brain produces a suppression of lymphocyte function[59] and an increase in the activity of the sympathetic nervous system with increased catecholamine turnover in the spleen.[61] Macrophages produce IL-1, and if the IL-1 release from macrophages crosses the blood brain–barrier, with a resultant activation of either the sympathetic nervous or the H-P-A axis, a feedback loop would exist leading to suppression of macrophage activity.

Using the presence of c-Fos as an indicator of neuronal activation, the areas of the brain activated by IL-1 injected into the ventricle of the brain or intravenously were determined.[54] Both routes of injection of IL-1 elevated plasma concentrations of ACTH but luteinizing hormone was only elevated when IL-1 was injected into the ventricle. Infusion of IL-1 into the ventricle stimulated c-Fos expression in the PVN and the arcuate nucleus of the hypothalamus. This finding is consistent with IL-1 activation of the H-P-A axis. However, intravenous injection of IL-1 did not activate cells of the PVN or arcuate nucleus. This suggests that if IL-1 participates in stressor-induced immune alterations, then its production within the CNS is essential.

In humans, IL-1 has been used as a biological response modifier for the treatment of malignancies. Infusion of high concentrations of IL-1 produces an increase in heart rate and cystolic blood pressure. These effects can be antagonized by a beta-adrenergic antagonist, indicating that catecholamines are involved in these changes.[24] Thus, in humans as in rodents, IL-1 is associated with sympathetic nervous system activation.

If cytokines which are produced during an immune response are found to be capable of influencing the activity of the brain, their role may be to restore a physiological balance (homeostasis). Indeed, the immune response does fight the presence of a foreign antigen and the antigen may be considered as an aversive event. Therefore, in considering the neuroendocrine response to stress, not only the effect of hormones on the immune system but also the effect of the immune system on the brain must be considered.

IX. METHODOLOGICAL ISSUES

Immunological alterations induced by a stressor have no analogy to an off-on switch. As described above there is a vast amount of literature which establishes that the hormonal alterations induced by stress are capable of modifying immune system function. However, as also indicated, the intensity of the stressor and even the time of day that the stressor is experienced can modify the effects of the stressor on the immune system. This review has emphasized that stress can suppress the function of the immune system. However, stress has also been shown capable of enhancing the immune response to a specific antigen.[4,43,65]

It is, of course, possible to interrelate a suppression of a component of the immune system with an enhancement of the activity of another portion of the immune system. For example, a decrease in the functional activity of the suppressor population of CD8 lymphocytes may increase the activity of CD4 lymphocytes. A decrease in the functional activity of Th1 lymphocytes may increase the functional activity of Th2 lymphocytes. A decrease in the phago-cytic activity of macrophages, secondary to a stressor at the time of antigen injection, may lead to an increase in the total number of macrophages which ingest the antigen because fewer would tend to be removed by macrophages at the site of antigen drainage. This may result in an increase of antigen presen-tation by antigen-presenting cells to CD4 lymphocytes. Thus, it is apparent that many aspects of stressor-induced immune alteration remain to be determined. Attention must be directed to the effects of stress on the various individual components of the immune system and then to the interactive aspects of immune system function.

Other considerations regarding how stress alters immune system function relate to the background level of stress that a subject has experienced prior to participating in a study. A stressor imposed on a subject who has had low levels of life events may produce different changes than a stressor imposed on an already highly stressed subject. Factors which assist in coping with the stressor such as a peer support group, the amount of sleep the individual has had, nutritional aspects of the subject, and physical fitness are additional factors which may modify a subject's response to stress. In addition, there are genetic aspects regarding activation of hormonal systems such as the H-P-A axis, which may influence the characteristics of the effect on the immune system of a stressor.[58] Even housing conditions can have an effect on the immune system with the density of animals housed in a cage being a factor which modifies immune system function.[51]

It is possible that stressors experienced by a pregnant female may have an influence on the ability of the offspring to cope with a stressor. Increases in the concentration of hormones which are present in the fetal circulation after having traversed the placenta may permanently alter the number of receptors for various ligands which are present on the external surface of membranes of cells of the immune system and of neurons. Alterations in the numbers of cell surface receptors may be associated with changes in behavior or biochemical processes. Several studies have demonstrated that exposure of a pregnant animal to a stressor will produce changes in the reactivity of the offspring to stress.[20,21,62] In addition, there are also alterations in the function of the H-P-A axis, particularly in female offspring of animals experiencing a stressor.[64] Postnatal handling of rodents has been reported to alter the development of the glucocorticoid receptor system in the hippocampus and frontal cortex.[41]

The response of lymphocytes to mitogenic stimulation differs between nursery reared and maternally reared infant nonhuman primates,[13] and these differences persist for at least 2 years of life. Other immune function differ-ences have been noted at the time of weaning of maternally or nursery-reared nonhuman primates, and a decrease of immune function has been induced by multiple separations of the offspring from the mother. These studies suggest that early rearing conditions can have a long-lasting effect on immune function. Obviously, in human research obtaining information regarding the above parameters would be difficult. However, they emphasize the difficulty of studying the mechanisms of stressor-induced immune alteration.

X. CONCLUSIONS

Characterization of the mechanism by which stress modifies immune function will be important if stressor-induced immune alteration has a negative impact on health. As this seems to be the case, it will be important to develop strategies that will alleviate the negative effects of stress on immune system function. Given that many background characteristics of an individual may influence how stress affects the immune system and that there are distinct differences between acute and chronic stress effects on the immune system, this will not be an easy task. However, as considerable information is already known regarding the nature of the hormones which are induced by stress and which modify immune system function, clear directions for future studies are apparent. The next decade should be one in which many significant advances are made in our understanding and modulation of stressor-induced immune alteration.

REFERENCES

1. Ackerman, K. D., Felten, S. Y., Bellinge, D. L., Livnat, S., and Felten, D. L., Noradrenergic sympathetic innervation of spleen and lymph nodes in relation to specific cellular components, in *Progress in Immunology IV,* Cinader, B. and Miller, R. G., Eds., Academic Press, Orlando, FL, 1987, 588.
2. Bachen, E. A., Manuck, S. B., Marsland, A. L., Cohen, S., Malkoff, S. B., Muldoon, M. F., and Rabin, B. S., Lymphocyte subsets and cellular immune responses to a brief experimental stressor, *Psychosom. Med.*, 54, 673, 1992.
3. Bachen, E. A., Manuck, S. B., Cohen, S., Muldoon, M. F., Raibel, R., Herbert, T. B., and Rabin, B. S., Adrenergic blockade ameliorates cellular immune responses to mental stress in humans, *Psychosom. Med.*, 57, 366, 1995.
4. Berkenbosch, F., Wolvers, D. A. W., and Derijk, R., Neuroendocrine and immunological mechanisms in stress-induced immunomodulation, *J. Steroid Biochem. Mol. Biol.*, 40, 639, 1991.
5. Besedovsky, H. O., Del Rey, A. E., Sorkin, E., Da Prada, M., Burri, R., and Honegger, C., The immune response evokes changes in brain noradrenergic neurons, *Science*, 221, 564, 1983.
6. Besedovsky, H. O., Sorkin, E., Felix, D., and Haas, H., Hypothalamic changes during the immune response, *Eur. J. Immunol.*, 7, 325, 1977.
7. Besedovsky, H. and Sorkin, E., Network of immune-neuroendocrine interactions, *Clin. Exp. Immunol.*, 27, 1, 1977.
8. Blalock, J. E., The syntax of immune-neuroendocrine communication, *Immunol. Today*, 15, 504, 1994.
9. Breneman, S. M., Moynihan, J. A., Grota, L. J., Felten, D. L., and Felten, S. Y., Splenic norepinephrine is decreased in MRL-lpr mice, *Brain Behav. Immunity*, 7, 135, 1993.
10. Brooks, W. H., Cross, R. J., Roszman, T. L., and Markesbery, W. R., Neuroimmunomodulation: neural anatomical basis for impairment and facilitation, *Ann. Neurol.*, 12, 56, 1982.

11. Carlson, S. L., Brooks, W. H., and Roszman, T. L., Neurotransmitter-lymphocyte interactions: dual receptor modulation of lymphocyte proliferation and cAMP production, *J. Neuroimmunol.*, 24, 155, 1989.
12. Clarke, B. L. and Bost, K. L., Differential expression of functional adrenocorticotropic hormone receptors by subpopulations of lymphocytes, *J. Immunol.*, 143, 464, 1989.
13. Coe, C. L., Lubach, G. R., Ershler, W. B., and Klopp, W., Influence of early rearing on lymphocyte proliferation responses in juvenile Rhesus monkeys, *Brain Behav. Immunity*, 3, 47, 1989.
14. Cohen, S., Tyrrell, D. A. J., and Smith, A. P., Psychological stress and susceptibility to the common cold, *N. Eng. J. Med.*, 325, 606, 1991.
15. Coussons-Read, M. E., Maslonek, K. A., Fecho, K., Perez, L., and Lysle, D. T., Evidence for the involvement of macrophage-derived nitric-oxide in the modulation of immune status by a conditioned aversive stimulus, *J. Neuroimmunol.*, 50, 51, 1994.
16. Crary, B., Borysenko, M., Sutherland, D. C., Kutz, I., Borysenko, J. S., and Benson, H., Decrease in mitogen responsiveness of mononuclear cells from peripheral blood after epinephrine administration in humans, *J. Immunol.*, 130, 694, 1983.
17. Cross, R. J., Markesbery, W. R., Brooks, W. H., and Roszman, T. L., Hypothalamic-immune interactions. I. The acute effect of anterior hypothalamic lesions on the immune response, *Brain Res.*, 196, 79, 1980.
18. Cunnick, J. E., Lysle, D. T., Armfield, A., and Rabin, B. S., Shock induced modulation of lymphycte responsiveness and natural killer cell activity: differential mechanisms of induction, *Brain Behav. Immunity*, 2, 102, 1988.
19. Cunnick, J., Lysle, D. T., Kucinski, B. J., and Rabin, B. S., Evidence that shock induced immune suppression is mediated by adrenal hormones and peripheral beta-adrenergic receptors, *Pharmacol. Biochem. Behavior*, 36, 645, 1990.
20. Fride, E. and Weinstock, M., Prenatal stress increases anxiety-related behavior and alters cerebral lateralization of dopamine activity, *Life Sci.*, 42, 1059, 1988.
21. Fride, E., Han, Y., Feldon, J., Halevy, G., and Weinstock, M., Effects of prenatal stress on vulnerability to stress in prepubertal and adult rats, *Psychol. Behav.*, 37, 681, 1986.
22. Glaser, R., Kiecolt-Glaser, J. K., Stout, J. C., Tarr, K. L., Speicher, C. E., and Holliday, J. E., Stress-related impairments in cellular immunity, *Psychiatr. Res.*, 16, 233, 1985.
23. Graham, N. M. H., Douglas, R. M., and Ryan, P., Stress and acute respiratory infection, *Am. J. Epidemiol.*, 124, 389, 1986.
24. Haefeli, W. E., Bargetzi, M. J., Starnes, H. F., Blaschke, T. F., and Hoffman, B. B., Evidence for activation of the sympathetic nervous system by recombinant human interleukin-1 in humans, *J. Immunother.*, 13, 136, 1993.
25. Hatfield, S. M., Petersen, B. H., and DiMicco, J. A., Beta adrenoceptor modulation of the generation of murine cytotoxic T lymphocytes in vitro, *J. Pharm. Exper. Ther.*, 23, 460, 1986.
26. Herbert, T. B., Cohen, S., Marsland, A. L., Bachen, E. A., Rabin, B. S., Muldoon, M. F., and Manuck, S. B., Cardiovascular reactivity and the course of the immune response to an acute psychological stressor, *Psychosom. Med.*, 56, 337, 1994.
27. Herbert, T. and Cohen, S., Stress and immunity in humans: a meta-analytic review, *Psychosom. Med.*, 55, 364, 1993.
28. Hoffman, G. E., Smith, M. S., and Verbalis, J. G., C-Fos and related immediate-early gene-products as markers of activity in neuroendocrine systems, *Front. Neuroendocrinol.*, 14, 173, 1993.
29. Irwin, M., Brown, M., Patterson, T., Hauger, R., Mascovich, A., and Grant, I., Neuropeptide Y and natural killer cell activity: findings in depression and Alzheimer caregiver stress, *Fed. Soc. Exp. Biol. Med. J.*, 5, 3100, 1991.
30. Khan, M. M., Sansoni, P., Silverman, E. D., Engleman, E. G., and Melmon, K. I., Beta-adrenergic receptors on human suppressor, helper, and cytolytic lymphocytes, *Biochem. Pharmacol.*, 35, 1137, 1986.

31. Kiecolt-Glaser, J. K., Speicher, C. E., Holliday, J. E., and Glaser, R., Stress and the transformation of lymphocytes by Epstein-Barr virus, *J. Behav. Med.*, 7, 1, 1984.
32. Kiecolt-Glaser, J. K., Malarkey, W. B., Cacioppo, J. T., Mao, H. Y., and Glaser, R., Stressful personal relationships. Immune and endocrine function, in *Handbook of Human Stress and Immunity*, Glaser, R. and Kiecolt-Glaser, J. K., Eds., Academic Press, San Diego, 1994, 321.
33. Kiecolt-Glaser, J. K., Malarkey, W. B., Chee, M., Newton, T., Cacioppo, J. T., Mao, H. Y., and Glaser, R., Negative behavior during marital conflict is associated with immunological down-regulation, *Psychosom. Med.*, 55, 395, 1993.
34. Koff, W. C. and Dunegan, M. A., Modulation of macrophage-mediated tumoricidal activity by neuropeptides and neurohormones, *J. Immunol.*, 135, 350, 1985.
35. Kusnecov, A. W. and Rabin, B. S., Stressor-induced alterations of immune function: mechanisms and issues, *Int. Arch. Allergy Immunol.*, 105, 107, 1994.
36. Lysle, D. T., Cunnick, J. E., Kucinski, B. J., Fowler, H., and Rabin, B. S., Characterization of immune alterations induced by a conditioned aversive stimulus, *Psychobiology*, 18, 220, 1990.
37. Madden, K. S. and Felten, D. L., Experimental basis for neural-immune interactions, *Physiol. Rev.*, 75, 77, 1995.
38. Maisel, A. S., Knowlton, K. U., Fowler, P., Reardon, A., Ziegler, M. G., Motulsky, H. J., Insel, P. A., and Michel, M. C., Adrenergic control of circulating lymphocyte subpopulations. Effects of congestive heart failure, dynamic exercise, and terbutaline treatment, *J. Clin. Invest.*, 85, 462, 1990.
39. Maisel, A. S., Fowler, P., Rearden, A., Motulsky, H. J., and Michel, M. C., A new method for isolation of human lymphocyte subsets reveals differential regulation of beta-adrenergic receptors by terbutaline treatment, *Clin. Pharmacol. Ther.*, 46, 429, 1989.
40. Manuck, S. B., Cohen, S., Rabin, B. S., Muldoon, M. F., and Bachen, E. A., Individual differences in cellular immune responses to stress, *Psychol. Sci.*, 2, 1, 1991.
41. Meaney, M. J., Aitken, D. H., Bodnoff, S. R., Iny, L. J., and Tatarewicz, J. E., Early postnatal handling alters glucocorticoid receptor concentrations in selected brain regions, *Behav. Neurosci.*, 99, 765, 1985.
42. Miller, A. H., Spencer, R. L., Husain, A., Rhee, R., McEwen, B. S., and Stein, M., Differential expression of type-i adrenal-steroid receptors in immune tissues is associated with tissue-specific regulation of type-ii receptors by aldosterone, *Endocrinology*, 133, 2133, 1993.
43. Moynihan, J. A., Ader, R., Grota, L. J., Schachtman, T. R., and Cohen, N., The effects of stress on the development of immunological memory following low-dose antigen priming in mice, *Brain Behav. Immunity*, 4, 1, 1990.
44. Naliboff, B. D., Benton, D., Solomon, G. F., Morley, J. E., Fahey, J. L., Bloom, E. T., Makinodan, T., and Gilmore, S. L., Immunological changes in young and old adults during brief laboratory stress, *Psychosom. Med.*, 53, 121, 1991.
45. Nance, D., Rayson, D., and Carr, R., The effects of lesions in the lateral septal and hippocampal areas on the humoral immune response of adult female rats, *Brain Behav. Immunity*, 1, 292, 1987.
46. Ogarra, A. and Murphy, K., Role of cytokines in determining t-lymphocyte function, *Curr. Opinion Immunol.*, 6, 458, 1994.
47. Pernow, J., Schwieler, J., Kahan, T., Hjemdahl, P., Oberle, J., Gunnar Wallin, B., and Lundberg, J. M., Influence of sympathetic discharge pattern on norepinephrine and neuropeptide Y release, *Am. J. Physiol.*, 257, H866, 1989.
48. Pezzone, M. A., Lee, W. S., Hoffman, G. E., Pezzone, K. M., and Rabin, B. S., Activation of brainstem catecholaminergic neurons by conditioned and unconditioned aversive stimuli as revealed by c-Fos immunoreactivity, *Brain Res.*, 608, 310, 1993.

49. Pezzone, M., Dohanics, J., and Rabin, B. S., Effects of footshock stress upon spleen and peripheral blood lymphocyte mitogenic responses in rats with lesions of the paraventricular nuclei, *J. Neuroimmunol.*, 53, 39, 1994.

50. Pezzone, M. A., Lee, W. S., Hoffman, G. E., and Rabin, B. S., Induction of c-Fos immunoreactivity in the rat forebrain by conditioned and unconditioned aversive stimuli, *Brain Res.*, 597, 41, 1992.

51. Rabin, B., Cohen, S., Ganguli, R., Lysle, D. T., and Cunnick, J. E., Bidirectional interaction between the brain and the immune system, *CRC Crit. Rev. Immunol.*, 9, 279, 1989.

52. Rabin, B. S., Pezzone, M. A., Kusnecov, A. W., and Hoffman, G. E., Identification of stressor-activated areas in the central nervous system, in *Methods Neurosci. Methods*, 24, 185, 1995.

53. Rabin, B. S., Cunnick, J. E., and Lysle, D. T., Stress induced alteration of immune function, *Prog. Neuroendocrinol. Immunol.*, 3, 116, 1990.

54. Rivest, S., Torres, G., and Rivier, C., Differential effects of central and peripheral injection of interleukin-1 on brain c-Fos expression and neuroendocrine functions, *Brain Res.*, 587, 13, 1992.

55. Shavit, Y., Stress-induced immune modulation in animals: Opiates and endogenous opioid peptides, in *Psychoneuroimmunology*, Ader, R., Felten, D. L., and Cohen, N., Academic Press, New York, 1991, 789.

56. Sibinga, N. E. S. and Goldstein, A., Opioid peptides and opioid receptors in cells of the immune system, *Ann. Rev. Immunol.*, 6, 219, 1988.

57. Spencer, R. L., Miller, A. H., Moday, H., Stein, M., and McEwen, B. S., Diurnal differences in basal and acute stress levels of type I and type II adrenal receptor steroid activation in neural and immune tissues, *Endocrinology*, 122, 1941, 1993.

58. Sternberg, E. M., Hill, J. M., Chrousos, G. P., Kamilaris, T., Listwak, S. J., Gold, P. W., and Wilder, R., Inflammatory mediator-induced hypothalamic-pituitary-adrenal axis activation is defective in streptococcal cell wall arthritis-susceptible Lewis rats, *Proc. Natl. Acad. Sci.*, 86, 2374, 1989.

59. Sundar, S. K., Becker, K. J., Cierpial, M. A., Carpenter, M. D., Rankin, L. A., Fleener, S. L., Ritchie, J. C., Simson, P. E., and Weiss, J. M., Intracerebroventricular infusion of interleukin-1 rapidly decreases peripheral cellular immune responses, *Proc. Natl. Acad. Sci.*, 86, 6398, 1989.

60. van Tits, L. J. H. and Graafsma, S. J., Stress influences CD4+ lymphocyte counts, *Immunol. Lett.*, 30, 141, 1991.

61. Vriend, C. Y., Zuo, L., Dyck, D. G., Nance, D. M., and Greenberg, A. H., Central administration of interleukin-1 increases norepinephrine turnover in the spleen, *Brain Res. Bull.*, 31, 39, 1993.

62. Wakshlak, A. and Weinstock, M., Neonatal handling reverses behavioral abnormalities induced in rats by prenatal stress, *Physiol. Behav.*, 48, 289, 1990.

63. Wan, W., Vriend, Y., Wetmore, L., Gartner, J., Greenberg A., and Nance, D., The effect of stress on splenic immune function are mediated by the splenic nerve, *Brain Res. Bull.*, 30, 101, 1993.

64. Weinstock, M., Matlina, E., Maor, G. I., Rosen, H., and McEwen, B. S., Prenatal stress selectively alters the reactivity of the hypothalamic-pituitary adrenal system in the female rat, *Brain Res.*, 595, 195, 1992.

65. Wood, P. G., Karol, M. H., Kusnecov, A. W., and Rabin, B. S., Enhancement of antigen specific humoral and cell mediated immunity by electric footshock stress in rats, *Brain Behav. Immunity*, 7, 121, 1993.

Chapter 3

EXERCISE AND THE ACUTE PHASE RESPONSE

Joseph G. Cannon

CONTENTS

I. THE ACUTE PHASE RESPONSE

A. HISTORICAL OBSERVATIONS

Long before human beings knew of the existence of bacteria, they had empirically developed antiseptic procedures. Three thousand years ago, ancient Egyptians appear to have treated wounds with copper compounds.[61] Egg white (containing the iron chelator conalbumin) was apparently applied for the same purposes as early as the sixteenth century.[103] At the beginning of this century, Wagner-Jauregg[100] intentionally infected patients with malaria, which was clinically manageable, in order to induce fever and cure neurosyphilis which was not treatable in any other way at the time. It is now known that these early remedies mimic endogenous mechanisms that alter trace metal concentrations, produce binding proteins, and induce fever as part of host defense against microorganisms: these mechanisms are known collectively as the acute phase response. Mobilization and activation of phagocytic cells, and production of immunomodulating factors such as complement and cytokines are also part of the acute phase response. These adaptations develop relatively quickly (minutes to hours), compared to B and T cell responses that generally take several days to develop. On the other hand, the acute phase response acquires no memory and thus does not react to a second challenge with an augmented response in the manner of lymphocytes.

B. EARLY OBSERVATIONS OF ACUTE PHASE MANIFESTATIONS FOLLOWING EXERCISE

Increases in circulating white blood cell numbers were carefully studied after the 1900 through 1902 Boston marathons as part of a comprehensive medical study of the finishers;[7] moreover, the phenomenon had been described even earlier.[87] Elevated excretion of acute phase proteins after a marathon was observed by Poortmans and Jeanloz in the late 1960s.[78] The influences of both chronic and acute exercise on circulating concentrations of acute phase proteins and trace metals such as copper were reported in a series of papers by Haralambie and co-workers[43,44] in the late 1960s through the mid-70s, as well as Rocker et al.[80] and Liesen et al.[59] In 1972, Haight and Keatinge reported a delayed alteration in thermoregulation after exercise that had attributes of a fever.[40]

The present review will first describe the mechanisms and the potential adaptive value of the acute phase response in its conventional context of injury and infection. Next, evidence for manifestations of an acute phase response following exercise will be reviewed along with a discussion of whether these manifestations are mechanistically the same as a classical acute phase response. Last, the question of whether these changes have any adaptive value in association with exercise will be discussed.

II. THE ACUTE PHASE RESPONSE TO INFECTION OR INJURY

A. COMPLEMENT

Pathogenic microorganisms or cell fragments from damaged host cells can trigger the proteolytic cleavage of circulating inactive precursor molecules belonging to the complement system.[68] These cleavage products become proteolytic enzymes themselves, cleaving other complement precursors. Other activated products participate in the assembly of membrane attack complexes that disrupt the membranes of foreign cells. The result is a rapid, autocatalytic response similar to the blood clotting cascade. Other end products of this cascade recruit neutrophils into the bloodstream (C3e); draw leukocytes to the site of infection or injury (a process known as chemotaxis, promoted by C3a and C5a); activate phagocytic cells (C3a, C4a, and C5a); and coat foreign particles to facilitate phagocytosis (a process known as opsonization, performed by C3b).[36] Complement activation occurs within minutes of an injury or infection.

B. CYTOKINES

Pathogenic organisms and their products stimulate a wide variety of cells, notably blood monocytes and tissue macrophages, to produce small molecular weight proteins (most ~8 to 30 kDa) known collectively as cytokines.[24] These cytokines, like protein hormones, serve as intercellular signals. Nevertheless, unlike classical protein hormones which have relatively discrete sources, targets, and consistent biological actions, cytokines are produced by and act on a wide variety of cells; and the biological activity of each cytokine can be radically altered by the presence of other cytokines.[91] Several cytokines act in an endocrine manner and can be detected in the circulation; however, a great deal of cytokine-mediated activity probably occurs through paracrine and autocrine interactions at the tissue level.[57]

The cytokines interleukin-1β (IL-1β), tumor necrosis factor (TNFα), and interleukin-6 (IL-6) have been most extensively studied in terms of the acute phase response. Injection of these cytokines into laboratory animals[23] or humans[98,101] will induce most if not all aspects of the acute phase response. On the other hand, circulating concentrations of these cytokines have not consistently correlated with the magnitude of various aspects of the acute phase response. This inconsistency is due, in part, to binding proteins and antagonists that affect cytokine activity *in vivo* and hinder the ability to measure circulating cytokines with either bioassays or immunoassays.[17] Furthermore, these cytokines can induce production of each other and often act in a synergistic manner.

C. WHITE BLOOD CELLS

The white blood cell count increases severalfold within a few hours of infection, due primarily to increases in the neutrophil subpopulation. Normally, about half of the mature neutrophils released from the bone marrow circulate: the other half known as marginated neutrophils adhere to vessel walls where they can be recruited rapidly during infection or injury[21]. Other mature neutrophils, along with less mature forms such as band cells, are stored in the bone marrow. These are recruited during injury or infection through the action of C3e and several cytokines. The flux of neutrophils through the vascular compartment is accelerated during infection as the cells are recruited from bone marrow and marginated stores, and then drawn by chemoattractive bacterial toxins, complement components, and cytokines to the site of injury.[93] Neutrophils phagocytize pathogens and cellular fragments, and then break them down with degradative enzymes (including elastase and lysozyme) and reactive oxygen species secreted into the phagosome.[21]

Neutrophils represent the first wave of the cellular defense response. Over a longer period of time — days rather than hours — monocytes begin to appear at the site of injury. Monocytes are also phagocytic cells capable of secreting catabolic enzymes and reactive oxygen species. Moreover, monocytes and their differentiated forms in tissue (macrophages) are primary sources of cytokines.[71]

The catabolic enzymes and reactive oxygen species released by phagocytic cells do not discriminate between foreign and host cells. For the most part, these substances remain within the phagosome, but there is some release into extracellular fluid. To some extent this release is adaptive since breaking down basement membranes of the microvasculature near a site of injury will increase vascular permeability and promote influx of leukocytes.[67] In addition, pathogen-induced destruction of host tissue must be cleared in advance of tissue repair. However, these processes can also lead to damage of healthy innocent bystander host tissues if they are not kept focused and controlled at the site of infection or injury.[62]

D. ACUTE PHASE PROTEINS

A primary mechanism that keeps catabolic products of phagocytic cells focused and controlled is the synthesis of the acute phase proteins.[57] Most acute phase proteins are circulating globulins produced by hepatocytes in response to cytokines, principally IL-6 and IL-1β.[35] Glucocorticoids appear to have little direct stimulatory effect on acute phase protein synthesis, but do enhance the action of cytokines.[2] Cytokine-induced gene expression and subsequent *de novo* protein synthesis take time; thus significant elevations of acute phase plasma proteins require 12 to 24 h to occur. Several acute phase proteins including ceruloplasmin are oxygen radical scavengers that help limit the destruction of host tissue by reactive oxygen species.[35] Other acute phase proteins including α_1-protease inhibitor provide protection from proteolytic enzymes that may stray from the site of injury.[57] Not all acute phase proteins are hepatic-derived plasma proteins. Intracellular proteins such as manganous superoxide dismutase, metallothionein, and catalase are induced in various cells by IL-1β and TNFα and provide further antioxidant protection.[50,104,107]

Other acute phase proteins possess antimicrobial properties. Certain complement precursor proteins are among those synthesized at accelerated rates.[35] C-reactive protein opsonizes foreign substances as well as necrotic host tissue,[35] and participates in cytotoxic reactions against parasites.[9] Haptoglobin, by virtue of its iron/heme-binding activity, has antibacterial properties for reasons described in the next section.[29]

E. TRACE METALS

The changes in trace metal metabolism are intimately linked to acute phase protein synthesis. During infection, plasma iron and zinc concentrations fall, while plasma copper concentrations increase. These changes are associated with antimicrobial as well as antioxidant adaptations.[76]

The mechanism for iron redistribution involves changes in the expression of iron-binding proteins.[103] Normally, senescent red blood cells are phagocytized by reticuloendothelial cells and the heme iron is recycled via the extracellular transport protein transferrin. During infection, a rapid down-regulation of hepatic transferrin production is accompanied by up-regulation of ferritin, the intracellular iron storage protein in hepatocytes and other cells[103]. The reciprocal changes in these iron-binding proteins are induced by IL-1β.[77,81] Activated neutrophils also release lactoferrin which binds to extracellular iron and is subsequently cleared from extracellular fluid by macrophages.

Iron catalyzes the formation of destructive hydroxyl radicals; therefore sequestration of iron reduces the potential for oxidative stress. *In vitro* studies have shown that unsaturated lactoferrin can inhibit lipid peroxidation in experimental liposome preparations.[39] Furthermore, iron sequestration in intracellular depots during infection reduces the availability of this nutrient to bacteria that require it for growth and replication.[103] Food distribution programs in developing countries have encountered unforeseen outbreaks of infectious disease because the high iron content of the food enabled subclinical pathogen burdens to grow to virulent levels in the food recipients.[70]

Although zinc is also an important nutrient for pathogen growth, and zinc is a cofactor in many bacterial proteases that enhance virulence,[45] the movement of zinc from extracellular to intracellular compartments (especially the liver) may promote host cell function more than hinder pathogen growth. Zinc is a cofactor in several enzymes involved in transcription and protein synthesis,[49] which is accelerated in hepatocytes during an acute phase response. The antimicrobial properties of copper are well established; however, it is not clear whether the increase in plasma copper during an acute phase response serves such a purpose or whether it merely reflects the increased plasma concentration of the copper-bearing antioxidant protein ceruloplasmin.[76]

F. FEVER

Body temperature is regulated at a set point, nominally 37°C, but this differs among individuals and varies with a circadian rhythm.[47] The fever brought about by infection is not caused by an impairment of the thermoregulatory system by pathogens or toxins, but rather represents a shift of the set point and a regulated increase in body temperature.[52] The shift in set point is mediated by host-derived endogenous pyrogens which appear to include IL-1β, TNFα, IL-6, and possibly several other cytokines.[53]

Fever appears to have adaptive value as evidenced by Wagner-Jauregg's work with neurosyphilis as well as other more recent clinical studies in which pharmacological inhibition of fever prolonged recovery from chicken pox.[25] One mechanism involves a direct antibacterial effect of elevated temperature, especially in conjunction with lowered iron concentrations.[54] Another is a synergistic augmentation of lymphocyte proliferation by elevated temperature in association with IL-1 and IL-2.[28]

G. EXPERIMENTAL INDUCTION OF THE ACUTE PHASE RESPONSE

Intravenous injection of bacterial lipopolysaccharide (LPS) has been used for decades as an experimental approach for studying the acute phase response in humans.[106] Both the number of acute phase reactants expressed and the magnitude of the expression are dose dependent. For example, doses of LPS too low to cause fever will induce significant changes in circulating leukocytes.[105]

In response to 4 ng/kg LPS, there is no significant increase in body core temperature for the first hour, but then a rapid increase occurs, reaching a maximum (~1.8°C increase) at about 3 h postinjection. Circulating TNFα concentrations rise earliest, peaking at approximately 90 min. Plasma IL-1β reaches maximal concentrations approximately 180 min after injection of LPS, and IL-6 has a slightly longer time course. The maximal cytokine concentrations differ by orders of magnitude: IL-1β at 0.1 ng/ml, TNFα at 1 ng/ml, and IL-6 at >10 ng/ml (reviewed in Reference 11).

Plasma C3a des arg concentrations increase 60 to 70% in human volunteers after infusion of bacterial endotoxin.[74] Neutrophil counts can increase threefold, with about one third of these in the form of band cells.[10] C-reactive protein concentrations can increase >sixfold and iron concentrations fall by approximately 50% (reviewed in Reference 11). Experimental endotoxin infusion represents a relatively mild stimulus: a serious infection can induce much greater increases: for example, C-reactive protein can increase 1000-fold.[35]

III. MANIFESTATIONS OF AN ACUTE PHASE-LIKE RESPONSE FOLLOWING EXERCISE

A. METHODOLOGICAL CONSIDERATIONS

Studying the influence of exercise on host defense responses presents various challenges to the investigator. Both exercise and host defense are dynamic processes such that several independent parameters can change simultaneously. This can sometimes make normalization and interpretation of data difficult. Exercise causes rapid shifts in fluid volumes: changes in the plasma compartment can be corrected to hemoglobin/hematocrit concentrations,[19] and changes in urinary concentration can usually be normalized to creatinine excretion. However, since increased sympathetic drive during exercise increases total protein secretory rates into saliva independent of reductions in salivary water secretion,[3,22] there is no simple way to interpret changes in the salivary concentration of an individual protein. Urinary pH can change during or after exercise[65] which will affect antigen-antibody binding in immunoassays. Finally, recovery of leukocytes from various biological fluids may be influenced by whether the cells are activated *in vivo*, which will affect their adhesion and aggregation characteristics.

As described in the last section, increasing doses of endotoxin cause increases not only in the magnitude of each manifestation of the acute phase response, but also in the number of different manifestations that can be detected. A similar dose-response relationship may hold true for the acute phase-like responses following exercise. In this case the dose of exercise is the product of exercise intensity multiplied by duration. For example, running a marathon[102] or triathlon[97] induces many characteristics of an acute phase response, but a VO_2max test may elicit few such responses. In addition, the various components of the acute phase response are transient and sequential. Some are maximal within minutes (such as complement activation); others require hours (neutrophils) or days (trace metals and acute phase proteins) to reach full expression. Thus, the sampling schedule has a fundamental influence on whether a response is observed.

B. COMPLEMENT

Moderate-duration exercise consisting of 30 min of level running can cause an immediate ~25% increase in plasma concentrations of C3a,[89] whereas longer duration exercise (2.5 h of level running) causes larger (~70%) increases.[27] The complement system can be activated by antigen-antibody complexes through a process of enzymatic reactions known as the classical pathway. Dufaux et al.[26] found increased circulating immune complexes (~10%) after 2.5 h of running consistent with complement activation through this pathway. Classical pathway activation is further indicated by significant increases in enzymatic products (C4a) that are specific for this pathway.[27,89]

Eccentric exercise consisting of 45 min of downhill running also caused an immediate ~20% increase in C3a.[14] This protocol, which causes quadricep muscles to lengthen as they develop tension, has been shown to induce significant ultrastructural damage to sarcomeres.[32] Thus, tissue fragments released by mechanical damage to contractile or connective elements may activate the complement cascade through a different set of enzymatic reactions known as the alternative pathway.

C. CYTOKINES

In 1983, endogenous pyrogen-like activity was demonstrated in human plasma after exercise by injecting the plasma into rats: this increased the body temperature, and depressed the plasma iron concentrations of the rats.[16] As previously mentioned, IL-1β, TNFα, IL-6, and several other cytokines are now known to act as endogenous pyrogens. Other studies have detected circulating factors, or factors released from blood mononuclear cells isolated after exercise, that caused increased proliferation of responder cells in bioassays.[31,102] Due to the overlapping activities of cytokines, the results of these experiments may be due to additive or synergistic actions of several cytokines. This postexercise proliferation-inducing activity was neutralized using specific antibodies against IL-1, supporting the concept that IL-1 was one of the cytokines involved[13].

Using specific immunoassays, conflicting reports have been published regarding the presence of circulating TNFα (e.g., Reference 30 vs. Reference 88) and IL-6 (e.g., Reference 92 vs. Reference 88) following exercise. This is not surprising, in view of the widely varying performance characteristics of immunoassay kits with plasma or serum samples.[5] Another contributing factor is that, in general, immunoassays are less sensitive than bioassays. Immunoassay evidence for significant postexercise increases in circulating IL-1β has been consistently negative. However, immunoassay evidence for elevated plasma levels of an individual cytokine cannot tell the whole story because biological activity depends on the balance of each cytokine with synergists and endogenous counterregulatory factors.[23]

Enhanced secretion of cytokines by unstimulated or LPS-stimulated mononuclear cells isolated after exercise has been reported. Cultures that do not intentionally include LPS are not strictly unstimulated since isolation procedures, contact with plastic surfaces during incubation, and trace contaminants can prime or partially activate the cells. Nevertheless, an exercise-associated priming effect on LPS-induced cytokine production is sometimes observed that may be related to the production of reactive oxygen species or lipid peroxides generated during exercise.[20] Dietary supplements that attenuate or exacerbate lipid peroxide generation can eliminate or intensify exercise-enhanced secretion of IL-1β.[15] These observations are consistent with reports that superoxide anions induce IL-1-like activity from human mononuclear cells, and superoxide dismutase or vitamin E blocks this response.[51] In addition, lipid oxidation products of low-density lipoproteins induced IL-1β secretion *in vitro* in a dose-related manner.[56]

It is possible that circulating mononuclear cells may not represent the most relevant cell population. Increased flux of bacterial products from the gut during exercise[8] may activate macrophages in the liver to produce cytokines. Even during systemic endotoxemia, portal blood contains higher cytokine concentrations than systemic venous blood, suggesting that the fixed hepatic macrophages may be the primary producer cells.[33] Moreover, epinephrine enhances LPS-induced IL-6 release from isolated perfused liver.[58] Finally, it has been suggested that increased circulating cytokine activity following exercise may be the result of enhanced lymphatic flow into the circulation,[99] thus relevant cellular sources of cytokines may be in secondary lymphoid tissue.

D. WHITE BLOOD CELLS

As previously mentioned, increased numbers of circulating leukocytes, primarily neutrophils, have been observed after marathons.[7] Leukocytosis has also been noted after exercise of less intensity or duration, such as 5 min of gymnastics[63] or 10 min of running upstairs.[60,94] Several mechanisms may be involved in the mobilization of these cells, and the relative contribution of each may depend on the type and intensity of exercise.

After short-duration exercise, immediate, transient increases may be caused by epinephrine or hemodynamic shear forces that release marginated neutrophils from blood vessel walls (especially lung vasculature). Intravenous injection of epinephrine can cause similar increases,[95] and several studies have correlated postexercise increases in epinephrine with leukocytosis, but beta blockers do not substantially reduce postexercise leukocytosis.[34,79]

Longer duration exercise causes more prolonged increases in circulating neutrophils with peak increases of >100% observed 4 to 6 h after exercise and a modest increase in immature forms such as band cells (usually <10%).[42,66] Such increases in total neutrophils are more than threefold higher than the rise that occurs due to circadian rhythm.[46] Pharmacological administration of glucocorticoids will induce a neutrophilia of similar time course including similar increases in immature forms;[6] however, conflicting data have been reported regarding correlations between postexercise plasma cortisol concentrations and leukocytosis.[42,64] It may be that other neutrophil-mobilizing factors, such as activated complement components and cytokines, contribute to a greater or lesser degree depending on the nature of the exercise.

Neutrophil increases observed after damaging eccentric exercise were greater than those observed after normal concentric exercise in the same subjects at similar levels of oxygen consumption.[90] Since the eccentric exercise is associated with greater tissue damage, it is possible that increased complement activation occurs which in turn mobilizes more neutrophils.[82] Another study involving only eccentric exercise found a correlation between increases in complement activation and increases in circulating neutrophils.[14]

There is also evidence of neutrophil activation during exercise. *In vivo* activation can be monitored by measuring plasma concentrations of enzymes normally stored in neutrophil granules that are released when the cells are activated. Several studies have reported such evidence of neutrophil activation following exercise, including increased plasma concentrations of lactoferrin[97] and elastase.[15,37,55]

E. ACUTE PHASE PROTEINS

The early studies documenting appearance of acute phase plasma proteins after exercise were discussed in a preceding section. Induction of acute phase protein synthesis appears to require a considerable dose of exercise, usually >2-h duration, and concentrations are not significantly increased until approximately 24 h after exercise. Among the proteins that increase are C-reactive protein (three- to tenfold), fibrinogen (twofold) and haptoglobin (10 to 25% increase).[59,97,102]

F. TRACE METALS

Plasma iron concentrations usually do not change significantly following a single exercise session.[1,97,102] Since exercise is often associated with some degree of hemolysis, the steady plasma iron concentrations observed may indicate that an iron-sequestering mechanism is upregulated.[97] Chronically lower plasma iron concentrations[41] along with lower plasma zinc[4] and higher plasma copper concentrations[43] in trained subjects are consistent with the pattern expected during an acute phase response.

G. FEVER

Studying the possibility that a true fever (i.e., change in set point) is induced by exercise is complicated by the increased metabolic heat production that occurs. During exercise, body temperature increases in proportion to metabolic rate and independent of ambient temperature (within the limits of 8 to 29°C).[72] The difference between the new body temperature and thermoregulatory set point, called the load error, is the signal that elicits heat dissipation mechanisms such as vasodilation and sweating. If the set point were to change after the onset of exercise, a relatively small change might be insignificant compared to the load error. Thus most evidence does not support a change in set point during exercise (see Reference 96).

However, there is a lag time of ~180 min between endotoxin infusion and peak fever. Furthermore, the febrile response is a facet of the acute phase response that requires higher doses of endotoxin, as described earlier. Is it possible that a putative exercise-induced fever would be detectable after exercise and that it would require a large dose of exercise? Haight and Keatinge[40] found that after prolonged (8 to 10 h), low-intensity exercise involving walking and climbing, human subjects exhibited slightly increased core temperatures (0.36°C) associated with altered thresholds for heat production and heat dissipation that suggested a fever.[40] More recently, it has been demonstrated that hamsters given access to exercise wheels had higher body temperatures during their inactive diurnal periods than hamsters who were not able to voluntarily exercise.[18] In further studies conducted in rats, it was shown that antiserum to TNFα did not block this response,[85] but antibodies against corticotropin-releasing hormone (CRH) did block the response.[86] CRH has been implicated in the central nervous system pathway that mediates IL-1β-induced fever.[83]

IV. DO ACUTE PHASE RESPONSES AFTER EXERCISE HAVE ADAPTIVE VALUE?

Without knowing all the essential elements involved in a stressful situation, it is impossible to state whether a particular, isolated variation in host function is beneficial or detrimental. A decrease in a particular parameter is not necessarily disadvantageous. As described earlier, raising plasma iron levels toward normal in the wrong circumstances can increase susceptibility to infection. Likewise, increases in phagocytic cell activity are not necessarily always in the host's best interests. The proximal causes of tissue necrosis in sepsis and trauma are often overactive host phagocytes.[75] It is clear that during an infectious episode, a great many elements of the acute phase response are directed at keeping the destructive power of host effector cells under control.[57,69]

Although systemic changes similar to an acute phase response after a single exercise session tend to be small and transient, local tissue responses may be of sufficient magnitude and duration to have biological relevance. For example, neutrophils rapidly infiltrate eccentric contraction-damaged muscle tissue, with the magnitude of infiltration proportional to the extent of z-band damage.[32] Monocytes follow, accumulating in muscle tissue over the course of the next several days.[48,84] These phagocytic cells may promote clearance of damaged tissue and secrete several factors that stimulate tissue repair.[12,71]

Likewise, chronic training-induced changes in trace metal distribution and acute phase protein concentrations may represent a significant adaptation to exercise-induced oxidative stress. Iron catalyzes the production of reactive oxygen species and transforms lipid peroxides to cytotoxic aldehydes.[38] Since exercise increases oxygen radical formation,[20] lowering plasma iron may limit damage to tissues during exercise. In addition, increased concentrations of the circulating antioxidant ceruloplasmin and the intracellular antioxidant metallothionein may be other adaptations aimed at preventing oxidative damage.[73]

Although these may be plausible adaptive values for an exercise-induced acute phase response, at present they are merely speculative. Designing experiments that examine these processes in appropriate contexts while simultaneously assessing relevant physiological or pathological outcomes is the formidable challenge for future research.

ACKNOWLEDGMENTS

The research studies of the author have been supported by NIH grants AR39595 and AI33414.

REFERENCES

1. Aruoma, O. I., Reilly, T., MacLaren, D., and Halliwell, B., Iron, copper and zinc concentrations in human sweat and plasma; the effect of exercise, *Clin. Chim. Acta*, 177, 81, 1988.
2. Baumann, H., Richards, C., and Gauldie, J., Interaction among hepatocyte-stimulating factors, interleukin 1 and glucocorticoids for regulation of acute phase plasma proteins in human hepatoma (HepG2) cells, *J. Immunol.*, 139, 4122, 1987.
3. Ben-Aryeh, H., Roll, N., Lahav, M., Dlin, R., Hanne-Paparo, N., Szargel, R., Shein-Orr, C., and Laufer, D., Effect of exercise on salivary composition and cortisol in serum and saliva in man, *J. Dent. Res.*, 68, 1495, 1989.
4. Berg, A., Kieffer, F., and Keul, J., Acute and chronic effects of endurance exercise on serum zinc levels, in *Biochemical Aspects of Physical Exercise*, Benzi, G., Packer, L., and Siliprandi, N., Eds., Elsevier, Amsterdam, 1986, 201.
5. Bienvenu, J., Coulon, L., Gutowski, M. C., and Grau, G. E., Comparison of the analytical performances of commercial ELISA kits for TNFα, IL-6 and IL-2 measurements. a WHO study, *Lymphokine Cytokine Res.*, 12, (Abstr.), 393, 1993.
6. Bishop, C. R., Athens, J. W., Boggs, D. R., Warner, H. R., Cartwright, G. E., and Wintrobe, M. M., Leukokinetic studies. XIII. A non-steady-state kinetic evaluation of the mechanism of cortisone-induced granulocytosis, *J. Clin. Invest.*, 47, 249, 1968.
7. Blake, J. B. and Larrabee, R. C., Observations upon long-distance runners, *Boston Med. Surg. J.*, 148, 195, 1903.
8. Bosenberg, A. T., Brock-Utne, J. G., Gaffin, S. L., Wells, M. T. B., and Blake, G. T. W., Strenuous exercise causes systemic endotoxemia, *J. Appl. Physiol.*, 65, 106, 1988.
9. Bout, D., Joseph, M., Pontet, M., Vorng, H., Deslee, D., and Capron, A., Rat resistance to schistosomiasis: platelet-mediated cytotoxicity induced by C-reactive protein, *Science*, 231, 153, 1986.
10. Brown, C. C., Malech, H. L., and Gallin, J. I., Intravenous endotoxin recruits a distinct subset of human neutrophils, defined by monoclonal antibody 31D8, from bone marrow to the peripheral circulation, *Cell. Immunol.*, 123, 294, 1989.
11. Cannon, J. G., Endotoxin and cytokine responses in human volunteers, in *Bacterial Endotoxic Lipopolysaccharides*, Ryan, J. L. and Morrison, D. C., Eds., CRC Press, Boca Raton, FL, 311, 1992.
12. Cannon, J. G., Cytokines in muscle homeostasis and disease, in *Clinical Applications of Cytokines*, Oppenheim, J. J., Rossio, J. L., and Gearing, A. J. H., Eds., Oxford University Press, New York, 1993, 329.
13. Cannon, J. G., Evans, W. J., Hughes, V. A., Meredith, C. N., and Dinarello, C. A., Physiological mechanisms contributing to increased interleukin-1 secretion, *J. Appl. Physiol.*, 61, 1869, 1986.
14. Cannon, J. G., Fiatarone, M. A., Fielding, R. A., and Evans, W. J., Aging and stress-induced changes in complement activation and neutrophil mobilization, *J. Appl. Physiol.*, 76, 2616, 1994.
15. Cannon, J. G., Fiatarone, M. A., Meydani, M., Scott, L., Blumberg, J. B., and Evans, W. J., Aging and dietary modulation of elastase and interleukin-1β secretion, *Am. J. Physiol.*, 268, R208, 1995.
16. Cannon, J. G. and Kluger, M. J., Endogenous pyrogen activity in human plasma after exercise, *Science*, 220, 617, 1983.
17. Cannon, J. G., Nerad, J. L., Poutsiaka, D. D., and Dinarello, C. A., Measuring circulating cytokines, *J. Appl. Physiol.*, 75, 1897, 1993.
18. Conn, C. A., Borer, K. T., and Kluger, M. J., Body temperature rhythm and response to pyrogen in exercising and sedentary hamsters, *Med. Sci. Sports Exerc.*, 22, 636, 1990.
19. Costill, D. L. and Fink, W. J., Plasma volume changes following exercise and thermal dehydration, *J. Appl. Physiol.*, 37, 521, 1974.

20. Davies, K. J. A., Packer, L., and Brooks, G. A., Free radicals and tissue damage produced by exercise, *Biochem. Biophys. Res. Commun.*, 107, 1198, 1982.

21. Davis, J. M. and Gallin, J. I., The neutrophil, in *Cellular Functions in Immunity and Inflammation*, Oppenheim, J. J., Rosenstreich, D. L., and Potter, M., Eds., Elsevier North Holland, New York, 1981, 77.

22. Dawes, D., The effects of exercise on protein and electrolyte secretion in parotid saliva, *J. Physiol. (London)*, 320, 139, 1981.

23. Dinarello, C. A., Interleukin-1 and interleukin-1 antagonism, *Blood*, 77, 1627, 1991.

24. Dinarello, C. A., Cannon, J. G., and Wolff, S. M., New concepts on the pathogenesis of fever, *Rev. Infect. Dis.*, 10, 168, 1988.

25. Doran, T. F., Angelis, C. D., Baumgardner, R. A., and Mellits, E. D., Acetaminophen: more harm than good for chickenpox?, *J. Pediatrics*, 114, 1045, 1989.

26. Dufaux, B., Muller, R., and Hollmann, W., Assessment of circulating immune complexes by a solid-phase C_{1q}-binding assay during the first hours and days after prolonged exercise, *Clin. Chim. Acta*, 145, 313, 1985.

27. Dufaux, B. and Order, U., Complement activation after prolonged exercise, *Clin. Chim. Acta*, 179, 45, 1989.

28. Duff, G. W. and Durum, S. K., The pyrogenic and mitogenic actions of interleukin-1 are related, *Nature (London)*, 304, 449, 1983.

29. Eaton, J. W., Brandt, P., and Mahoney, J. R., Haptoglobin: a natural bacteriostat, *Science*, 215, 691, 1982.

30. Espersen, G. T., Elbaek, A., Ernst, E., Toft, E., Kaalund, S., Jersild, C., and Grunnet, N., Effect of physical exercise on cytokines and lymphocyte subpopulations in human peripheral blood, *APMIS*, 98, 395, 1990.

31. Evans, W. J., Meredith, C. N., Cannon, J. G., Dinarello, D. A., Fronter, W. R., Hughes, V. A., Jones, B. H., and Knuttgen, H. G., Metabolic changes following eccentric exercise in trained and untrained men, *J. Appl. Physiol.*, 61, 1864, 1986.

32. Fielding, R. A., Manfredi, T. J., Ding, W., Fiatarone, M. A., Evans, W. J., and Cannon, J. G., Acute phase response in exercise. III. Neutrophil and IL-1β accumulation in skeletal muscle, *Am. J. Physiol.*, 265, R166, 1993.

33. Fong, U., Marano, M. A., Moldawer, L. L., Wei, H., Calvano, S. E., Kenney, J. S., Allison, A. C., Cerami, A. G., Shires, T., and Lowry, S. F., The acute splanchnic and peripheral tissue metabolic response to endotoxin in humans, *J. Clin. Invest.*, 85, 1896, 1990.

34. Foster, N. K., Martyn, J. B., Rangno, R. E., Hogg, J. C., and Pardy, R. L., Leukocytosis of exercise: role of cardiac output and catecholamines, *J. Appl. Physiol.*, 61, 2218, 1986.

35. Gauldie, J. and Baumann, H., Cytokines and acute phase protein expression, in *Cytokines and Inflammation*, Kimball, E. S., Ed., CRC Press, Boca Raton, FL, 1991, 275.

36. Goldstein, I. M., Complement: biologically active products, in *Inflammation: Basic Principles and Clinical Correlates*, Gallin, J. I., Goldstein, I. M., and Snyderman, R., Eds., Raven Press, New York, 1992, 63.

37. Gray, A. B., Telford, R. D., Collins, M., Baker, M. S., and Weidemann, M. J., Granulocyte activation induced by intense interval running, *J. Leuk. Biol.*, 53, 591, 1993.

38. Gutteridge, J. M. C., Role of free radicals and catalytic metal ions in human disease: an overview, *Methods Enzymol.*, 186, 1, 1990.

39. Gutteridge, J. M. C., Paterson, S. K., Segal, A. W., and Halliwell, B., Inhibition of lipid peroxidation by the iron-binding protein lactoferrin, *Biochem. J.*, 199, 259, 1981.

40. Haight, J. S. J. and Keatinge, W. R., Elevation in set point for body temperature regulation after prolonged exercise, *J. Physiol. (London)*, 229, 77, 1973.

41. Hallberg, L. and Magnusson, B., The etiology of "sports anemia", *Acta Med. Scand.*, 216, 145, 1984.

42. Hansen, J.-B., Wilsgard, L., and Osterud, B., Biphasic changes in leukocytes induced by strenuous exercise, *Eur. J. Appl. Physiol.*, 62, 157, 1991.

43. Haralambie, G. and Keul, J., Serum glycoprotein levels in athletes in training, *Experientia*, 26, 959, 1970.

44. Haralambie, G., Keul, J., and Theumert, F., Protein, eisen, und kupfer veranderungen im serum bei schwimmern vor und nach hohentraining, *Eur. J. Appl. Physiol.*, 35, 21, 1976.
45. Hase, C. C. and Finkelstein, R. A., Bacterial extracellular zinc-containing metalloproteases, *Microbiol. Rev.*, 57, 823, 1993.
46. Haus, E., Lakatua, D. J., Swoyer, J., and Sackett-Lundeen, L., Chronobiology in hematology and immunology, *Am. J. Anat.*, 168, 467, 1983.
47. Houdas, Y. and Ring, E. F. J., *Human Body Temperature: Its Measurement and Regulation*, Plenum Press, New York, 1982, 238.
48. Jones, D. A., Newham, D. J., Round, J. M., and Tolfree, S. E. J., Experimental human muscle damage: morphological changes in relation to other indicies of damage, *J. Physiol. (London)*, 375, 435, 1986.
49. Karin, M., Metallothioneins: proteins in search of a function, *Cell*, 41, 9, 1985.
50. Karin, M., Imbra, R. J., Heguy, A., and Wong, G., Interleukin-1 regulates human metallothionein gene expression, *Mol. Cell. Biol.*, 5, 2866, 1985.
51. Kasama, T., Kobayashi, K., Fukushima, T., Tabata, M., Ohno, I., Negishi, M., Ide, H., Takahashi, T., and Niwa, Y., Production of interleukin-1-like factor from human peripheral blood monocytes and polymorphonuclear leukocytes by superoxide anion: the role of interleukin 1 and reactive oxygen species in inflamed sites, *Clin. Immunol. Immunopathol.*, 53, 439, 1989.
52. Kluger, M. J., *Fever: Its Biology, Evolution, and Function*, Princeton University Press, Princeton, NJ, 1979, 195.
53. Kluger, M. J., Fever: role of pyrogens and cryogens, *Physiol. Rev.*, 71, 93, 1991.
54. Kluger, M. J. and Rothenburg, B. A., Fever and reduced iron: their interaction as a host defense response to bacterial infection, *Science*, 203, 374, 1979.
55. Kokot, K., Schaefer, R. M., Teschner, M., Gilge, U., Plass, R., and Heidland, A., Activation of leukocytes during prolonged physical exercise, *Adv. Exp. Med. Biol.*, 240, 57, 1988.
56. Ku, G., Thomas, C. E., Akeson, A. L., and Jackson, R. L., Induction of interleukin 1β expression from human peripheral blood monocyte-derived macrophages by 9-hydroxyoctadecadienoic acid, *J. Biol. Chem.*, 267, 14183, 1992.
57. Kushner, I., Regulation of the acute phase response by cytokines, *Perspect. Biol. Med.*, 36, 611, 1993.
58. Liao, J. F., Keiser, J. A., Scales, W. E., and Kluger, M. J., The role of epinephrine on TNF and IL-6 production in isolated perfused rat liver, *Am. J. Physiol.*, 268, R896, 1995.
59. Liesen, H., Dufaux, B., and Hollman, W., Modifications of serum glycoproteins the days following a prolonged physical exercise and the influence of physical training, *Eur. J. Appl. Physiol.*, 37, 243, 1977.
60. Loppnow, H. and Libby, P., Proliferating or interleukin-1-activated human vascular smooth muscle cells secrete copious interleukin-6, *J. Clin. Invest.*, 85, 731, 1990.
61. Majno, G., *The Healing Hand*, Harvard University Press, Cambridge, MA, 1975, 571.
62. Malech, H. L. and Gallin, J. I., Neutrophils in human diseases, *N. Engl. J. Med.*, 317, 687, 1987.
63. Martin, H. E., Physiological leukocytosis, *J. Physiol. (London)*, 75, 113, 1932.
64. McCarthy, D. A., Macdonald, I., Grant, M., Marbut, M., Watling, M., Nicholson, S., Deeks, J. J., Wade, A. J., and Perry, J. D., Studies on the immediate and delayed leucocytosis elicited by brief (30-min) strenuous exercise, *Eur. J. Appl. Physiol.*, 64, 513, 1992.
65. McKelvie, R. S., Lindinger, M. I., Heigenhauser, G. J. F., Sutton, J. R., and Jones, N. L., Renal responses to exercise-induced lactic acidosis, *Am. J. Physiol.*, 257, R102, 1989.
66. Moorthy, A. V. and Zimmerman, S. W., Human leukocyte response to and endurance race, *Eur. J. Appl. Physiol.*, 38, 271, 1978.
67. Movat, H. Z., Cybulsky, M. I., Colditz, I. G., Chan, M. K. W., and Dinarello, C. A., Acute inflammation in Gram-negative infection: endotoxin, interleukin 1, tumor necrosis factor and neutrophils, *Fed. Proc.*, 46, 97, 1987.

68. Muller-Eberhard, H. J., Complement: chemistry and pathways, in *Inflammation: Basic Principles and Clinical Correlates*, Gallin, J. I., Goldstein, I. M., and Snyderman, R., Eds., Raven Press, New York, 1992, 33.

69. Munck, A., Guyre, P. M., and Holbrook, N. J., Physiological functions of glucocorticoids in stress and their relation to pharmacological actions, *Endocr. Rev.*, 5, 25, 1984.

70. Murray, M. J., Murray, A. B., Murray, M. B., and Murray, C. J., The adverse effect of iron repletion on the course of certain infections, *Br. Med. J.*, 2, 1113, 1978.

71. Nathan, C. F., Secretory products of macrophages, *J. Clin. Invest.*, 79, 319, 1987.

72. Nielsen, M., Die regulation der korpertemperatur bei muskelarbeit, *Skand. Arch. Physiol.*, 79, 193, 1938.

73. Oh, S. H., Deagen, J. T., Whanger, P. D., and Weswig, P. H., Biological function of metallothionein. V. Its induction in rats by various stresses, *Am. J. Physiol.*, 3, E282, 1978.

74. Parrillo, J. E., Burch, C., Shelhamer, J. H., Parker, M. M., Natanson, C., and Schuette, W., A circulating myocardial depressant substance in humans with septic shock, *J. Clin. Invest.*, 76, 1539, 1985.

75. Parrillo, J. E., Parker, M. M., Natanson, C., Suffredini, A. F., Danner, R. L., Cunnion, R. E., and Ognibene, F. P., Septic shock in humans, *Ann. Intern. Med.*, 113, 227, 1990.

76. Pekarek, R. S. and Engelhardt, J. A., Infection-induced alterations in trace metal metabolism: relationship to organism virulence and host defense, in *Infection: The Physiologic and Metabolic Responses of the Host*, Powanda, M. C. and Canonico, P. G., Eds., Elsevier North-Holland, Amsterdam, 1981, 131.

77. Perlmutter, D. H., Dinarello, C. A., Punsal, P. I., and Colten, H. R., Cachectin/tumor necrosis factor regulates hepatic acute phase gene expression, *J. Clin. Invest.*, 78, 1334, 1986.

78. Poortmans, J. and Jeanloz, R. W., Quantitative immunological determination of 12 plasma proteins excreted in human urine collected before and after exercise, *J. Clin. Invest.*, 47, 386, 1968.

79. Rocker, L. and Franz, I.-W., Effect of chronic b-adrenergic blockade on exercise-induced leukocytosis, *Klin. Wochenschr.*, 64, 270, 1986.

80. Rocker, L., Kirsch, K. A., and Stoboy, H., Plasma volume, albumin and globulin concentrations and their intravascular masses. A comparative study in endurance athletes and sedentary subjects, *Eur. J. Appl. Physiol.*, 36, 57, 1976.

81. Rogers, J. T., Bridges, K. R., Durmowicz, G. P., Glass, J., Auron, P. E., and Munro, H. N., Translational control during the acute phase response, *J. Biol. Chem.*, 265, 14572, 1990.

82. Rother, K., Leukocyte mobilizing factor: a new biological activity derived from the third component of complement, *Eur. J. Immunol.*, 2, 550, 1972.

83. Rothwell, N. J., CRF is involved in the pyrogenic and thermogenic effects of interleukin-1β in the rat, *Am. J. Physiol.*, 256, E111, 1989.

84. Round, J. M., Jones, D. A., and Cambridge, G., Cellular infiltrates in human skeletal muscle: exercise induced damage as a model for inflammatory muscle disease?, *J. Neurol. Sci.*, 82, 1, 1987.

85. Rowsey, P. J., Borer, K. T., and Kluger, M. J., Tumor necrosis factor is not involved in exercise-induced elevation in core temperature, *Am. J. Physiol.*, 265, R1351, 1993.

86. Rowsey, P. J. and Kluger, M. J., Corticotropin releasing hormone is involved in exercise-induced elevation in core temperature, *Psychoneuroimmunology*, 19, 179, 1994.

87. Schultz G., Experimentelle untersuchungen uber das vorkommen und die diagnostische bedeutung der leukocytose, *Dtsch. Arch. Klin. Med.*, 51, 234, 1893.

88. Smith, J. A., Telford, R. D., Baker, M. S., Hapel, A. J., and Weidemann, M. J., Cytokine immunoreactivity in plasma does not change after moderate endurance exercise, *J. Appl. Physiol.*, 73, 1396, 1992.

89. Smith, J. K., Chi, D. S., Krish, G., Reynolds, S., and Cambron, G., Effect of exercise on complement activity, *Ann. Allergy*, 65, 304, 1990.

90. Smith, L. L., McCammon, M., Smith, S., Chamness, M., Israel, R. G., and O'Brien, K. F., White blood cell response to uphill walking and downhill jogging at similar metabolic loads, *Eur. J. Appl. Physiol.*, 58, 833, 1989.

91. Sporn, M. B. and Roberts, A. B., Peptide growth factors are multifunctional, *Nature (London)*, 332, 217, 1988.

92. Sprenger, H., Jacobs, C., Nain, M., Gressner, A. M., Prinz, H., Wesemann, W., and Gemsa, D., Enhanced release of cytokines, interleukin-2 receptors, and neopterin after long-distance running, *Clin. Immunol. Immunopathol.*, 63, 188, 1992.

93. Springer, T. A., Traffic signals for lymphocyte recirculation and leukocyte emigration: the multistep paradigm, *Cell*, 76, 301, 1994.

94. Steel, C. M., Evans, J., and Smith, M. A., Physiological variation in circulating B cell: T cell ratio in man, *Nature (London)*, 247, 387, 1974.

95. Steel, C. M., French, E. B., and Aitchison, W. R. C., Studies on adrenaline-induced leukocytosis in normal man, *Br. J. Haematol.*, 21, 413, 1971.

96. Stitt, J. T., Fever versus hyperthermia, *Fed. Proc.*, 38, 39, 1979.

97. Taylor, C., Rogers, G., Goodman, C., Baynes, R. D., Bothwell, T. H., Bezwoda, W. R., Kramer, F., and Hattingh, J., Hematologic, iron-related, and acute-phase protein responses to sustained strenuous exercise, *J. Appl. Physiol.*, 62, 464, 1987.

98. Tewari, A., Buhles, W. C., and Starnes, H. F., Preliminary report: effects of interleukin-1 on platelet counts, *Lancet*, 336, 712, 1990.

99. Viti, A., Muscettola, M., Paulesa, L., Bocci, V., and Almi, A., Effect of exercise on plasma interferon levels, *J. Appl. Physiol.*, 59, 426, 1985.

100. Wagner-Jauregg, J., The treatment of dementia paralytica by malaria inoculation, in *Nobel Lectures: Physiology or Medicine, 1922–1941*, Elsevier: New York, 1927.

101. Warren, R. S., Starnes, J. H. F., Gabrilove, J. L., Oettgen, H. F., and Brennan, M. F., The acute metabolic effects of tumor necrosis factor administration in humans, *Arch. Surg.*, 122, 1396, 1987.

102. Weight, L. M., Alexander, D., and Jacobs, P., Strenuous exercise: analogous to the acute phase response?, *Clin. Sci.*, 81, 67, 1991.

103. Weinberg, E. D., Iron withholding: a defense against infection and neoplasia, *Physiol. Rev.*, 64, 65, 1984.

104. White, C. W., Ghezzi, P., McMahon, S., Dinarello, C. A., and Repine, J. E., Cytokines increase rat lung antioxidant enzymes during exposure to hyperoxia, *J. Appl. Physiol.*, 66, 1003, 1989.

105. Wolff, S. M., Biological effects of bacterial endotoxins in man, in *Bacterial Lipopolysaccharides*, Kass, E. H. and Wolff, S. M., Eds., University of Chicago Press, Chicago, 1973, 251.

106. Wolff, S. M., Rubenstein, M., Mulholland, J. H., and Alling, D. W., Comparison of hematologic and febrile response to endotoxin in man, *Blood*, 26, 190, 1965.

107. Wong, G. H. W. and Goeddel, D. V., Induction of manganous superoxide dismutase by tumor necrosis factor: possible protective mechanism, *Science*, 242, 941, 1988.

Chapter 4

EXERCISE AND CYTOKINES: SPONTANEOUS AND ELICITED RESPONSES

Gregory J. Bagby
Larry D. Crouch
Raymond E. Shepherd

CONTENTS

I. INTRODUCTION

The primary function of the immune or host defense system, as with all other body systems, is the maintenance of homeostasis. The immune system supports homeostatic control through the recognition and elimination of invading pathogens, and the repair or elimination of damaged or abnormal cells. Our understanding of the complex intercellular communication between immunocompetent cells in accomplishing these tasks has been revolutionized by the discovery of an array of proteins now known as the cytokines. The host defense cytokines are produced by circulating and tissue-resident leukocytes, as well as other cell types. The cytokines include interleukins (IL), interferons (IFN), tumor necrosis factors (TNF), colony-stimulating factors (CSF), and growth factors.

When cellular elements of the host defense system are challenged by noxious stimuli (e.g., pathogens, abnormal or damaged cells, etc.), cytokines are synthesized and secreted to orchestrate a response that will eradicate the challenge or limit the extent of damage. The response mediated by these cytokines resides in their ability to alter cell functions both within and outside the host defense system. Cytokines regulate the overall host response by initiating an inflammatory cascade, potentiating elements of the specific immune system, communicating heightened host defense activity to the central nervous system (CNS), and promoting proliferation of selected cell populations needed to reinforce the response and to repair the process. Initially, proinflammatory cytokines (e.g., TNFα, IL-1α/ß, IL-6, IFNγ) work synergistically to mobilize host defense elements against invading pathogens or otherwise abnormal tissue. Localizing this cytokine-induced inflammatory response is vital to the successful resolution of the impairment. An exaggerated response is normally prevented via several mechanisms. The immune system itself can limit inflammatory responses through the production of antiinflammatory cytokines (IL-4 and IL-10) and mediators such as prostaglandin E$_2$. In addition to communication between immunocompetent cells, cytokines also provide communication between the immune system and virtually all other body systems. In this regard, proinflammatory cytokines have been shown to directly or indirectly activate both the hypothalamic-pituitary-adrenal (H-P-A) axis and the sympathoadrenergic system. Activation of these systems exert potent antiinflammatory actions that limit the further production of proinflammatory cytokines. When the host defense system functions appropriately, proinflammatory and antiinflammatory events are counterbalanced via an elaborate negative feedback system which effectively eradicates noxious stimuli in support of homeostasis. Unchecked the proinflammatory cytokines are powerful enough to result in a systemic inflammatory response that leads to multiorgan failure and death. Likewise, overprotection of endogenous immunosuppressive mediators can impair proper functioning of the host defense system thereby increasing the incidence of infection and compromising surveillance for cancerous cells.

Exercise affects both proinflammatory and antiinflammatory elements of this control system. Events taking place during exercise within active skeletal muscle, and possibly within the splanchnic bed and kidney, are proinflammatory in nature. In response to these exercise-derived signals, host defense cells or other cells within these stressed tissues may respond by producing cytokines, thus amplifying the inflammatory state. These proinflammatory events of exercise may be opposed by increased production of antiinflammatory modulators via increased sympathoadrenergic activity and activation of the H-P-A axis. It is possible that these pathways serve to curtail proinflammatory tendencies. However, exercise-induced antiinflammatory processes may impair the host defense system cytokine response to invading pathogens thereby increasing the incidence of infection after severe exercise and during intense training periods. Whereas exercise itself would be expected to increase the production of proinflammatory cytokines, the cytokine response to subsequent noxious stimuli might be impaired by exercise. In this chapter, we hope to demonstrate that elements of both scenarios are true.

II. THE SPONTANEOUS CYTOKINE RESPONSE TO EXERCISE

A. EARLY EVIDENCE OF CYTOKINE EXPRESSION

Prior to the discovery of cytokines, plasma obtained from endotoxemic, septic, or traumatized animals or patients was known to elicit an array of infection-like responses when administered to recipient animals.[31,51,56] These responses were not seen with normal plasma, and could not be reproduced by classical endocrine hormones. However, the incubation media from various leukocyte preparations possessed similar activities, suggesting that leukocytes produce and release soluble factors responsible for many of the host responses observed when invading pathogens or trauma conditions occur. Although these studies were viewed with some skepticism, they do represent early evidence that leukocyte-derived mediators exert a profound impact on the host during compromised states.

With this background, Cannon and Kluger[20] conducted experiments and found that plasma from exercised subjects elevated rectal temperature and depressed plasma zinc and iron concentrations when injected into rats, while plasma obtained prior to exercise failed to produce these responses. These activities were present in plasma collected immediately after or 3 h after exercise by a mediator that was heat labile and had an apparent molecular weight of 14 kDa. Furthermore, they demonstrated that media collected after *in vitro* incubation of peripheral blood mononuclear cells (PBMC) obtained immediately after exercise contained similar activities. Although other laboratories had already suggested that exercise produced elements of the acute phase response seen during infection and trauma,[34,35,44] this study represented the first evidence that exercise leads to the production of circulating molecules, potentially of leukocytic origin, capable of eliciting such a response.

B. PLASMA CYTOKINE RESPONSE
1. Interleukin-1 and -6

Interleukin-1 was believed to be the cytokine responsible for the exercise-induced plasma activities described by Cannon and Kluger.[20] Cannon et al.[18] and Evans et al.[30] used the murine thymocyte proliferation bioassay in combination with column chromatography to identify IL-1 activity in plasma after exercise. Interestingly, highly trained endurance runners tended to have elevated plasma IL-1 activity prior to exercise, but these values did not increase further in response to exercise.[30] An anti-IL-1 antibody was employed that effectively neutralized the ability of chromatographed fractions to stimulate thymocyte proliferation. This study was conducted prior to the availability of recombinant IL-1 proteins, and the antibody used was produced against a purified antigen. Thus, the possibility that other cytokines were present in the purified fraction used to immunize rabbits likely meant that cytokines other than IL-1 might have contributed to the detected activity. This possibility is supported by subsequent studies that demonstrate the difficulty of detecting IL-1 in human subjects under even severe inflammatory states.[12,22,49] On the other hand, IL-6, active in the thymocyte bioassay, is elevated under a variety of conditions.[3,7,12] Multiple forms of stress increase plasma IL-6 activity, a response that is temporally related to increases in plasma corticosterone values, and is attenuated by prior adrenalectomy.[80] These findings raise the possibility that the plasma component responsible for the proliferative response in the thymocyte bioassay used by Cannon et al.[18] was IL-6 instead of IL-1. Indeed, IL-6 may have been responsible for the fever-inducing properties of plasma from their earlier study.[20]

Despite the availability of more sensitive and specific assays for IL-1α and IL-1ß, subsequent studies have failed to detect IL-1 in plasma obtained during or after exercise with one possible exception.[21,54,67,72] Northoff and Berg[54] were unable to detect IL-1ß in the plasma at the completion of a marathon using either an enzyme-linked immunosorbent assay (ELISA) having a stated detection limit of 15 pg/ml or the thymocyte proliferation bioassay. Ullum et al.[72] failed to detect either IL-1α or IL-1ß in plasma obtained during or 2 and 4 h after subjects exercised for 60 min at 75% of their maximum oxygen uptake.

Finally, Smith et al.[67] were unable to see exercise-induced effect on plasma IL-1ß despite using an immunoassay capable of detecting this cytokine under resting conditions.

In contrast to IL-1, several studies have identified an exercise-induced increase in plasma IL-6 activity or concentration in response to exercise.[54,55,69,72] In a couple of instances, increased plasma IL-6 was not observed after exercise. However, the many studies that do demonstrate this response, add credence to the likelihood that exercise increases the plasma concentration of this cytokine.

2. Additional Cytokines in the Circulation

The effect of exercise on the plasma expression of other cytokines is even less clear. Several studies have failed to detect TNFα or GM-CSF in plasma during or after exercise.[61,67,72,73] However, other investigators have observed increased plasma TNFα and IFNα, and decreased IL-2 in response to exercise. Dufaux and Order[27] and Espersen et al.[29] reported an increased plasma TNFα response in trained subjects 2 h after completing exercise bouts of differing durations. Although both studies used immunoassays, some concern exists because the resting values were substantially greater than values typically reported. Plasma interferon activity was observed to be increased immediately after and 1 h after, but not 2 h after a 1-h exercise session at 70% VO$_2$max.[74] IFNα appeared to be responsible for this plasma activity since it was neutralized by antibody selective for IFNα, but not antibodies selective for IFNß or IFNγ.

The plasma IL-2 response to exercise has also been studied.[29] Immediately after exercise, plasma IL-2 concentration was decreased compared to the levels found in resting plasma or plasma obtained 2 or 24 h postexercise. To date, this is the only cytokine reported to decrease in response to exercise. Because CD4+ cells are the primary source of IL-2 and IL-2 is an important regulator of the specific immune response, a substantiation of this finding might indicate that this system is compromised under conditions of severe exercise.

C. URINARY CYTOKINE RESPONSE

Existing studies indicate that exercise has a minimal effect on circulating cytokine values relative to more extensive trauma states. This should not be taken to mean that exercise does not alter local production of cytokines. Many cytokines function in a paracrine fashion and only enter the circulation in large amounts during a severe inflammatory challenge, a condition that is fortunately not achieved with exercise. Thus, it is entirely possible that production of specific cytokines is altered by exercise, without affecting plasma concentrations in a meaningful way. Sprenger et al.[69] detected increased cytokine concentrations in the urine of long-distance runners at the completion of 20 km and over the subsequent 24 h. At the conclusion of exercise, urine contained increased IFNγ, TNFα, and IL-6. Urine IFNγ was only increased immediately after exercise, whereas TNFα and IL-6 were increased for 1 and 5 h after completion of exercise, respectively. IL-1ß was not elevated in urine obtained at the completion of exercise, but was increased in urine collected 1 h later and remained elevated for at least 24 h postexercise. This study is the clearest indication to date that the cytokine cascade is activated as a consequence of exercise. However, the source of these host defense modulators is not known.

D. POTENTIAL SOURCES
1. Skeletal Muscle

To date, few studies have considered the tissue site of cytokine production in response to exercise. Ullum et al.[72] were unable to detect exercise-induced changes in blood mononuclear leukocyte mRNA for IL-1α, IL-1ß, IL-6, or TNFα. This infers a tissue rather than a blood origin. One likely source is the active muscle where proinflammatory events can occur. Cannon et al.[19] observed increased immunohistochemical staining for IL-1ß in muscle sections treated with rabbit anti-IL-1ß IgG. Tissue sections treated with nonimmune rabbit serum, anti-IL-1ß antibody preabsorbed with IL-1ß recombinant protein, anti-IL-1α, or anti-TNFα exhibited little staining. Increased staining intensity for IL-1ß was prolonged, being evident at both 45 min and 5 d after completing exercise. At 45 min postexercise staining was in the vicinity of capillaries and around plasma membranes; intracellular staining was minimal. However, the micrographs did not reveal the cell of origin. Macrophages are believed to be the primary source of the proinflammatory cytokines such as IL-1ß. Although muscle has few of these cells, they are such potent cytokine producers that few cells would be required. Moreover, exercise-damaged muscle accumulates monocytes which could serve as an additional source.[1,2] Alternatively, vascular endothelial cells are capable of producing IL-1 in response to inflammatory signals, and contain IL-1 receptors.[15,75] Thus, capillary endothelial cells within active muscle may respond to mechanical damage or other signals by producing IL-1ß as well as responding to IL-1ß in a autocrine or paracrine manner. This heightened proinflammatory state would enhance expression of adhesion proteins and increase the biosynthesis of other cytokines like IL-6 and TNFα.[23,37,47,66] In any event, the identification of IL-1ß in muscle and urine after exercise is a clear indication that this cytokine is increased in response to physical activity.

2. Splanchnic Bed

At present one cannot exclude the possibility that tissues other than muscle also increase cytokine production in response to exercise. *In vivo* studies have not identified a nonmuscle site of enhanced cytokine production to exercise, but one must consider lymphoid tissues and tissues rich in macrophages, i.e., the liver and barrier tissues, as possible sources. Exercise redistributes blood flow to active muscle and under severe conditions might compromise blood flow to the splanchnic bed sufficient to cause a relative ischemic state. Several studies demonstrate a cytokine response to hepatic ischemic reperfusion injury.[25,63,70] Of course, such insults are more severe than the reduced hepatic blood flow that might occur during exercise. Nonetheless, the splanchnic bed is rich with cells of the host defense system. The liver contains 85% of the tissue-resident macrophages, the gastrointestinal (GI) tract possesses macrophages and lymphocytes, and the spleen and lymph nodes house immunocompetent cells. Whether the blood flow disturbance to the splanchnic bed itself during exercise is sufficient to enhance cytokine production and secretion is not known. However, in addition to decreased blood flow, such disturbances might cause endotoxemia or gut wall bacterial translocation that could in turn upregulate cytokine expression by immunocompetent cells in the GI tract, liver, and lymph nodes.

Multiple studies report endotoxemia in response to exercise.[16,17] Endotoxin or lipopolysaccharide (LPS) is a cell wall component of Gram-negative bacteria, and is a potent macrophage stimulator that leads to the production of proinflammatory cytokines. The most likely source of endotoxin under these conditions would be micobes from the lumen of the GI tract. It is unknown whether the endotoxemia reported to occur with exercise is sufficient to cause the increased liberation of cytokines expected with intense exercise.

3. Kidney

During exercise, blood flow to the kidneys can also be compromised, and renal tissue has been demonstrated to produce cytokines to such stimuli.[33] Thus, it is possible that the cytokines observed in urine after exercise are produced by the cells within the kidney itself and not the clearance of circulating cytokines. In this regard, Sprenger et al.[69] identified the exercise performed by their subjects as nonexhaustive. Because of this, they inferred that the increased presence of cytokines in urine after exercise came from the circulation.

4. Immunocompetent Cells: *Ex Vivo* Studies

Another means of assessing the effect of exercise on cytokine production is by examining its impact on cytokine release by immunocompetent cells *ex vivo*. For this purpose, blood or tissue-resident leukocytes are obtained at rest, during exercise, or at varying intervals after exercise in order to compare their ability to produce cytokines during *ex vivo* incubations. Cannon and Kluger[20] found exercise to enhance the spontaneous appearance of "cytokine-like" activity into the media of mononuclear leukocytes. In their study, such media produced a febrile response when administered to recipient rats. However, such a spontaneous cytokine response by incubated blood leukocytes has not been observed in subsequent studies despite the use of more sophisticated and specific assays. Haahr et al.[52] were unable to detect IL-1 (α/ß), IL-2, IL-6, TNFα, or IFNγ in the media of 24-h incubated peripheral blood mononuclear cells (PBMC) obtained after exercise. Although Rivier et al.[61] were able to detect TNFα and IL-6 in 24 h conditioned media of adherent blood monocytes, they did not observe meaningful changes in cytokine production by cells obtained immediately after or 20 min after an exercise test in either young or master cyclists. These latter studies, together with the inability of Ullum et al.[72] to observe exercise-induced alterations of pre-mRNA for these cytokines in PBMC, cast doubt on the ability of exercise to induce intrinsic alterations in circulating mononuclear leukocytes that would modify cytokine expression of this particular cell population. As described above, exercise-induced cytokine producing cells are likely found in active muscle, the splanchnic bed, or the kidneys. However, obtaining cells that retain this enhanced production profile in culture has not been reported, and could prove difficult.

E. CONSEQUENCES OF THE CYTOKINE RESPONSE

Whereas an understanding of the cytokine response to exercise is beginning to take shape, the consequences of altered cytokine expression is essentially unknown. That is, although cytokine expression is altered by exercise, it is not clear whether these changes are responsible for the physiological changes associated with exercise. To date no study has demonstrated cytokines to be performing a physiological role postexercise. Indeed, such a role may be difficult to demonstrate because of the diminutive cytokine response. Rowsey et al.[62] attempted to identify TNF as the endogenous mediator responsible for alterations of 24-h body temperature patterns of voluntarily exercising rats. An administration of anti-TNFa antiserum failed to alter the body temperature pattern or wheel exercise activity over a 24-h period.

F. SUMMARY OF THE SPONTANEOUS CYTOKINE RESPONSE

Collectively, these studies indicate that exercise has the potential of increasing proinflammatory cytokine expression (Table 1). However, definitive conclusions with respect to most cytokines cannot be made without additional data. Indeed, many cytokines have not been studied at all. Because the effect of exercise on the plasma cytokine response is small, it is important that future studies: (1) utilize specific cytokine assays with sufficient sensitivity to detect concentrations in plasma under normal quiescent conditions, (2) examine multiple cytokines, and (3) consider the impact of exercise intensity and duration. As several studies indicate that certain cytokines peak in the plasma during the postexercise recovery period, it is imperative that assays be conducted on samples collected throughout this period if a complete picture is to be developed. Additional studies identifying tissue origin of cytokines and the mechanisms responsible for altering cytokine expression in response to exercise are also needed.

Table 1   Summary of Spontaneous *in vivo* Cytokine Expression in Response to Exercise

Cytokine	Muscle	Plasma	Urine	Conclusion
IL-1	↑ IL-1β; IL-1α ND	↑ IL-1 by bioassay, not verified by anti-IL-1α or -1β neutralization or immunoassay	↑ IL-1β	↑ IL-1β expression, but not sufficient to detect in plasma
IL-2	Not determined	↓	Not determined	↓ In plasma
IL-6	Not determined	↑ (Multiple studies)	↑	↑ Expression
TNF	ND	↑ (Inconsistent)	↑	↑ Expression
IFN	Not determined	↑ IFNα; IFNγ and IFNβ ND	↑ IFNγ	↑ Expression
GM-CSF	Not determined	ND	Not determined	Unknown
Other	Not determined	Not determined	Not determined	Unknown

Note: ↑ = Increased; ↓ = decrease; ND = not detected.

III. EXERCISE IMPACT ON ELICITED CYTOKINE RESPONSE

A. IMMUNOCOMPETENT CELLS: *EX VIVO* STUDIES
1. Isolated Cells

Ex vivo incubation experiments are generally conducted in the presence of an agent that stimulates cytokine production. Several investigators have utilized this approach to address the effect of exercise on the function of host defense cells. Such experiments speak to the potential of these cells to respond to adverse stimuli, and not necessarily to whether they produce cytokines in response to exercise itself. Lewicki et al.[43] examined the IL-1 and IL-2 response of monocytes and lymphocytes stimulated with LPS and phytohemagglutinin (PHA), respectively. In their study, twice as much IL-1-like activity was found in the media of adherent PBMC (monocyte/macrophages) obtained from subjects immediately after or 2 h after exercise as compared to media of cells obtained prior to exercise. In the same study, an exercise-induced decrease of IL-2 production by PHA-stimulated nonadherent cells (lymphocytes) was also observed. Because cell numbers were controlled, the results imply that exercise affects the ability of blood-derived monocytes and lymphocytes to respond to their respective stimulating agents. With respect to adherent cells, this may be true, because monocytes are the only cells among the PBMC that readily adhere. However, the composition within the nonadherent component of PBMC includes multiple lymphocyte subsets and natural killer (NK) cells, and the relative contribution of these subsets are altered with exercise.[10,43,57,58] With this in mind, the exercise-induced decrease in IL-2 production by nonadherent PBMC could have resulted from a reduced CD4+ cell percentage, cells known to be primary IL-2 producers among circulating leukocytes.[68]

Other investigators have also observed a decreased IL-2 response to mitogens although one study failed to see such an effect.[45,46,52] Tvede et al.[71] observed a decreased IL-2 response by PBMC to PHA stimulation, particularly when subjects exercised at 75% of maximal aerobic capacity, the highest exercise intensity they employed. Suppression was prevented by the addition of indomethacin, indicating that cyclooxygenase products may be involved. However, the reduced IL-2 response also paralleled a decrease in CD4+ lymphocytes. An exercise-induced parallel decrease in CD4+ cells and the IL-2 response of PBMC was also seen by Baj et al.[9]

Unlike Lewicki et al.,[43] others have failed to observe increased IL-1 production by LPS-stimulated PBMC when obtained during or immediately after exercise.[21,52] However, Haahr et al.[52] did find increased IL-1 and IL-6 production by LPS-stimulated PBMC when cells were obtained 2 h after exercise. In the same study, the TNFα response to LPS and IFNγ response to PHA were unchanged by exercise. Cannon et al.[21] observed an increased IL-1ß and TNFα production by LPS-stimulated PBMC 1 h after completion of 3×15-min bouts of downhill running, an exercise regimen designed to produce muscle damage. The relationship between urinary 3-methylhistidine excretion and IL-1ß was statistically significant but weak; no correlation was evident between muscle damage and TNFα. Also in this study, one group received vitamin E as a daily supplement for 7 weeks. This treatment prevented the exercise-induced increase in LPS-stimulated PBMC IL-1ß production, but it had no effect on the TNFα response. This finding implies that oxidative stress may in part be linked to increased cytokine production after exercise. These studies indicate that exercise induces alterations in the *ex vivo* cytokine response by mononuclear leukocytes stimulated by immunomodulators. However, it is premature to identify this effect as resulting from true intrinsic change in cell responsiveness or as a shift in the relative contribution of leukocyte subsets to the cell mixtures studied.

2. Whole Blood

In addition to the ability of a host defense cell to respond to noxious stimuli, these cells are also influenced by endogenous mediators which include hormones, neurotransmitters, cytokines, and other molecules produced by these and adjacent cells. For this reason, it is difficult to extrapolate from the *ex vivo* stimulated response of isolated cells to how these same cells would respond in the more complex *in vivo* environment. During exercise, immunocompetent cells are potentially exposed to both proinflammatory and antiinflammatory agents. As the cellular response to these agents may be differentially labile, the *in vivo* state may not be retained when cells are separated from their endogenous environment. The closest one can come to this endogenous state during *ex vivo* conditions is whole blood, in which the proximity between the cytokine-producing leukocytes and the extracellular milieu is retained. In this regard, Kvernmo et al.[40] observed a suppression of the LPS-induced TNFα response of whole blood obtained after exercise in three groups of subjects divided according to training intensity and frequency. This is contrary to the enhanced expression of proinflammatory cytokines observed by others with isolated PBMC from exercising subjects.[21,43,52] In addition, Kvernmo et al.[40] observed that as training intensity increased, the whole blood TNFα response decreased in blood obtained during resting conditions. Blood monocyte numbers typically increase in response to exercise.[42,59,76] Therefore, it is tempting to speculate that the altered milieu of the plasma rather than a change in the cell constituents within blood are responsible for this exercise effect.

3. Cytokine-Induced Cytotoxicity

Increased TNFα production may be involved in the ability of exercise to enhance macrophage killing of tumor cells. Woods et al.[77] found thioglycolate-elicited peritoneal macrophages from exercised animals to more effectively kill or inhibit growth of adenocarcinoma cells under coculturing conditions. Increased cytotoxicity was attenuated by including anti-TNFα antibody in the culture media, but not anti-IL-1ß. This result infers that exercise alters the ability of elicited macrophages to produce TNFα, or that macrophages from exercising rodents produce other mediators that sensitized tumor cells to TNFα killing. Similar experiments were conducted with macrophages after *in vivo* activation with *Propionibacterium acnes*.[78] During the 7-d activation period, mice remained sedentary or were exercised daily. Exercise enhanced the ability of *P. acnes*-activated macrophages to kill tumor cells. Although anti-TNFα abrogated cytotoxicity, it did so by macrophages from both control and exercised mice. Thus, unlike thioglycolate-elicited macrophages, exercise-induced differences in TNFα effectiveness were not evident.

It is possible for cell responsiveness to cytokines to change as a consequence of exercise. IFNγ addition to the media of elicited macrophages and tumor cells enhances tumor cell killing. Three daily bouts of exercise do not alter the magnitude of this IFNγ effect.[78] Blank et al.[13] also found the cytolytic activity of IL-2-activated splenocytes to be similar when obtained from either sedentary or treadmill-trained mice. In contrast, Hoffman-Goetz et al.[39] observed a differential response between splenocytes from sedentary and trained mice activated with IL-2. In this study mice were allowed to exercise voluntarily by having 24-h access to a running wheel. After completing 8 weeks of exercise, splenocyte natural killer (NK) cell activity did not differ between sedentary control and trained mice. However, if cells were stimulated with IL-2 for 3 d prior to performing the NK cytotoxicity assay, cells from trained animals exhibited significantly more enhanced killing ability than did cells from time-matched control mice. This study demonstrates in principle the possibility that exercise of a nonstressful nature cannot only affect cytokine production but also may alter the capacity of cells to respond to these immunomodulators.

B. THE *IN VIVO* ELICITED CYTOKINE RESPONSE

1. TNFα Response to Infection

The impact of exercise on the cytokine response to infections has not been adequately studied. In the single study published, Chao et al.[24] examined the impact of swimming exercise on the progression of *Toxoplasma gondii* infection in mice. On the day mice were inoculated with *T. gondii*, daily bouts of swimming were initiated and continued for 25 d. In infected mice, serum TNF activity was elevated 11 and 25 d after injection of *T. gondii*. The TNF response was attenuated in mice subjected to daily swims as compared to sedentary mice. The cause of the reduced serum TNF activity in exercising mice at this stage of infection is unclear. The exercise-induced lowering of serum TNF activity may have represented either a reduced pathogen burden at the time measurements were made or an impaired capacity to respond to the pathogen. With similar infections a complete abrogation of the TNF response with anti-TNF antibodies or soluble TNF receptors can impair host defense resulting in increasing pathogen burden and lethality.[36,41,53] In this study, exercised mice exhibited clinical signs of faster recovery from infection than did sedentary mice. Thus, it is evident that the TNF response observed in exercise mice was sufficient to mount an effect host response.

2. LPS-Induced Proinflammatory Cytokine Response

Normally, large quantities of proinflammatory cytokines enter the plasma of animals challenged with LPS.[11,14,38,81] Indeed, several studies demonstrate that this proinflammatory cytokine response is largely responsible for LPS-induced lethality.[5,26] However, it is also clear that proinflammatory cytokines are essential to the successful host response to many life-threatening infections.[4,28,53,79] Depending on the pathogen, otherwise sublethal infections progress to lethal ones when this cytokine cascade is inhibited. Thus, conditions that suppress the production of macrophage-derived cytokines might be expected to increase susceptibility to infections.

With these results in mind, we conducted experiments to determine the effect of exercise on the *in vivo* LPS-induced TNFα response. Similar to the whole blood experiment reported by Kvernmo et al.,[40] exercise dramatically suppressed the LPS-induced plasma TNFα response.[6] In these experiments rats were exercised to near exhaustion on a motor driven treadmill. At the completion of exercise, rats were administered LPS intravenously. Compared to time-matched nonexercise control rats, the plasma TNFα response was suppressed by greater than 90% with exercise. If exercised animals were allowed to recover prior to LPS challenge, the suppressed state waned but was still evident up to 6 h after completion of exercise. By 24-h postexercise the LPS-induced TNFα response returned to normal. In this study, TNFα was measured with the L929 cytotoxicity assay. Anti-TNFα antibodies completely neutralized the cytotoxic activity of post-LPS plasma. In subsequent experiments, exercise-induced suppression of the TNF response to i.v. LPS was also observed with immunoassay (Figure 1).

It is likely that the suppressive effect of exercise on the LPS-induced TNFα response extends to other proinflammatory cytokines since TNF is in part responsible for the increased IL-1, IL-6, and IFNγ production that is observed following LPS challenge.[26,32] We have found that prior exercise also suppresses of the plasma IFNγ response to subsequent LPS challenge (Figure 1). Thus, prior exercise causes a substantial suppression of the LPS-induced proinflammatory response, a condition that returns to normal within hours after recovery from exercise.

Further studies reveal that the suppressive effect of near exhaustive exercise on the LPS-induced TNFα response is also present in trained rats. Rats trained for 10 weeks on a motor driven treadmill (5 d/week, 30 m/min, 60 min/d) had normal plasma TNFα responses to LPS when challenged 48 h after the last exercise bout (Figure 2). However, when trained rats were

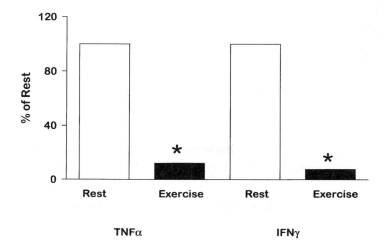

FIGURE 1   Effect of exercise on plasma TNFα and IFNγ determined by immunoassay (Biosource International, Camarello, CA). Time-matched nonexercised control rats (rest) and exercised rats received 1 mg/kg LPS i.v. immediately after near exhaustive exercise (n = 8 per group). Serial arterial blood samples were obtained from an indwelling vascular catheter 1.5 and 4 h post-LPS for determination of plasma TNFα and IFNγ, respectively. Data are expressed as percent of nonexercised control (rest). * $p < 0.05$ compared to rest group.

exercised prior to LPS challenge, the plasma TNFα response was blunted to a similar degree as observed in similarly exhausted sedentary animals (Figure 2). In this study, sedentary and trained rats ran to similar states of exhaustion. This required vastly different amounts of exercise with the trained rats running more than twice the distance compared to previously sedentary animals. It is possible that training would alter the degree of suppression if animals were subjected to the same absolute exercise intensity.

We have found the exercise-induced suppression of the plasma TNF response to i.v. LPS challenge to likely involve the liver. The liver contains approximately 80% of the tissue-resident macrophages, and a majority of LPS is cleared by the liver when administered intravenously.[48] When livers from exercised rats were perfused 90 min after i.v. LPS challenge, TNFα output from the liver was reduced 90 to 98% compared to that of nonexercised control animals (Figure 3).

Studies are underway to identify the endogenous mediators responsible for suppressing the LPS-induced TNF response to prior exercise. In subsequent experiments we found that the LPS-induced TNF response was suppressed with as little as 5 min of exercise (Figure 4). Several studies indicate that glucocorticoids and agents that elevate macrophage cyclic adenosine 5′-monophosphate (cAMP) (e.g., PGE_2, adenosine, and catecholamines) suppress the

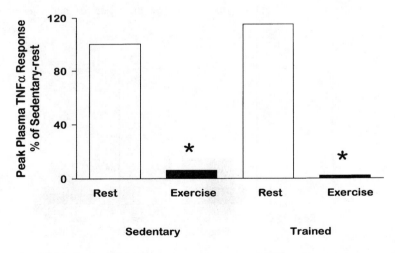

FIGURE 2   Effect of physical training on exercise-induced suppression of the TNFα response to i.v. LPS. Trained or sedentary rats were implanted with indwelling catheters the day before receiving 1 mg/kg LPS i.v. Prior to LPS challenge half the rats were exercised to near exhaustion. Rats not subjected to acute exercise (rest) were placed on top of the treadmill lane dividers during the exercise period. Serial arterial blood samples were obtained for determination of TNFα by L929 bioassay. Cytolytic activity was completely neutralized with a goat anti-TNFα antibody. Data are expressed as percent of resting sedentary rats that were not exercised (n = 9 per group). * $p < 0.05$ compared to sedentary-rest group.

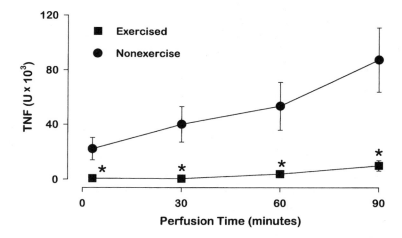

FIGURE 3 Effect of exercise on the release of TNFα during liver perfusion. Time-matched nonexercised control rats (rest) and exercised rats received 1 mg/kg LPS i.v. immediately after exercise (n = 6 per group). Rats were anesthetized 90 min after LPS to initiate liver perfusion. After a few minutes of nonrecirculating perfusion to wash out blood, livers were perfused an additional 90 min by recirculating 150 ml of media. TNFα in the media was determined by the L929 bioassay. * $p < 0.05$ compared to nonexercised group.

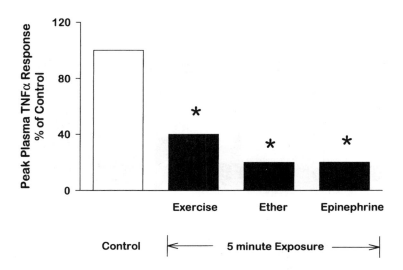

FIGURE 4 Effect of 5-min exercise, ether vapor exposure, or epinephrine infusion (1 μg/min/kg) on the plasma TNFα response to 1 mg/kg LPS i.v. Data are expressed as percent of time-matched control (n = 10 to 15 per group). * $p < 0.05$ compared to appropriate control group.

LPS-induced TNF response both *in vitro* and *in vivo*.[8,60,64,82] Whether such mechanisms perform this role during exercise remains to be determined, but it is well known that exercise increases plasma glucocorticoids and catecholamines.

To date, we have focused our attention on the sympathoadrenergic pathway. Rats stressed by 5 min ether vapor exposure prior to LPS challenge have a suppressed plasma TNFα response (Figure 4). Plasma catecholamine concentrations, but not corticosterone, are elevated by this stress; and epinephrine infusion suppressed the LPS-induced TNF response (Figure 4). For this reason, we conducted experiments to determine whether adrenergic antagonists would prevent the suppressive effect of ether stress on this response. These studies demonstrated that short-term ether stress suppresses the TNF response to i.v. LPS via a β_2-adrenergic pathway (Figure 5).

With this background, we then turned our attention to the role performed by catecholamines in short-term exercise. In a manner similar to ether stress, 5 min of exercise elevated plasma catecholamine concentrations and suppressed the LPS-induced TNF response. This suppression was prevented by the β_2-adrenergic antagonist ICI 118551 (Figure 6). These findings are consistent with *in vitro* experiments using isolated macrophages where β-adrenergic receptors agonists suppress the TNFα response to LPS.[50,65] Short-term stresses, like exercise, that are sufficient to increase plasma catecholamine concentrations are clearly capable of attenuating the proinflammatory cytokine response to LPS. Because similar stresses also increase sympathoadrenergic activity in

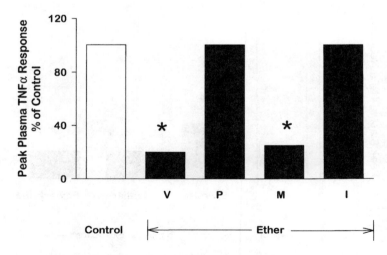

FIGURE 5 Effect of pretreatment with beta-adrenergic receptor antagonists on the plasma TNFα response to 1 mg/kg LPS i.v. Rats were pretreated with vehicle or antagonist 1 h before LPS challenge. V = vehicle; P = 1 mg/kg propranolol (mixed β), M = 0.5 mg/kg metoprolol (β_1), I = 1 mg/kg ICI118551 (β_2). Data are expressed as percent of time-matched control (n = 10 to 15 per group). * $p < 0.05$ compared to vehicle treated control group.

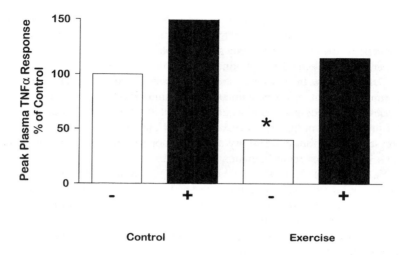

FIGURE 6 Effect of β_2-adrenergic receptor antagonist on 5-min exercise-induced suppression of the TNFα response to 1 mg/kg LPS i.v. Rats were pretreated with vehicle (-) or 1 mg/kg ICI 118551 (+). Data are expressed as percent of time-matched control (n = 6 to 8 per group). * $p < 0.05$ compared to vehicle-treated nonexercised control group.

human beings, one would expect a similar response although such studies have not been performed. Further studies on the modulators responsible for the suppressive effect of exercise on cytokine responses to pathogens and their products are clearly needed.

IV. CONCLUSIONS

The inflammatory nature of exercise results in the increased expression of proinflammatory cytokines. However, exercise results in a cytokine response that is minute relative to those observed in response to more severe challenges of the host defense system. IL-6 is the predominate cytokine expressed in plasma, but increases in circulating concentrations of TNFα and IFNα have also been reported. The presence of IL-1ß in muscle and the appearance of multiple cytokines in urine following exercise show that the expression of a broad spectrum of cytokines in response to exercise is possible. Tissue sources have not been resolved, but muscle, kidney, and tissue-resident leukocytes in the splanchnic bed are likely candidates. The exercise-induced cause of cytokine production has not been identified. Possibilities include mechanical disturbances or injury within muscle, hypoperfusion of the splanchnic tissues or kidneys in favor of blood flow to active muscles or endotoxemia. Because the exercise-induced expression of cytokines is minute, resolving the source and responsible mechanisms will prove to be difficult. To date, the physiological consequences of altered cytokine expression with exercise have not been identified. IL-1ß may be important to the inflammatory response within muscle damaged by exercise. Again the small cytokine response to exercise will hamper efforts to elucidate cytokine effects during exercise.

Cytokine induction by exercise may play a role in tumor cell surveillance. Macrophages from exercised animals impair tumor cell grow more effectively than cells from sedentary animals, a property that involves TNFα under some conditions. Also, mild forms of exercise may enhance the ability of IL-2 to increase natural killer cell activity against tumor cell targets. The *in vivo* role of cytokines in this regard remains to be established.

Exercise also alters the response of immunocompetent cells to immunomodulators via antiinflammatory pathways. Isolated host defense cells often exhibit enhanced proinflammatory cytokine production to LPS or mitogens like PHA. In contrast, *in vivo* experiments reveal suppressed proinflammatory cytokine expression in response to LPS or pathogens, a condition that can be mimicked by whole blood of exercised subjects. Exercise-induced suppression of the plasma TNFα response to i.v. LPS challenge is transient, but is retained for at least 6 h after completion of near exhaustive exercise. As little as 5 min of exercise is sufficient to suppress the LPS-induced TNFα response in rats. The suppressive effect of short-term exercise on this response is prevented by increased sympathoadrenergic activity through β_2-adrenergic receptors. Thus, the neuroendocrine response to exercise may have a profound impact of the ability of the host defense system to respond to noxious stimuli. The suppressed ability to elicit a proinflammatory cytokine response to LPS may relate to the increased incidence of infection after intense exercise or training.

REFERENCES

1. Armstrong, R. B., Muscle damage and endurance events, *Sports Med.*, 3, 370, 1986.
2. Armstrong, R. B., Olgilvie, R. W., and Schwane, J. A., Eccentric exercise-induced injury to rat skeletal muscle, *J. Appl. Physiol.*, 54, 80, 1983.
3. Ayala, A., Wang, P., Ba, Z. F., Perrin, M. M., Ertel, W., and Chaudry, I. H., Differential alterations in plasma IL-6 and TNF levels after trauma and hemorrhage, *Am. J. Physiol. Regul. Integr. Comp. Physiol.*, 260, R167, 1991.
4. Bagby, G. J. and Nelson, S., The role of tumor necrosis factor in the host's response to infection, *Crit. Care Rep.*, 2, 176, 1991.
5. Bagby, G. J., Plessala, K. J., Wilson, L. A., Thompson, J. J., and Nelson, S., Divergent efficacy of anti-TNFα antibody in intravascular and peritonitis models of sepsis, *J. Infect. Dis.*, 163, 83, 1991.
6. Bagby, G. J., Sawaya, D. E., Crouch, L. D., and Shepherd, R. E., Prior exercise suppresses the plasma tumor necrosis factor response to bacterial lipopolysaccharide, *J. Appl. Physiol.*, 77, 1542, 1994.
7. Baigrie, R. J., Lamont, P. M., Kwiatkowski, D., Dallman, M. J., and Morris, P. J., Systemic cytokine response after major surgery, *Br. J. Surg.*, 79, 757, 1992.

8. Bainton, B. G., Nelson, S., Chidiac, C., Bagby, G. J., and Summer, W. R., Anti-inflammatory agents in sepsis and acute lung injury, *Crit. Care Rep.*, 1, 201, 1990.

9. Baj, Z., Kantorski, J., Majewska, E., Zeman, K., Pokoca, L., Fornalczyk, E., Tchórzewski, H., Sulowska, Z., and Lewicki, R., Immunological status of competitive cyclists before and after the training season, *Int. J. Sports Med.*, 15, 319, 1994.

10. Berk, L. S., Nieman, D., Tan, S. A., Nehlsen-Cannarella, S., Kramer, J., Eby, W. C., and Owens, M., Lymphocyte subset changes during acute maximal exercise, *Med. Sci. Sports Exerc.*, 18, 706, 1986.

11. Billiau, A. and Vandekerckhove, F., Cytokines and their interactions with other inflammatory mediators in the pathogenesis of sepsis and septic shock, *Eur. J. Clin. Invest.*, 21, 559, 1991.

12. Bitterman, H., Kinarty, A., Lazarovich, H., and Lahat, N., Acute release of cytokines is proportional to tissue injury induced by surgical trauma and shock in rats, *J. Clin. Immunol.*, 11, 184, 1991.

13. Blank, S. E., Johansson, J.-O., Origines, M. M., and Meadows, G. G., Modulation of NK cell activity by moderate intensity endurance training and chronic ethanol consumption, *J. Appl. Physiol.*, 72, 8, 1992.

14. Block, M. I., Berg, M., McNamara, M. J., Norton, J. A., Fraker, D. L., and Alexander, H. R., Passive immunization of mice against D factor blocks lethality and cytokine release during endotoxemia, *J. Exp. Med.*, 178, 1085, 1993.

15. Boraschi, D., Rambaldi, A., Sica, A., Ghiara, P., Colotta, F., Wang, J. M., De Rossi, M., Zoia, C., Remuzzi, G., Bussolino, F., Scapigliati, G., Stoppacciaro, A., Ruco, L., Tagliabue, A., and Mantovani, A., Endothelial cells express the interleukin-1 receptor type I, *Blood*, 78, 1262, 1991.

16. Bosenberg, A. T., Brock-Utne, J. G., Gaffin, S. L., Wells, M. T. B., and Blake, G. T. W., Strenuous exercise causes systemic endotoxemia, *J. Appl. Physiol.*, 65, 106, 1988.

17. Brock-Utne, J. G., Gaffin, S. L., Wells, M. T., Gathiram, P., Sohar, E., James, M. F., Morrell, D. F., and Norman, R. J., Endotoxaemia in exhausted runners after a long-distance race, *S. Afr. Med. J.*, 73, 533, 1988.

18. Cannon, J. G., Evans, W. J., Hughes, V. A., Meredith, C. N., and Dinarello, C. A., Physiological mechanisms contributing to increased interleukin-1 secretion, *J. Appl. Physiol.*, 61, 1869, 1986.

19. Cannon, J. G., Fielding, R. A., Fiatarone, M. A., Orencole, S. F., Dinarello, C. A., and Evans, W. J., Increased interleukin 1ß in human skeletal muscle after exercise, *Am. J. Physiol.*, 257, R451, 1989.

20. Cannon, J. G. and Kluger, M. J., Endogenous pyrogen activity in human plasma after exercise, *Science*, 220, 617, 1983.

21. Cannon, J. G., Meydani, S. N., Fielding, R. A., Fiatarone, M. A., Meydani, M., Farhangmehr, M., Orencole, S. F., Blumberg, J. B., and Evans, W. J., Acute phase response in exercise. II. Associations between vitamin E, cytokines, and muscle proteolysis, *Am. J. Physiol. Regul. Integr. Comp. Physiol.*, 260, R1235, 1991.

22. Cannon, J. G., Tompkins, R. G., Gelfand, J. A., Michie, H. R., Stanford, G. G., Van der Meer, J. W. M., Endres, S., Lonnemann, G., Corsetti, J., Chernow, B., Wilmore, D. W., Wolff, S. M., Burke, J. F., and Dinarello, C. A., Circulating interleukin-1 and tumor necrosis factor in septic shock and experimental endotoxin fever, *J. Infect. Dis.*, 161, 79, 1990.

23. Cendan, J. C., Moldawer, L. L., Souba, W. W., Copeland, E. M., III, and Lind, D. S., Endotoxin-induced nitric oxide production in pulmonary artery endothelial cells is regulated by cytokines, *Arch. Surg. (Chicago)*, 129, 1296, 1994.

24. Chao, C. C., Strgar, F., Tsang, M., and Peterson, P. K., Effects of swimming exercise on the pathogenesis of acute murine *Toxoplasma gondii* Me49 infection, *Clin. Immunol. Immunopathol.*, 62, 220, 1992.

25. Colletti, L. M., Remick, D. G., Burtch, G. D., Kunkel, S. L., Strieter, R. M., and Campbell, D. A., Jr., Role of tumor necrosis factor-α in the pathophysiologic alterations after hepatic ischemia/reperfusion injury in the rat, *J. Clin. Invest.*, 85, 1936, 1990.

26. Doherty, G. M., Lange, J. R., Langstein, H. N., Alexander, H. R., Buresh, C. M., and Norton, J. A., Evidence for IFN-gamma as a mediator of the lethality of endotoxin and tumor necrosis factor-α, *J. Immunol.*, 149, 1666, 1992.

27. Dufaux, B. and Order, U., Plasma elastase-α1-antitrypsin, neopterin, tumor necrosis factor, and soluble interleukin-2 receptor after prolonged exercise, *Int. J. Sports Med.*, 10, 434, 1989.

28. Echtenacher, B., Falk, W., Männel, D. N., and Krammer, P. H., Requirement of endogenous tumor necrosis factor/cachectin for recovery from experimental peritonitis, *J. Immunol.*, 145, 3762, 1990.

29. Espersen, G. T., Elbaek, A., Ernst, E., Toft, E., Kaalund, S., Jersild, C., and Grunnet, N., Effect of physical exercise on cytokines and lymphocyte subpopulations in human peripheral blood, *Acta Pathol. Microbiol. Immunol. Scand.*, 98, 395, 1990.

30. Evans, W. J., Meredith, C. N., Cannon, J. G., Dinarello, C. A., Frontera, W. R., Hughes, V. A., Jones, B. H., and Knuttgen, H. G., Metabolic changes following eccentric exercise in trained and untrained men, *J. Appl. Physiol.*, 61, 1864, 1986.

31. Filkins, J. P., Monokines and the metabolic pathophysiology of septic shock, *Fed. Proc.*, 44, 300, 1985.

32. Fong, Y., Tracey, K. J., Moldawer, L. L., Hesse, D. G., Manogue, K. B., Kenney, J. S., Lee, A. T., Kuo, G. C., Allison, A. C., Lowry, S. F., and Cerami, A., Antibodies to cachectin/tumor necrosis factor reduce interleukin 1ß and interleukin 6 appearance during lethal bacteremia, *J. Exp. Med.*, 170, 1627, 1989.

33. Goes, N., Urmson, J., Ramassar, V., and Halloran, P. F., Ischemic acute tubular necrosis induces an extensive local cytokine response: evidence for induction of interferon-gamma, transforming growth factor-ß1, granulocyte-macrophage colony-stimulating factor, interleukin-2, and interleukin-10, *Transplantation*, 59, 565, 1995.

34. Haight, J. S. J. and Keatinge, W. R., Elevation in set-point for body temperature regulation after prolonged exercise, *J. Physiol. (London)*, 229, 77, 1973.

35. Haralambie, G., Serum zinc in athletes in training, *Int. J. Sports Med.*, 2, 135, 1981.

36. Havell, E. A., Production of tumor necrosis factor during murine listeriosis, *J. Immunol.*, 139, 4225, 1987.

37. Hawrylowicz, C. M., Howells, G. L., and Feldmann, M., Platelet-derived interleukin 1 induces human endothelial adhesion molecule expression and cytokine production, *J. Exp. Med.*, 174, 785, 1991.

38. Hesse, D. G., Tracey, K. J., Fong, Y., Manogue, K. R., Palladino, M. A., Cerami, A., Shires, G. T., and Lowry, S. F., Cytokine appearance in human endotoxemia and primate bacteremia, *Surg. Gynecol. Obstet.*, 166, 147, 1988.

39. Hoffman-Goetz, L., Arumugam, Y., and Sweeny, L., Lymphokine activated killer cell activity following voluntary physical activity in mice, *J. Sports Med. Phys. Fitness*, 34, 83, 1994.

40. Kvernmo, H., Olsen, J. O., and Osterud, B., Changes in blood cell response following strenuous physical exercise, *Eur. J. Appl. Physiol.*, 64, 318, 1992.

41. Langermans, J. A. M., Van der Hulst, M. E. B., Nibbering, P. H., and van Furth, R., Endogenous tumor necrosis factor alpha is required for enhanced antimicrobial activity against *Toxoplasma gondii* and *Listeria monocytogenes* in recombinant gamma interferon-treated mice, *Infect. Immun.*, 60, 5107, 1992.

42. Lewicki, R., Tchorzewski, H., Denys, A., Kowalska, M., and Golinska, A., Effect of physical exercise on some parameters of immunity in conditioned sportsmen, *Int. J. Sports Med.*, 8, 309, 1987.

43. Lewicki, R., Tchorzewski, H., Majewska, E., Nowak, Z., and Baj, Z., Effect of maximal physical exercise on t-lymphocyte subpopulations and on interleukin 1 (IL 1) and interleukin 2 (IL 2) production in vitro, *Int. J. Sports Med.*, 9, 114, 1988.
44. Liesen, H., Dufaux, B., and Hollman, W., Modifications of serum glycoproteins the days following prolonged physical exercise and the influence of physical training, *Eur. J. Appl. Physiol. Occup. Physiol.*, 37, 243, 1977.
45. Lin, Y. S., Jan, M. S., and Chen, H. I., The effect of chronic and acute exercise on immunity in rats, *Int. J. Sports Med.*, 14, 86, 1993.
46. Lin, Y. S., Jan, M. S., Tsai, T. J., and Chen, H. I., Immunomodulatory effects of acute exercise bout in sedentary and trained rats, *Med. Sci. Sports Exerc.*, 27, 73, 1995.
47. Loppnow, H. and Libby, P., Adult human vascular endothelial cells express the IL6 gene differentially in response to LPS or IL1, *Cell. Immunol.*, 122, 493, 1989.
48. Mathison, J. C. and Ulevitch, R. J., The clearance, tissue distribution, and cellular localization of intravenously injected lipopolysaccharide in rabbits, *J. Immunol.*, 123, 2133, 1979.
49. Michie, H. R., Manogue, K. R., Spriggs, D. R., Revhaug, A., O'Dwyer, S., Dinarello, C. A., Cerami, A., Wolff, S. M., and Wilmore, D. W., Detection of circulating tumor necrosis factor after endotoxin administration, *N. Engl. J. Med.*, 318, 1481, 1988.
50. Monastra, G. and Secchi, E. F., ß-Adrenergic receptors mediate in vivo the adrenaline inhibition of lipopolysaccharide-induced tumor necrosis factor release, *Immunol. Lett.*, 38, 127, 1993.
51. Moore, R. N. and Berry, L. J., Endocrinelike activities of the RES. An overview, in *The Reticuloendothelial System: A Comprehensive Treatise*, Reichard, S. M. and Filkins, J. P., Eds., Plenum Press, New York, 1985, 3.
52. Haahr, P. M., Pedersen, B. K., Fomsgaard, A., Tvede, N., Diamont, M., Klarlund, K., Halkjær-Kristensen, J., Effect of physical exercise on *in vitro* production of interleukin 1, interleukin 6, tumor necrosis factor-α, interleukin 2, and interferon-gamma, *Int. J. Sports Med.*, 12, 223, 1991.
53. Nauciel, C. and Espinasse-Maes, F., Role of gamma interferon and tumor necrosis factor alpha in resistance to *Salmonella typhimurium* infection, *Infect. Immun.*, 60, 450, 1992.
54. Northoff, H. and Berg, A., Immunologic mediators as parameters of the reaction to strenuous exercise, *Int. J. Sports Med.*, 12, S9, 1991.
55. Northoff, H., Flegel, W. A., Männel, D. N., Baumstark, M., and Berg, A., Increased levels of interleukin-6 (IL-6) and/or IL-7 in sera of long-distance runners, in *The Physiological and Pathological Effects of Cytokines*, Powanda, M. C., Oppenheim, J. J., Kluger, M. J., and Dinarello, C. A., John Wiley & Sons/Alan R. Liss, New York, 1990, 75.
56. Old, L. J., Tumor necrosis factor, *Sci. Am.*, May, 59, 1988.
57. Oshida, Y., Yamanouchi, K., Hayamizu, S., and Sato, Y., Effect of acute physical exercise on lymphocyte subpopulations in trained and untrained subjects, *Int. J. Sports Med.*, 9, 137, 1988.
58. Pedersen, B. K., Influence of physical activity on the cellular immune system: mechanism of action, *Int. J. Sports Med.*, 12, S23, 1991.
59. Pedersen, B. K., Tvede, N., Hansen, F. R., Andersen, V., Bendix, T., Bendixen, G., Bendtzen, K., Galbo, H., Haahr, P. M., Klarlund, K., Sylvest, J., Thomsen, B. S., and Halkjær-Kristensen, J., Modulation of natural killer cell activity in peripheral blood by physical exercise, *Scand. J. Immunol.*, 27, 673, 1988.
60. Peters, T., Karck, U., and Decker, K., Interdependence of tumor necrosis factor, prostaglandin E_2, and protein synthesis in lipopolysaccharide-exposed rat Kupffer cells, *Eur. J. Biochem.*, 191, 583, 1990.
61. Rivier, A., Pène, J., Chanez, P., Anselme, F., Caillaud, C., Préfaut, C., Godard, P., and Bousquet, J., Release of cytokines by blood monocytes during strenuous exercise, *Int. J. Sports Med.*, 15, 192, 1994.

62. Rowsey, P. J., Borer, K. T., and Kluger, M. J., Tumor necrosis factor is not involved in exercise-induced elevation in core temperature, *Am. J. Physiol. Regul. Integr. Comp. Physiol.*, 265, R1351, 1993.
63. Sakr, M. F., McClain, C. J., Gavaler, J. S., Zetti, G. M., Starzl, T. E., and Van Thiel, D. H., FK 506 pre-treatment is associated with reduced levels of tumor necrosis factor and interleukin 6 following hepatic ischemia/reperfusion, *J. Hepatol.*, 17, 301, 1993.
64. Scales, W. E., Chensue, S. W., Otterness, I., and Kunkel, S. L., Regulation of monokine gene expression: prostaglandin E_2 suppresses tumor necrosis factor but not interleukin-1α or ß-mRNA and cell-associated bioactivity, *J. Leukocyte Biol.*, 45, 416, 1989.
65. Severn, A., Rapson, N. T., Hunter, C. A., and Liew, F. Y., Regulation of tumor necrosis factor production by adrenaline and ß-adrenergic agonists, *J. Immunol.*, 148, 3441, 1992.
66. Shalaby, M. R., Waage, A., and Espevik, T., Cytokine regulation of interleukin 6 production by human endothelial cells, *Cell. Immunol.*, 121, 372, 1989.
67. Smith, J. A., Telford, R. D., Baker, M. S., Hapel, A. J., and Weidemann, M. J., Cytokine immunoreactivity in plasma does not change after moderate endurance exercise, *J. Appl. Physiol.*, 73, 1396, 1992.
68. Smith, K. A., Interleukin 2, *Annu. Rev. Immunol.*, 2, 319, 1984.
69. Sprenger, H., Jacobs, C., Nain, M., Gressner, A. M., Prinz, H., Wesemann, W., and Gemsa, D., Enhanced release of cytokines, interleukin-2 receptors, and neopterin after long-distance running, *Clin. Immunol. Immunopathol.*, 63, 188, 1992.
70. Suzuki, S. and Toledo-Pereyra, L. H., Interleukin 1 and tumor necrosis factor production as the initial stimulants of liver ischemia and reperfusion injury, *J. Surg. Res.*, 57, 253, 1994.
71. Tvede, N., Kappel, M., Halkjoer-Kristensen, J., Galbo, H., and Pedersen, B. K., The effect of light, moderate and severe bicycle exercise on lymphocyte subsets, natural and lymphokine activated killer cells, lymphocyte proliferative response and interleukin 2 production, *Int. J. Sports Med.*, 14, 275, 1993.
72. Ullum, H., Haahr, P. M., Diamant, M., Palmo, J., Halkjaer-Kristensen, J., and Pedersen, B. K., Bicycle exercise enhances plasma IL-6 but does not change IL-1α, IL-1ß, IL-6, or TNF-α pre-mRNA in BMNC, *J. Appl. Physiol.*, 77, 93, 1994.
73. Ullum, H., Palmo, J., Halkjaer-Kristensen, J., Diamant, M., Klokker, M., Kruuse, A., LaPerriere, A., and Pedersen, B. K., The effect of acute exercise on lymphocyte subsets, natural killer cells, proliferative responses, and cytokines in HIV-seropositive persons, *J. Acquired Immune Deficiency Syndr.*, 7, 1122, 1994.
74. Viti, A., Muscettola, M., Paulesu, L., Bocci, V., and Almi, A., Effect of exercise on plasma interferon levels, *J. Appl. Physiol.*, 59, 426, 1985.
75. Warner, S. J. C., Auger, K. R., and Libby, P., Interleukin 1 induces interleukin 1. II. Recombinant human interleukin 1 induces interleukin 1 production by adult human vascular endothelial cells, *J. Immunol.*, 139, 1911, 1987.
76. Weight, L. M., Alexander, D., and Jacobs, P., Strenuous exercise: analogous to the acute-phase response, *Clin. Sci.*, 81, 677, 1991.
77. Woods, J. A., Davis, J. M., Mayer, E. P., Ghaffar, A., and Pate, R. R., Exercise increases inflammatory macrophage antitumor cytotoxicity, *J. Appl. Physiol.*, 75, 879, 1993.
78. Woods, J. A., Davis, J. M., Mayer, E. P., Ghaffar, A., and Pate, R. R., Effects of exercise on macrophage activation for antitumor cytotoxicity, *J. Appl. Physiol.*, 76, 2177, 1994.
79. Wu-Hsieh, B. A., Lee, G.-S., Franco, M., and Hofman, F. M., Early activation of splenic macrophages by tumor necrosis factor alpha is important in determining the outcome of experimental histoplasmosis in mice, *Infect. Immun.*, 60, 4230, 1992.
80. Zhou, D., Kusnecov, A. W., Shurin, M. R., DePaoli, M., and Rabin, B. S., Exposure to physical and psychological stressors elevates plasma interleukin 6: relationship to the activation of hypothalamic-pituitary-adrenal axis, *Endocrinology*, 133, 2523, 1993.

81. Zuckerman, S. H., Evans, G. F., and Butler, L. D., Endotoxin tolerance: independent regulation of interleukin-1 and tumor necrosis factor expression, *Infect. Immun.*, 59, 2774, 1991.
82. Zuckerman, S. H., Evans, G. F., Snyder, Y. M., Shellhaas, J., and Roeder, W. D., Macrophage-endotoxin interactions: regulation of TNF levels by glucocorticoid and nonglucocorticoid dependent mechanisms, *Cytokine*, 1, 135, 1989.

Chapter 5

IMMUNE RESPONSES TO ACUTE EXERCISE

Bente Klarlund Pedersen

CONTENTS

0-8493-8190-8/96/$0.00+$.50
© 1996 by CRC Press Inc.

I. INTRODUCTION

Understanding the mechanisms behind the changes in the immune system in relation to acute time-limited exercise stress is of interest from several points of view. In the first place, in order to understand how physical activity may influence resistance to infections, knowledge about the influence of training on resting levels of the immune system and the influence of acute exercise on the immune system are of importance.[52] Second, it has been suggested that the immunological responses to exercise are a subset of physical stress reactions that include surgery, thermal and traumatic injury, hemorrhagic shock, and acute myocardial infarction.[61] Therefore, acute exercise can be viewed as a prototype for studying the effects of physical factors on the immune system.[24] Third, several types of exercise induce muscle damage, and eccentric exercise may serve as a model for studying the pathogenesis of muscle inflammation.[5]

II. ACUTE TIME-LIMITED EXERCISE STRESS AND THE IMMUNE SYSTEM

A. EXERCISE LEUKOCYTOSIS

The basal level of circulating leukocytes is rapidly increased by physical activity.[5] The first English language publication reporting exercise-leukocytosis is from 1902 by Larrabee.[38] The leukocytosis is due to increased concentrations of neutrophils, monocytes, and lymphocytes. The neutrophil concentration increases during exercise and it continues to increase following exercise.[47,59] During exercise natural killer (NK), B, and T cells are recruited to the blood, reflected in an elevated total lymphocyte count. The composition of T cells is altered, thus the CD4:CD8 ratio decreases, because the CD8 count increases more than the CD4 count. Following severe exercise the lymphocyte concentration decreases below baseline value, and the duration of this suppression depends on the intensity and duration of the exercise stress.[61]

B. NATURAL KILLER CELLS

NK cells are a heterogeneous population of cells that mediate killing of a broad range of target cells;[22] they express a characteristic array of surface markers including CD56 and CD16, but by definition they do not express the CD3 marker.[22] The NK cell activity is determined as the percentage lysis[51] of Cr-labeled tumor cells, e.g., K562 target cells. They are thought to play an important role in the first line of defense against acute and chronic virus infections and tumor spread.[22] NK cells are highly sensitive to physical exercise and are recruited immediately to the blood during acute exercise. The modulation of the NK cell activity in response to exercise has been investigated extensively.[9-38] During physical exercise the absolute concentration and the relative fraction of blood mononuclear cells (BMNC) expressing characteristic NK cell markers are markedly enhanced. Simultaneously, the NK cell activity (the cytotoxic activity of the NK cells) increases. Following intense exercise the NK cell activity is suppressed (see References 4, 9, 10, 12, 14-16, 18, 19, 21, 23, 25, 33, 35, 42, 43, 51, 53-55, 57, 62-64, 68, 70, 75, 77, 80).

In some exercise models the suppressed NK cell activity is due to decreased percentages of NK cells postexercise;[53] in other models the NK cell activity has been suggested to involve a mechanism of prostaglandin-mediated suppression.[63,75]

C. ANTIBODY PRODUCTION

The secretory immune system of mucosal tissues such as the upper respiratory tract is considered to be the first barrier to colonization by pathogenic microorganisms causing upper respiratory tract infection (URTI).[71,73] In mucosal secretions immunoglobulin A (IgA) is the major class of immunoglobulins, and the level of IgA in mucosal fluids correlates more closely with resistance to URTI than to serum antibodies.[39] Tomasi et al.[73] reported suppressed levels of the salivary IgA in cross-country skiers after a race. This finding was confirmed by a 70% decrease in salivary IgA for several hours after 2 h intense ergometer cycling.[44] Decreased salivary IgA was found after swimming[71] and salivary IgA was low for several hours after marathon running.[49] In order to study the mechanism behind the suppression of immunoglobulins a plaque-forming cell (PFC) assay was used. This assay allows an identification of the individual immunoglobulin-secreting cells of blood. Stimulation of cells with pokeweed mitogen (PWM), interleukin-2 (IL-2), and Epstein–Barr virus (EBV) resulted in significantly decreased numbers of IgG-, IgA-, and IgM-secreting blood cells during as well as 2 h postexercise, with recovery after 1 d. The fraction of CD20+ B cells does not change in relation to exercise, suggesting that the suppression of immunoglobulin-secreting cells was not due to changes in numbers of B cells. Purified B cells produce plaques only after stimulation with EBV, and in these cultures no exercise-induced suppression was found. Addition of indomethacin to IL-2 stimulated cultures of BMNC partly reversed the postexercise-suppressed B cell function. Altogether it was concluded that the exercise-induced suppression of the PFC response was mediated by monocytes.[74]

D. LYMPHOCYTE PROLIFERATION

There has been much focus on the fact that the ability of lymphocytes to proliferate following stimulation with mitogens, antigens and interleukins changes in relation to exercise and other stress forms. Phytohemagglutinin (PHA) and concanavalin A (ConA) are T lymphocyte mitogens; on the other hand, pokeweed mitogen (PWM) is a T and B cell mitogen, which nonspecifically stimulates DNA synthesis, blast transformation, and proliferation of lymphocytes. The ability of lymphocytes to proliferate following stimulation with ConA and PHA decreases, whereas the proliferative response to IL-2, lipopolysaccharide (LPS), or PWM increases.[10,16,24,59,77] The low PHA response of cells isolated during bicycle exercise was shown to be due to a decreased contribution to the BMNC-pool of the CD4+ cell subfraction rather than to a changed proliferative response per CD4+ T cell;[77] and the increased ability of cells to proliferate following stimulation with IL-2 was caused by an increased fraction of CD16+ cells, and not by an increased expression of IL-2 receptors (N. Tvede et al., unpublished results). Thus the changes in proliferative response during exercise are not a result of altered function or activation of the individual lymphocytes.

E. CYTOKINES

The complex interactions among lymphoid cells, inflammatory cells, and other cells are mediated by a group of secreted low-molecular weight proteins that are designated cytokines. Cytokines serve as messengers of the immune system, but unlike endocrine hormones (the messengers of the endocrine system), which exert their effects over large distances, the cytokines generally act locally.[3] Physical exercise including eccentric muscle contractions increases the production of some cytokines. Increased interleukin-1ß (IL-1ß) in muscle tissue was found for up to 5 d following eccentric exercise.[5] The IL-1 activity increased following eccentric exercise in plasma from untrained subjects.[12] Following long-distance running, increased concentrations of interleukin-6 (IL-6) in plasma were found,[56] and others have found increased plasma tumor necrosis factor-alpha (TNFα).[11] Theoretically, increased production of monokines in response to dynamic exercise could be a result of an elevated number of monocytes.[59] Furthermore, increased *in vitro* production of IL-1, IL-6, and TNFα was found in supernatants from LPS-stimulated BMNC isolated from untrained persons 2 h following cycling.[51] Increased endogenous pyrogen activity in plasma following concentric exercise was shown several years ago.[52] We have recently investigated the effects of aerobic, concentric exercise on plasma levels of IL-1α, IL-1ß, IL-6, and TNFα; and the presence of pre-mRNA for these cytokines in BMNC. Moderately trained, healthy young men performed ergometer cycling exercise for 1 h at 75% of VO_2max. The levels of plasma-IL-6 increased significantly during exercise, but IL-1α, IL-1ß, and TNFα were not reliably detected in plasma. Pre-mRNA for IL-1α,

IL-1ß, IL-6, and TNFα could be detected in BMNC, but the amounts did not change in relation to exercise.[53] These results indicate that, although the concentrations of CD14+ monocytes increase following exercise, the increased plasma-IL-6 during exercise may not be a result of activated monocytes in peripheral blood.

F. IMMUNE ACTIVATION MARKERS

Most of the exercise-induced changes that have been described employing functional immune assays can be ascribed to changes in the composition of blood mononuclear cells; for example, the increased NK cell activity during exercise is due to increased percentage of NK cells, the decreased PHA response was due to decreased fraction of the CD4+ cells, and the increased IL-2-induced proliferation was due to increased fraction of CD16+ cells. However, the increased levels of cytokines in the blood could not be ascribed to redistribution of monocytes. Tilz et al.[54] found increased plasma concentrations of soluble IL-2 receptors, CD8, intercellular adhesion molecule 1 (ICAM1), CD23, TNF receptor, and neopterin in 18 individuals during or after a long duration of exercise. These results suggest that there is some immune system activation during intense exercise of long duration. However, in another study the levels of colony-stimulating factor (GM-CSF) and neopterin remained unchanged after concentric exercise.[55] Gabriel et al.[17] found increased CD45RA+45RO+ cells after endurance exercise, and suggested that this might reflect activation of the T cells.

III. VARIOUS FORMS OF ACUTE EXERCISE

A. INTENSITY AND DURATION

In relation to short-term exercise of very high intensity, as represented by rowing for 6 min, the concentration of NK cells increased sixfold, but there was no postexercise suppression of the NK cell activity.[51] Following a marathon the NK cell activity is severely suppressed.[53] When the duration of exercise was fixed to 1 h, and the intensity of exercise varied (25, 50, and 75% of VO_2 max), it was found that all exercise intensities caused increase in the NK and LAK cell activity, whereas the NK cell activity was suppressed only following bicycle exercise at 75% of VO_2 max. Furthermore, only the latter induced a postexercise monocytosis.[75] In a recent review[61] we concluded from the results on different types of exercise (see References 4, 9, 10, 12, 14-16, 18, 19, 21, 23, 25, 33, 35, 42, 43, 51, 53-55, 57, 62-64, 68, 70, 75, 77, 80) that the intensity of exercise more than the duration of exercise is responsible for the degree of increment in number of NK cells and other lymphocyte subpopulations. On the other hand, the concentrations of lymphocytes and especially the NK cell activity are only suppressed following intense exercise of a certain duration.[61]

B. CONCENTRIC VS. ECCENTRIC EXERCISE

The exercise-related effect on NK cells and other lymphocyte subpopulations has been studied in relation to whole body exercise concerning concentric exercise (e.g., bicycling) and combinations of concentric and eccentric exercise (e.g., running). The isolated effect of eccentric exercise has been investigated in exercise involving a small muscle mass.[57] In this study one leg exercise increased %CD16+ cells and NK cell cytotoxic activity per fixed number of BMNC, whereas the NK cell activity per NK cell did not change. In the same study it was shown that the plasma level of neutrophils increased during and after exercise, whereas the level of monocytes only raised during exercise. Concerning BMNC we hypothesize that recruitment during physical activity may be due to the same mechanisms (e.g., increases in stress hormones) in eccentric and concentric exercise. The effect of eccentric work on the level and production of cytokines was described above. We hypothesize that high-intensity eccentric exercise causes a more pronounced increase in the muscle and plasma levels of cytokines involved in acute inflammatory responses (IL-1, TNF, and IL-6) during and after exercise than concentric exercise because of the more pronounced damage of the muscle. The cells responsible for an increased synthesis of cytokines may be macrophages, endothelial cells, and fibroblasts in the muscle.

IV. MECHANISMS OF ACTION

A. REDISTRIBUTION OF CELLS

The exercise-related neutrocytosis is thought to be due to movement of neutrophils from marginal pools located intravascularly and from extravascular storage pools. The role of the lung vasculature in neutrophilic granulocyte sequestration has been repeatedly demonstrated.[48,65] Concerning lymphocytes the concept of margination is less clear. It has been suggested that rapid transfer of lymphocytes into the intravascular compartment of the spleen might contribute to selectively increasing the number of circulating lymphocytes. However, in a recent article the increase in neutrophils and lymphocytes and their subpopulations were similar in the splenectomized subjects and the controls.[27] Thus, exercise-induced leukocytosis can take place in the absence of the spleen.

B. ROLE OF STRESS HORMONES

Physical stress increases the concentrations of a number of stress hormones in the blood, including catecholamines, growth hormone, beta endorphins, and cortisol.

1. Catecholamines

The expression of beta adrenoceptors on T, B, and NK cells; macrophages; and neutrophils in numerous species provides the molecular basis for these cells to be targets for catecholamine signaling.[46] Beta receptors on lymphocytes are linked intracellularly to the adenyl cyclase system for generation of cyclic adenosine 5′-monophosphate (cAMP) as a second messenger,[7] and the beta-adrenoceptor density appears to change in concert with lymphocyte activation and differentiation.[1] Dynamic exercise upregulates the beta-adrenoceptor density, especially on NK cells.[41] In humans, a single epinephrine injection induced transient increases in the number of circulating blood lymphocytes and monocytes and decreased the response to T cell mitogens.[8]

Selective administration of adrenaline to obtain plasma concentrations identical to those obtained during concentric bicycle exercise, 1 h, 75% of VO$_2$max, mimicked the exercise-induced effect on BMNC subsets, NK cell activity, and lymphocyte function. However, adrenaline infusion caused a significant smaller increase in neutrophil concentration than that observed following exercise.[33,76] The finding that adrenaline infusion was capable of mimicking the effect of exercise especially regarding recruitment of cells mediating NK and lymphokine activated killer (LAK) cell activity is compatible with the finding that exercise induces upregulation of beta-adrenoceptor cells on NK cells, but not on other lymphocyte subsets.[41]

2. Growth Hormone

In several species growth hormone (GH) deficiency is associated with small lymphoid organs with abnormal morphology; and reconstitution with growth hormone has reconstituted the lymphoid organs, suggesting that GH is important for normal development of the immune system.[46] In agreement with this, there are studies showing that growth hormone reconstitution may modulate the immune system of growth hormone-deficient patients.[60] Addressing the question of a possible role of growth hormone in mediating acute exercise-induced immune changes, Kappel et al.[29] administered an *in vivo* injection of growth hormone in humans to obtain blood concentrations of growth hormone comparable with those observed during exercise. An intravenous bolus injection of growth hormone had no effect on BMNC subsets, NK cell activity, cytokine production, or lymphocyte function, but induced a highly significant neutrocytosis.[29]

3. Beta Endorphin

Functional evidence for opioid receptors on human T lymphocytes was first reported by Wybrand,[81] and since then numerous reports have appeared (reviewed by Madden and Felten[46]). At present, a clear functional role has not yet emerged for the opioid peptides. The reasons for this lack of agreement may be related to the heterogeneity of the opioid peptides and receptors. Furthermore, some effects of opioids are blocked by opioid receptor blockers such as naloxone, whereas other effects are not.[46] In order to explore the possibility that the rise in beta endorphin during exercise was responsible for the exercise-induced increase in NK cell activity, Fiatarone et al.[14] administered naloxone *in vivo* to young women who underwent a maximal cycle ergometer test. In the naloxone experiment the rise in NK cell activity was no longer significant. However, the exercise-induced increase in cells expressing the CD16 marker (NK cells) was not significantly altered compared with the group receiving placebo. In another study healthy young men were given epidural analgesia that blocked the afferent nerve impulses and inhibited increase in beta endorphins and adrenocorticotropin (ACTH) during exercise; the exercise-induced increase in NK cell function, and percentage of NK cells and NK cell concentration were significantly enlarged.[37] Thus, blocking the beta-endorphin receptor and blocking the increase in concentration of beta endorphin during exercise exerts differential effects on the immune system.

4. Cortisol

Only a minor increase in the concentrations of plasma cortisol has been described in acute time-limited exercise stress of 1 h,[37,59,62] and it is unlikely that such modest increments alone can account for the magnitude of exercise-induced immunomodulation. Furthermore, unlike catecholamines, cortisol exerts its effect with a time-lag of several hours. However, this does not preclude an immunomodulatory role for cortisol in chronic exercise stress, and in maintaining the neutrocytosis after prolonged, intense exercise as e.g., a marathon.

C. ROLE OF HYPERTHERMIA AND HYPOXIA

Exercise induces elevated core temperature and arterial hypoxemia. *In vitro* hyperthermia and hypoxemia have numerous effects on the immune system.[31,61] The selective effects of *in vivo* hyperthermia and hypoxia on the human immune system have been investigated. To examine the selective effect of hyperthermia on the human immune system, Kappel et al.[28,30-32] immersed young healthy volunteers in a hot water bath after which their rectal temperature raised to 39.5°C. On another day they served as their own control and were immersed in thermoneutral water. The *in vivo* effect of hypoxia on the human immune system was evaluated by Klokker et al.[36] who placed young health volunteers in a decompression chamber for 20 min with oxygen supplementation and on another day without the supplementation of oxygen. Both hyperthermia and hypoxia induced recruitment of the lymphocytes, especially the CD16+ NK cells, and the neutrophils to the blood, but had little or no effect on the lymphocyte proliferative responses and the antibody production. Furthermore, the levels of cytokines did not increase in response to hyperthermia and hypoxia. When exercise was performed during hypoxic conditions, a significantly larger increase in concentrations of NK cells was seen compared to exercise performance during normoxic conditions.[37]

D. ROLE OF GLUTAMINE

Glutamine is required for *in vitro* mitogen-stimulated proliferation of lymphocytes from the rat[2] and man.[58] It was proposed that *in vivo* the glutamine pathway in lymphocytes may be under external regulation and that this may be with respect to the supply of glutamine itself. The major tissue involved in glutamine production is skeletal muscle: it contains a high concentration of glutamine, it has the enzymatic capacity to synthesize glutamine, and it is known to release glutamine into the bloodstream at a high rate.[78] Muscle, therefore, plays a vital role in maintenance of the rate of the key process of glutamine utilization in the immune cells; and, consequently, skeletal muscle can be considered as part of the immune system.[50] The so-called glutamine hypothesis says that under physical exercise the demands on muscles for glutamine is such that the immune system is forced into a glutamine depth and thereby immunosuppression.

V. ACUTE EXERCISE IN PATIENTS WITH CHRONIC IMMUNE DISORDERS

A. HUMAN IMMUNODEFICIENCY SYNDROME

Infection with the human immunodeficiency virus type 1 (HIV) results in progressive and profound immunosuppression. The primary defect is the depletion of CD4+ cells, but depletions and defects in the function of other lymphocyte subpopulations including NK and LAK cells and altered cytokine production are also involved.[13,63,78] HIV seropositive subjects have been shown to possess an impaired ability to mobilize neutrophils and NK and LAK cells to the blood in response to acute time-limited exercise stress (bicycling at 75% of VO_2max, 1 h).[80] The mechanisms behind the impaired recruitment are unknown, but may be ascribed to altered stress response, lower expression of beta receptors on the surface of NK cells, and/or smaller reservoir of cells available for recruitment.

B. CHRONIC FATIGUE SYNDROME

The chronic fatigue syndrome (CFS) is a disorder characterized by sudden onset of an influenza-like disease followed by the presence of fatigue and abnormal exercise-induced exhaustion for more than 6 months.[26] It has been proposed that the pathogenic mechanism is a persisting viral infection triggering an imbalance in the immune system; however, different studies have shown very different results concerning the investigation of immunological parameters in this group of patients.[66] A recent study[40] showed no differences in the level of IFNγ, IL-1β, and TNFα between patients with CFS and controls performing isometric handgrip exercise utilizing dynamometers for 30 min at 40% of the maximal voluntary contraction.

VI. CONCLUSIONS

During exercise, lymphoid cells, especially NK cells, are recruited to the blood; and if muscle damage occurs, the cytokine level is enhanced. Following intense exercise of long duration, the concentration of lymphocytes in the blood is suppressed and the function of NK and B cells is inhibited. The mechanisms underlying exercise-induced immunomodulation are probably multifactorial and include adrenaline, growth hormone, and probably also exercise-induced hyperthermia and hypoxia. Furthermore, lack of glutamine has been suggested to contribute to impaired lymphocyte function after muscular activity. During the time of immunodepression, often referred to as the open window, the host may be more susceptible to microorganisms bypassing the first line of defense. However, moderate exercise, which induces increase in the concentration of immunocompetent cells in the blood, without causing postexercise immunosuppression, may improve host defense to infections. Regarding patients with chronic diseases such as HIV infection or CFS, there are no reports showing that acute exercise is harmful to the immune system or worsens disease activity.

ACKNOWLEDGMENT

The work was supported by the Danish National Research Foundation No. 504-14.

REFERENCES

1. Ackerman, K. D, Bellinger, D. L., Felten, S. Y., and Felten, D. L., Ontogeny and senescence of noradrenergic innervation of the rodent and spleen, in *Psychoneroimmunology*, Vol. 2, Ader, R., Felten, D. L., and Cohen, N., Eds., Academic Press, San Diego, CA, 1991, 71.
2. Ardawi, M. S. M. and Newsholme, E. A., Glutamine metabolism in lymphocytes in the rat, *Biochem. J.*, 21, 835, 1983.
3. Balkwill, F. R. and Burke, F., The cytokine network, *Immunol. Today*, 10, 299, 1989.
4. Brahmi, Z., Thomas, J. E., Park, M., and Dowdeswell, I. R. G., The effect of acute exercise on natural killer cell activity of trained and sedentary human subjects, *J. Clin. Immunol.*, 5, 321, 1985.
5. Cannon, J. G., Fielding, R. A., Fiatarone, M. A., Orencole, S. F., Dinarello, C. A., and Evans, W. J., Increased interleukin 1 beta in human skeletal muscle after exercise, *Am. J. Physiol.*, 26, R451, 1989.
6. Cannon, J. G. and Kluger, M. J., Endogenous pyrogen activity in human plasma after exercise, *Science*, 220, 617, 1983.
7. Carlson, S. L. and Brooks, W. H., Neurotransmitter-lymphocyte interactions: dual receptor modulation of lymphocyte proliferation and cAMP production, *J. Neuroimmunol.*, 24, 155, 1989.

8. Crary, B., Hauser, S. L., Borysenko, M., Kutz, I., Hoban, C., Ault, K. A., Weiner, H. L., and Benson, H., Decreased mitogen responsiveness of mononuclear cells from peripheral blood after epinephrine administration in humans, *J. Immunol.*, 130, 694, 1983.

9. Deuster, P. A., Curiale, A. M., Cowan, M. L., and Finkelman, F. D., Exercise-induced changes in population of peripheral blood mononuclear cells, *Med. Sci. Sports Exerc.*, 20, 276, 1988.

10. Edwards, A. J., Bacon, T. H., Elms, C. A., Verardi, R., Felder, M., and Knight, S. C., Changes in the populations of lymphoid cells in human peripheral blood following physical exercise, *Clin. Exp. Immunol.*, 58, 420, 1984.

11. Espersen, G. T., Elbaek, A., Ernst, E., Toft, E., Kaalund, S., Jersild, C., and Grunnet, N., Effect of physical exercise on cytokines and lymphocyte subpopulations in human peripheral blood, *APMIS*, 98, 395, 1990.

12. Evans, W. J., Meredith, C. N., and Cannon, J. G., Metabolic changes following eccentric exercise in trained and untrained men, *J. Appl. Physiol.*, 61, 1864, 1986.

13. Fauci, A. S., Immunologic abnormalities in the acquired immunodefiency syndrome (AIDS), *Clin. Res.*, 32, 491, 1984.

14. Fiatarone, M. A., Morley, J. E., Bloom, E. T., Donna, M., Makinodan, T., and Solomon, G. F., Endogenous opioids and the exercise-induced augmentation of natural killer cell activity, *J. Lab. Clin. Med.*, 112, 544, 1988.

15. Field, C. J., Gougeon, R., and Marliss, E. B., Circulating mononuclear cell numbers and function during intense exercise and recovery, *J. Appl. Physiol.*, 71, 1089, 1991.

16. Fry, R. W., Morton, A. R., Crawford, G. P. M., and Keast, D., Cell numbers and in vitro responses of leukocytes and lymphocyte subpopulations following maximal exercise and interval training sessions of different intensities, *Eur. J. Appl. Physiol.*, 64, 218, 1992.

17. Gabriel, H., Schmitt, B., Urhausen, A., and Kindermann. W., Increased CD45RA+CD45RO+ cells indicate activated T cells after endurance exercise, *Med. Sci. Sports Exerc.*, 25, 1352, 1993.

18. Gabriel, H., Schwartz, L., Born, P., and Kinderman, W., Differential mobilization of leucocyte and lymphocyte subpopulations into the circulation during endurance exercise, *Eur. J. Appl. Physiol.*, 65, 529, 1992.

19. Gabriel, H., Urhausen, A., and Kindermann, W., Mobilization of circulating leucocyte and lymphocyte subpopulations during and after short, anaerobic exercise, *Eur. J. Appl. Physiol.*, 65, 164, 1992.

20. Haahr, P. M., Fomsgaard, A., Tvede, N., Diamant, M., Halkjaer Kristensen, J., and Pedersen, B. K., Effect of physical exercise on the in vitro production of IL-1, IL-6, TNF-α, IL-2 and IFN-γ, *Int. J. Sports. Med.*, 12, 223, 1991.

21. Haq, A., Al-Hussein, K., Lee, J., and Al-Sedairy, S., Changes in peripheral blood lymphocyte subsets associated with marathon running, *Med. Sci. Sports Exerc.*, 25, 186, 1993.

22. Hercend, T. and Schmidt, R. E., Characteristics and uses of natural killer cells, *Immunol. Today*, 9, 291, 1988.

23. Hoffman-Goetz, L., MacNeil, B., Arumugam, Y., and Randall-Simpson, J., Differential effects of exercise and housing condition on murine natural killer cell activity and tumor growth, *Int. J. Sports Med.*, 13, 167, 1992.

24. Hoffman-Goetz, L. and Pedersen B. K., Exercise and the immune system: a model of the stress response?, *Immunol. Today*, 15, 382, 1994.

25. Hoffman-Goetz, L., Simpson, J. R., Cipp, N., Arumugam, Y., and Houston, M. E., Lymphocyte subset responses to repeated submaximal exercise in med, *J. Appl. Physiol.*, 68, 1069, 1990.

26. Holmes, G. P., Kaplan, J. E., Gantzm N. M., Komaroff, A. L., Schonberger, L. B., and Straus, S. E., Chronic fatigue syndrome: a working case definition, *Ann. Intern. Med.*, 108, 387, 1988.

27. Iversen, P. O., Arvesen, B. L., and Benestad, H. B., No mandatory role for the spleen in the exercise-induced leucocytosis in man, *Clin. Sci.*, 86, 505, 1994.

28. Kappel, M., Barington, T., Gyhrs, A., and Pedersen, B. K., Influence of elevated body temperature on circulating immunoglobulin-secreting cells, *Int. J. Hyperthermia*, 10, 653, 1995.

29. Kappel, M., Hansen, M. B., Diamant, M., Jørgensen, J. O., Gyhrs, A., and Pedersen, B. K., Effects of an acute bolus growth hormone infusion on the human immune system, *Horm. Metab. Res.*, 11, 593, 1993.

30. Kappel, M., Kharazmi, A., Nielsen, H., Gyhrs, A., and Pedersen, B. K., Modulation of the counts and functions of neutrophils and monocytes under in vivo hyperthermia conditions, *Int. J. Hyperthermia*, 10, 165, 1994.

31. Kappel, M., Stadeager, C., Diamant, M., Hansen, M., Klokker, H., and Pedersen, B. K., Effects of hyperthermia in vitro on proliferative responses of individual blood mononuclear cell subsets, interferon lymphotoxin, tumor necrosis factor, interleukin 1,2 and 6, *Immunology*, 73, 304, 1991.

32. Kappel, M., Stadeager, C., Tvede, N., Galbo, H., and Pedersen, B. K., Effect of in vivo hyperthermia on natural killer cell activity, in vitro proliferative responses and blood mononuclear cell subpopulations, *Clin. Exp. Immunol.*, 84, 175, 1991.

33. Kappel, M., Tvede, N., Galbo, H., Haahr, P.M., Kjaer, M., Linstouw, M., Klarlund, K., and Pedersen, B. K., Evidence that the effect of physical exercise on NK cell activity is mediated by epinephrine, *J. Appl. Physiol.*, 70, 2530, 1991.

34. Kappel, M., Tvede, N., Hansen, M. B., Stadeager, C., and Pedersen, B. K., Cytokine production ex vivo: effect of raised body temperature, *Int. J. Hyperthermia*, 11, 329, 1995.

35. Keast D., Cameron K., and Morton A. R., Exercise and the immune response, *Sports Med.*, 5, 248, 1988.

36. Klokker, M., Galbo, H., Kharazmi, A., Bygbjerg, I., and Pedersen, B. K., Influence of in vivo hypobaric hypoxia on function of lymphocytes, neutrocytes, natural killer cells, and cytokines, *J. Appl. Physiol.*, 74, 1100, 1993.

37. Klokker, M., Kjaer, M., Secher, N. H., Hanel, B., Worm, L., Kappel, M., and Pedersen, B. K., Natural killer cell response to exercise in humans: effect of hypoxia and epidural anesthesia, *J. Appl. Physiol.*, 78, 709, 1995.

38. Larrabee, R. C., Leukocytosis after violent exercise, *J. Med. Res.*, 7, 76, 1902.

39. Liew, F. Y., Russell, S. M., Appleyard, G., Brand, G. M., and Beale, J., Cross-protection in mice infected with influenza A virus by the respiratory route is correlated with local IgA antibody rather than serum antibody or cytotoxic T cell reactivity, *Eur. J. Immunol.*, 14, 350, 1984.

40. Lloyd, A., Gandevia, S., Brockman, A., Hales, J., and Wakefield, D., Cytokine production and fatigue in patients with chronic fatigue syndrome and healthy control subjects in response to exercise, *Clin. Infect. Dis.*, 18 (Suppl. 1), 142, 1994.

41. Maisel, S. A., Harris, T., Rearden, C. A., and Michel, M. C., ß-adrenergic receptors in lymphocyte subsets after exercise, *Circulation*, 82, 2003, 1990.

42. MacKinnon L. T., Exercise and natural killer cells. What is the relationship?, *Sports Med.*, 7, 141, 1989.

43. MacKinnon, L. T., Chick T. W., van As, A., and Tomasi T. B., Effects of prolonged intense exercise on natural killer cells, *Med. Sci. Sports Exerc.*, 19, S10, 1987.

44. MacKinnon, L. T., Chick, A., van As, A., and Tomasi, T. B., The effect of exercise on secretory and natural immunity, *Adv. Exp. Med. Biol.*, 216A, 869, 1987.

45. Mackinnon, L. T. and Hooper, S., Mucosal (secretory immune system responses to exercise of varying intensity and during overtraining, *Int. J. Sports Med.*, 15, S179, 1994.

46. Madden, K. and Felten, D. L., Experimental basis for neural-immune interactions, *Physiol. Rev.*, 75, 77, 1995.

47. McCarthy, D. A. and Dale, M. M., The leucocytosis of exercise: a review and model, *Sports Med.*, 5, 282, 1988.

48. Muir, A. L., Cruz, M., Martin, B. A., Thomasen, H., Belzberg, A., and Hogg, J. C., Leucocyte kinetics in the human lung: role of exercise and catecholamines, *J. Appl. Physiol.*, 57, 711, 1984.
49. Muns, G., Liesen, H., Riedel, H., and Bergman, K. Ch., Influence of long-distance running on IgA in nasal secretion and saliva, *Dtsch. Z. Sportsmed.*, 40, 94, 1989.
50. Newsholme, E. A. and Parry-Billings, M., Properties of glutamine release from muscle and its importance for the immune system, *J. Parenteral Enteral Nutr.*, 63S, 1990.
51. Nielsen, H. B., Secher, N. H., Kappel, M., Hanel, B., and Pedersen, B. K., Lymphocyte, NK, and LAK cell responses to maximal exercise, *Int. J. Sports Med.*, in press, 1995.
52. Nieman, D. C., Exercise, infection, and immunity, *Int. J. Sports Med.*, 15, S131, 1994.
53. Nieman, D. C. and Henson, D. A., Role of endurance exercise in immune senescence, *Med. Sci. Sports Exerc.*, 26, 172, 1994.
54. Nieman, D. C., Henson, D. A., Johnson, R., Lebeck, L., Davis, J. M., and Nehlsen-Canarella, S. L., Effects of brief, heavy exertion on circulating lymphocyte subpopulations and proliferative response, *Med. Sci. Sports Exerc.*, 24, 1339, 1992.
55. Nieman, D. C., Nehlsen-Cannarella, S. L., Donohue, K. M., Chritton, D. B. W., Haddock, B. L., Stout, R. W., and Lee, J. W., The effects of acute moderate exercise on leukocyte and lymphocyte subpopulations, *Med. Sci. Sports Exerc.*, 23, 578, 1991.
56. Northoff, H. and Berg, A., Immunologic mediators as parameters of the reaction to strenous exercise, *Int. J. Sports Med.*, 12, S9, 1991.
57. Palmø, J., Asp, S., Daugaard, J., Richter, E., and Pedersen, B. K., Effect of eccentric exercise on natural killer cell activity, *J. Appl. Physiol.*, 78, 1442, 1995.
58. Parry-Billings, M., Evans, J., Calder, P. C., and Newsholme, E. A., Does glutamine contribute to immunosuppression after major burns?, *Lancet*, 336, 523, 1990.
59. Pedersen, B. K., Influence of physical activity on the cellular immune system: mechanisms of action, *Int. J. Sports Med.*, 1, S23, 1991.
60. Pedersen, B. K., Modulation of natural killer cell activity in patients with immuno-inflammatory diseases, *Dan. Med. Bull.*, 35, 315, 1988.
61. Pedersen, B. K., Kappel, M., Klokker, M., Nielsen, H. B., and Secher, N. H., The immune system during exposure to extreme physiologic conditions, *Int. J. Sports Med.*, 15, S116, 1994.
62. Pedersen, B. K., Tvede, N., Hansen, F. R., Andersen, V., Bendix, T., Bendixen, G., Bendtzen, K., Galbo, H., Haahr, P. M., Klarlund K., Sylvest J., Thomsen B., and Halkjaer-Kristensen, J., Modulation of natural killer cell activity in peripheral blood by physical exercise, *Scand. J. Immunol.*, 26, 673, 1988.
63. Pedersen B. K., Tvede N., Klarlund K., Christensen L. D., Hansen, F. R., Galbo H., Kharazmi A., and Halkjaer-Kristensen, J., Indomethacin in vitro and in vivo abolishes postexercise suppression of natural killer cell activity in peripheral blood, *Int. J. Sports Med.*, 11, 127, 1990.
64. Pedersen, B. K. and Ullum, H., NK cell response to physical activity: possible mechanisms of action, *Med. Sci. Sports Exerc.*, 26, 140, 1994.
65. Peters, A. M., Allsop, P., Stuttle, A. W. J., Armot, R. N., Gwilliam, M., and Hall, G. M., Granulocyte margination in the human lung and its response to strenuous exercise, *Clin. Sci.*, 82, 237, 1992.
66. Rasmussen, Å. K., Nielsen, H., Andersen, V., Barington, T., Bendtzen, K., Hansen, M. B., Nielsen, L., Pedersen, B. K., and Wiik, A., Chronic fatigue syndrome — a controlled cross sectional study, *J. Rheumatol.*, 21, 1527, 1994.
67. Rosenberg, Z. F. and Fauci, A. S., Immunopathogenic mechanisms of HIV expression: cytokine induction of HIV expression, *Immunol. Today*, 11, 176, 1990.
68. Shinkai S., Shore S., Shek P. N., and Shephard, R. J., Acute exercise and immune function, *Int. J. Sports Med.*, 13, 452, 1992.

69. Smith, J. A., Telford, R. D., Baker, M. S., Mapel, A. J., and Wiedemann, M. J., Cytokine immuno reactivity in plasma does not change after moderate endurance exercise, *J. Appl. Physiol.*, 73, 1396, 1992.

70. Targan, S., Britvan, L., and Dorey, F., Activation of human NKCC by moderate exercise increased frequency of NK cells with enhanced capability of effector-target lytic interactions, *Clin. Exp. Immunol.*, 45, 352, 1981.

71. Tharp, G. D. and Barnes, M. W., Reduction of salivary immunoglobulin levels by swim training, *Eur. J. Appl. Physiol.*, 60, 61, 1990.

72. Tilz, G. P., Domej, W., Diez-Ruiz, A., Weiss, G., Brezinschek, R., Brezinschek, H. P., Huttl, E., Pristautz, H., Wachter, H., and Fuchs, D., Increased immune activation during and after exercise, *Immunobiology*, 188, 194, 1993.

73. Tomasi, F., Trudeau, D., Czerqinski, D., and Erredge, S., Immune parameters in athletes before and after strenous exercise, *J. Clin. Immunol.*, 2, 173, 1982.

74. Tvede, N., Heilmann, C., Halkjaer Kristensen, J., and Pedersen, B. K., Mechanisms of B-lymphocyte suppression induced by acute physical exercise, *J. Clin. Lab. Immunol.*, 30, 169, 1989.

75. Tvede, N., Kappel, M., Halkjaer-Kristensen, J., Galbo, H., and Pedersen, B. K., The effect of light, moderate and severe exercise on lymphocyte subsets, natural and lymphokine activated killer cells, lymphocyte proliferative response and interleukin 2 production, *Int. J. Sports Med.*, 14, 275, 1993.

76. Tvede, N., Kappel, M., Klarlund, K., Duhn, S., Halkjaer-Kristensen, J., Kjaer, M., Galbo, H., and Pedersen, B. K., Evidence that the effect of bicycle exercise on blood mononuclear cell proliferative responses and subsets is mediated by epinephrine, *Int. J. Sports Med.*, 15, 100, 1994.

77. Tvede, N., Pedersen, B. K., Hansen, F. R., Bendix, T., Christensen, L. D., Galbo, H., and Halkjaer Kristensen, J., Effect of physical exercise on blood mononuclear cell subpopulations and in vitro proliferative responses, *Scand. J. Immunol.*, 29, 382, 1989.

78. Ullum, H., Gotzsche, P., Victor, J., Dickmeiss, E., Skinhøj, P., and Pedersen, B. K., Defective natural immunity — an early manifestation of HIV, *J. Exp. Med.*, 182, 789, 1995.

79. Ullum, H., Haahr, P. M., Diamant, M., Palmø, J., Halkjaer-Kristensen, J., and Pedersen, B. K., Bicycle exercise enhances plasma-IL-6, but does not change pre-MRNA for IL-1α, IL-1ß, IL-6 or TNF-α in blood mononuclear cells, *J. Appl. Physiol.*, 77, 93, 1994.

80. Ullum, H., Palmø, J., Halkjaer-Kristensen, J., Diamant, M., Klokker, M., Kruuse, A., La Perriere, A., and Pedersen, B. K., The effect of acute exercise on lymphocyte subsets, natural killer cells, proliferative response and cytokines in HIV seropositive persons, *J. AIDS*, 7, 1122, 1994.

81. Wybrand, J. T., Appelboom, T., Famaey, J. P., and Govaerts, A., Suggestive evidence for receptors for morphine and methionine-enkephalin on normal human blood T lymphocytes, *J. Immunol.*, 123, 1068, 1979.

Chapter 6

EXERCISE TRAINING AND IMMUNE FUNCTION

Roy J. Shephard
Pang N. Shek

CONTENTS

0-8493-8190-8/96/$0.00+$.50
© 1996 by CRC Press Inc.

I. INTRODUCTION

Although a program of moderate endurance exercise seems to have beneficial effects on immune function,[65,116] very heavy and prolonged training can have adverse consequences; this is best documented as an increased vulnerability to viral infections[7,27,30,55,85-87] but possibly also comprising accelerated aging, increased vulnerability to neoplasms and autoimmune diseases, and more rapid progression of human immunodeficiency virus (HIV) infections.[116] There is thus a need to document the response of various elements of the immune system to graded doses of training, with a view to setting appropriate limits to both athletic training and clinical rehabilitation programs. However, because exercise immunology is a recent specialization, only a limited amount of information is as yet available. Many authors have been content to examine acute responses to exercise; and even where experimental subjects have undertaken training, few investigators have compared the responses to differing amounts of training.

Available information includes epidemiological studies, cross-sectional comparisons between athletes and sedentary individuals, observations conducted on athletes during preparation for major competitions, and studies completed during the deliberate training or overtraining of animals and human subjects.

II. EPIDEMIOLOGICAL STUDIES

A. ISSUES OF METHODOLOGY

It is sometimes possible to link the adoption of a particular pattern of exercise training to the incidence of specific infections. The usual approach has been to ask athletic competitors to complete a respiratory symptom questionnaire, rather than to make a more direct determination of vulnerability to infection. This leaves a study open to the criticism that respiratory symptoms were increased by greater body awareness,[79] respiratory muscle fatigue,[72] or inhalation of air pollutants[28] rather than by a specific infection of the upper respiratory tract. Further, if the reported incidence of respiratory symptoms is compared with anticipated infection rates for the general population, there may be a response bias; thus, in the study of Nieman et al.,[87] only 46.9% of questionnaires were returned, and the respondents may have been those individuals who developed symptoms. Finally, it is difficult to exclude the possibility that a given training program has modified the risk of infection through some factors extraneous to the immune system, such as exposure to virally contaminated air or water,[49] an overall increase of inspired volume, a switch from nasal to oronasal breathing,[90] a depression of tracheal ciliary activity by the inhalation of cold or polluted air,[110] or an associated change of lifestyle (such as the cessation of smoking).[114]

B. CROSS-SECTIONAL COMPARISONS

Heavy training before or subsequent to infection seems to increase the susceptibility of animals to viruses. Reyes and Lerner[102] inoculated mice with Coxsackie B3 virus, finding 75 times more viremias and a 1000-fold increase of viral titers in the hearts of exercised animals. Likewise, Elson and Abelmann [22] found more severe parasitic and cellular infiltration of the heart and an increased mortality when mice were forced to swim for 6 weeks following infection with *Trypanosoma cruzi*. On the other hand, moderate exercise prior to experimentally induced infection has improved the survival of mice exposed to *Salmonella typhimurium*.[13]

Human comparisons between active and sedentary individuals, whether retrospective or prospective in type, have yielded divergent results.[7] This may be because of differences in the timing or the amounts of activity undertaken; the active groups have ranged from young, high-level athletic competitors to elderly people undertaking light exercise.

Some authors have reported an increase in the incidence, duration, and/or severity of upper respiratory infections in rowers,[20] orienteers,[62] marathoners,[100] and recreational swimmers[112] (Table 1). Horstmann[47] also noted an increased severity of infection and subsequent paralysis if subjects had been engaged in strenuous physical activity at the time of infection with anterior poliomyelitis. Others have suggested that children,[92] university athletes,[124] and international competitors[4,8] suffer from respiratory infections no more frequently than would be anticipated in the general population. In a few studies, including both marathoners[38] and average active young adults,[111] the incidence of respiratory infections has even appeared to be reduced.

Nieman et al.[86,87] made cross-sectional comparisons among distance runners. One study showed that the incidence of respiratory complaints was greater in runners training more than 42 km/week than in those training less than 12 km/week, and in a second study the prevalence was doubled in subjects training more than 97 km/week relative to subjects who trained less than 32 km/week. A further analysis suggested that risk factors for infection included living alone, a low body mass index, and a training distance of over

Table 1   Influence of Training on Resistance to Respiratory Infections

Method	Sample Size	Finding	Ref.
Comparisons Between Athletes (A) and Sedentary Subjects (S)			
Diary record	121 M, 53 F Nordic A skiers	Incidence no greater than general population	4
Questionnaire	69 Rowers	Incidence no greater than general population	8
Survival against *Salmonella typhimurium*	Mice: 20 T, 20 UT	Increased survival with moderate exercise	13
Symptom checklist	61 A (rowers), 126 S	Symptoms more severe and more frequent in A	20
Parasitic and cell infiltration	Mice: 33 swimming, 30 active, 29 UT	6 weeks swimming causes more severe infiltration, increased mortality	22
Lymphocyte subsets	64 M, 28 F	Low CD3, CD4, monocytes in T subjects	32
Questionnaire	20 Marathoners	9/20 thought risk of respiratory infection less than peers	38
Questionnaire	447 M, 83 F runners	Risk rises at 15 km/week	42
Vulnerability	100 nonparalytic 248 paralytic, 63 bulbar cases	Increased severity of infection and increased likelihood of bulbar paralysis	47
Diary record	42 A (orienteers), 41 S	2.5 vs. 1.7 episodes 7.9 vs. 6.4 days per episode	62
Questionnaire	9 M, 1 F marathon runners	Infections more severe with increased volume training	87
Interview	62 A, 75 S (children)	Similar incidence in gymnasts, swimmers, ice hockey 4 times/week, and sedentary	92
Questionnaire and interview	150 Marathoners, 150 S	33.3% vs. 15.3% respiratory symptoms 2 weeks after run	100

Table 1 (continued)   Influence of Training on Resistance to Respiratory Infections

Method	Sample Size	Finding	Ref.
Viremia, viral titers in heart muscle	Mice: 180 swimming, 360 controls	75-Fold increase of viremia, 1000-fold increase of viral titer in heart	102
Questionnaire	92M, 107 F subjects in growth study	Incidence and duration of infection unrelated to total activity or to $\dot{V}O_2$ max	111
Questionnaire and telephone	8000 Recreational swimmers, 8000 S	7.0% vs. 3.0% overall morbidity	112
Weekly interviews	87 University A	Incidence as expected in S	124
Longitudinal Comparisons			
Questionnaire	16 Seniors trained 3 times/week	Respiratory symptoms reduced over 9–12 months	51
Medical charts, symptom checklist	102 Air Force cadets	No increase of infections during basic training	58
Physician diagnosed	482 Trainee-months special warfare training	High incidence of muscoskeletal injuries and respiratory infections	63
Questionnaire	700 Masters athletes	Critical mileage	117
Weekly interviews	87 University A	Incidence highest during first 5 weeks training	124
Interview	10 Distance runners	2/10 Infections with 38% training increase for 3 weeks	132

Note: M = male; F = female; T = trained; UT = untrained.

15 km/week.[42] In contrast, Schouten et al.[111] examined a population of average young men and women. No relationship was found between the incidence or the duration of respiratory infections and the volume of habitual physical activity or the resulting maximal oxygen intake.

C. LONGITUDINAL COMPARISONS

There are few longitudinal studies looking at the effect of training on resistance to infections (Table 1). Strauss et al.[124] found that upper respiratory infections were most prevalent during the first 5 weeks of preparation for intercollegiate athletics. Linenger et al.[63] also observed a high incidence of both musculoskeletal injuries and respiratory infections when military recruits underwent heavy training. Verde et al.[132] commented that two of ten distance runners developed respiratory infections when they deliberately increased an initial heavy training program by a substantial 38%. Many of the Masters athletes questioned by Shephard et al.[117] were also aware that when they exceeded a certain running distance (often as much as 100 km/week), their risk of respiratory infections increased.

Nevertheless, more moderate physical activity programs have generally had beneficial effects. Nieman et al.[88] randomly allocated middle-aged women to an exercise or a control group. The exercised group undertook five 45 min sessions of walking at 60% of heart rate reserve per week. Relative to the controls, they showed no difference in the number of infectious episodes, but the duration of symptoms was only a half of the control value. Karper and Borschen[51] also found that seniors who completed 9 to 12 months of aerobic training reduced their incidence of respiratory symptoms relative to their preprogram experience.

III. RESTING IMMUNE FUNCTION OF ATHLETES VS. SEDENTARY SUBJECTS

A. EXPERIMENTAL CONSIDERATIONS

Cross-sectional comparisons between athletes and sedentary subjects have one major advantage. In most instances, training has been prolonged, and the individuals concerned have thus had adequate opportunity to demonstrate their potential for adaptation to the physical demands of heavy work. However, there are also many problems in the interpretation of cross-sectional data.

In addition to issues surrounding the selection of athletes by body build and other genetic characteristics, it is often difficult to persuade athletes to stop training. Supposed resting data may thus be distorted by the residual effects of recent hard training (which can persist for a week or longer),[113] and by microtraumata (which can provoke the secretion of prostaglandins and suppress various aspects of immune function such as B cell proliferation[33,35,36] and natural killer [NK] cell activity).[98] The quality and quantity of food ingested differ markedly between athletes and sedentary individuals, and endurance athletes suffer periodic depletion of muscle glycogen reserves; the resulting metabolism of branch-chain amino acids may have adverse consequences for lymphocyte proliferation.[1,95] Moreover, the immune system is quite vulnerable to psychological influences,[10] and findings in an athlete may be modified by the stresses associated with exposure to unaccustomed environments, jet lag, sleep deprivation, impending competition, or a poor response to training.

Finally, when comparing the responses of athletic and sedentary subjects to an acute bout of exercise, it is important to match individuals in terms of the relative rather than the absolute intensity of work to be performed.

B. RESTING STATUS

It has been argued that because immunological responses to a single bout of exercise are generally quite transient, long-term adaptations to a training program are unlikely to be demonstrated.[12,118] In support of this hypothesis, the resting immune status of athletes seems relatively normal unless they are training very hard.[6,38,41,91] (Table 2).

C. CELLULAR COMPONENTS

When comparing cellular elements of the immune system between athletes and sedentary individuals, it is important to take into account the expansion of blood volume that usually accompanies endurance training. Counts can also be altered by trafficking of cells between the bloodstream and peripheral reservoirs such as the spleen, liver, and lungs, although such exchanges are more critical in acute than in chronic responses to exercise. Finally, in terms of immunocompetence, a small number of active cells may be as effective as a larger count of less active cells.

D. LYMPHOCYTES

Circulating lymphocyte counts are usually lower in at least a proportion of trained subjects than in sedentary controls[19,38,75,104] although some authors have not found this.[41,91] Liesen et al.[60] and Gabriel et al.[32] both commented that relative to healthy untrained men, athletes undergoing basic, controlled intensity training showed lower total lymphocyte, pan T cell and T helper cell counts, as well as a lower CD4/CD8 cell ratio. Any training-related decrease in cell counts and proliferative responses may reflect a chronic increase of cortisol levels in the athlete, encouraging leukocytes to migrate out of the circulation and toward injured tissues, rather than a specific down-regulation of immune function.[23,30,31] Thus, Verde et al.[133] saw a further decrease in CD4:CD8 ratio when runners who were already training hard increased their training volume by a further 38%.

With a moderate exercise regimen, Rhind et al.[104] found higher leukocyte counts in trained than in untrained individuals (5.80 ± 0.83 vs. $4.63 \pm 0.21 \times 10^9$/l). Counts for T cells (CD3+), B cells (CD19+), and the CD4+:CD8+ ratio did not differ significantly between active and sedentary groups; and total lymphocyte counts were somewhat lower in trained than in untrained subjects (1.90 ± 0.22 vs. $2.26 \pm 0.25 \times 10^9$ cells/l).

An increased number of insulin receptors suggests an increase of metabolic activity in the leukocytes of trained individuals. However, experimental

Table 2   Comparison of Resting Immune Status Between Trained (T) and Untrained (UT) Subjects

Variable	Subject Numbers	Findings	Ref.
	Cross-Sectional Comparisons		
Splenic NK activity	20 T, 20 UT mice	10 weeks strenuous straining suppresses activity	5
NK activity against K562	10 T, 5 UT humans	No differences	6
NK activity	7 T, 7 UT elderly F	Greater in T	15
Leukocyte, lymphocyte, granulocyte count	37 F, 216 M	Leukocyte count inversely related to peak power (w/kg)	19
C-reactive protein	459 T, 85 UT	CRP lower in T, especially swimmers	21
IL-1 levels	5 T, 4 UT	Higher in T	24
CRP, IgA, IgM IgG	14 Cyclists	Normal Low	29
Leukocyte phagocytosis	20 Marathoners	Normal limits	38
Lymphocyte count		Low in 10/20 T	
IgG, IgA, IgM		Normal limits	
Neutrophil count, activity, chemotaxis	20 T, 10 UT	No differences	40
Leukocyte subpopulations Immunoglobulins Complement	6 Well-trained runners	Normal limits Normal limits Normal limits	41
NK activity, rIL-2 LAK of splenocytes	20 T, 20 UT mice	No change resting activity, rIL-2 LAK activity increased in T	43
Serine esterase activity	Mice	Training increases NK activity but not serine esterase	44
Lymphocyte proliferation		Greater in fit subjects	54
NK cell activity	62 Men	NK activity correlated with healthy lifestyle (including exercise)	56

Table 2 (continued) **Comparison of Resting Immune Status Between Trained (T) and Untrained (UT) Subjects**

Variable	Subject Numbers	Findings	Ref.
Cell counts	20 Cyclists, 19 UT	No differences in neutrophil, eosinophil or monocyte counts; neutrophil adhesion decreased in T	59
T cells and subsets		Pan T cells, CD4, CD4/CD8; T subjects lower counts than UT	60
Leukocyte count	10 Active men	Normal limits	75
NK activity	Weightlifters	No difference from controls	89
Lymphocytes, NK cells, neutrophils, subsets, PHA response	6 Athletes, 5 UT	No significant differences;	91
Pokeweed stimulated	7 Water polo players	65% decrease in CD25% compared to UT	94
NK cell% and activity	13 Cyclists and 8 UT	Increased NK%, MPh%, monocytes% and NK activity in T	98
Leukocytes and subsets, IL-2 receptors	7 T, 6 UT young M	Higher leukocytes, NK and granulocytes lower lymphocytes in T, increased IL-2β receptors	104
Immunoglobulins	153 Athletes	Low lysozymes in 48% of subjects	106
Lysozyme, trace minerals		Low Zn and Mg, high A2 macroglobulin	
Lymphocytes	66 Athletes, 20 UT	Decrease of T cells, increased null cells in T subjects	107
Salivary IgA	84 M, 91 F	Unrelated to total activity, weak correlation to sports in F only	111
Serum IL-1	32 Men	Unchanged by exercise in fit subjects	119

Table 2 (continued)   Comparison of Resting Immune Status Between Trained (T) and Untrained (UT) Subjects

Variable	Subject Numbers	Findings	Ref.
Phagocytic activity	11 Cyclists, 9 UT	Reduced oxidative capacity in T	120
Cytokines	8 T, 8 UT, 6 runners, 7 swimmers	Training does not alter resting levels of TNFα, IL-1β, IL-6, CSF	121
Lymphocyte proliferation	10 T, 10 UT	Lesser mitogen response in T	126
Salivary IgA	8 Nordic skiers 8 controls	Values low in athletes	129
T cell count and function	Elite cyclists, UT	No differences	131
Immunoglobulins		Values low in athletes	135

findings are inconsistent. Kono et al.[54] and MacNeil et al.[70] both reported greater mitogen-stimulated lymphocyte proliferation in individuals with a larger maximal oxygen intake. Verde et al.[133] also found increased mitogen-stimulated proliferation when runners deliberately increased an initial heavy-training program by 38%. Others found that the proliferative response to mitogens was no greater in distance runners[38,91] or cyclists[130] than in sedentary individuals. Papa et al.[94] found reduced T cell function in water polo players; and Telgenhoff and Renk[126] also found that conditioned individuals had lesser responses to concanavalin A (Con A), phytohemagglutinin (PHA), and pokeweed mitogen (PWM) than did their sedentary peers.

E. NATURAL KILLER CELLS

Top-level athletes generally show no advantage of resting natural killer cell percentages or total NK activity relative to sedentary controls,[6,38,60,67,89] although Pedersen et al.[96,97] did find high NK counts and resting NK activity in highly trained cyclists. At the peak of the training season, the NK activity per NK cell was also increased in this study. Studies of resting function in subjects involved in more moderate activity programs have shown an increase in either total or per cell NK activity relative to sedentary peers.[15,81,88]

We found that relative to untrained subjects, individuals who had undergone 12 weeks of moderate training showed higher NK (CD16+) counts (0.32 ± 0.14 vs. $0.16 \pm 0.05 \times 10^9$ per liter[104]). We observed[104] only an insignificant trend toward a higher p55 IL-2α receptor expression in moderately trained vs. untrained subjects. We also observed that the p70–75 IL-2β receptor expression was greater in the active group (mik-beta-1, 0.42 ± 0.09 vs. 0.20 ± 0.06;

TU27+, 0.36 $\pm$ 0.08 vs. 0.17 $\pm$ 0.07). The expression of the beta receptor was strongly correlated with aerobic power (r = 0.91 for mik-beta-1, r = 0.88 for TU27), and it was also related to the increase in NK count. Papa et al.[94] compared high-level water polo players with sedentary controls, finding the athletes had a lower IL-2α expression after PWM stimulation.

F. LYMPHOKINE-ACTIVATED KILLER CELLS

Hoffman-Goetz[43] and Hoffman-Goetz et al.[46] found that relative to control animals, the lymphokine activated killer (LAK) cell activity stimulated by rIL-2 was greater in the splenocytes of mice that had undergone moderate wheel training for 8 weeks. However, Blank et al.[5] found that relative to controls, the LAK activity of mouse splenocytes was suppressed by 30% if resting data were collected 48 h following 10 weeks of strenuous training.

G. NEUTROPHILS

We observed higher granulocyte counts in subjects who had undergone moderate training than in their untrained peers (3.14 $\pm$ 0.72 vs. 1.90 $\pm$ 0.30 $\times$ 10^9 cells per liter[104]). There seem to be no differences in the numbers of neutrophils, phagocytic activity,[40,59] ingestion capacity, and production of superoxide or chemotaxis[40] between athletes who are training moderately and sedentary controls, although the adherence of the neutrophils may be enhanced in the athletes.[59]

Very vigorous training seemingly has a more adverse effect. Davidson et al.[16] reported neutropenia in 4 of 90 male marathoners, and in 3 of 25 female competitors. Smith et al.[120] also commented that the ability of neutrophils to produce reactive species of oxygen and thus to kill invading microorganisms was lower in athletes who had undertaken intensive training.

H. MONOCYTES AND MACROPHAGES

Monocyte and macrophage activity is probably modified by the extent of subclinical muscle damage incurred during training. Gabriel et al.[32] found lower monocyte counts in subjects with the largest aerobic power, and Lewicki et al.[59] reported no difference in monocyte counts between trained cyclists and untrained subjects. In contrast, Pedersen et al.[98] reported higher percentages of macrophages in highly trained cyclists than in untrained individuals.

The antibody-dependent cytotoxicity of peritoneal macrophages does not differ between trained and untrained animals.[64]

I. SOLUBLE FACTORS

Interleukin-1 (IL-1) is released by macrophages in response to tissue injury. Athletes may thus show an increase in plasma interleukin-1-like activity, particularly if they have been involved in recent eccentric activity.[24]

However, Simpson and Hoffman-Goetz[119] and Smith et al.[120] found no differences in resting levels of IL-1 between moderately trained athletes and sedentary controls.

Normal resting levels of serum immunoglobulins have been reported in distance runners[38,41] and other athletes.[68] However, Verde et al.[132] noted that very heavy training suppressed mitogen-stimulated immunoglobulin synthesis. Thus much depends on the individual's level of competition and the duration of recovery from the most recent bout of exercise. Tomasi et al.[129] found lower resting salivary IgA levels in elite cross-country skiers than in controls, and Frenkl et al.[29] found low levels of IgG (but not IgA, IgM, or C-reactive protein [CRP]) in competitive cyclists. Von Weiss et al.[135] and Ricken and Kindermann[106] have also noted low immunoglobulin levels, with an increased risk of infection in elite athletes.

Hanson and Flaherty[41] found normal complement levels in six well-trained runners, but Nieman et al.[86] have reported lower levels of complement C3 and C4 in well-trained individuals. Serum levels of C-reactive protein were also lower in an assorted population of top-level athletes than in controls.[21]

IV. RESPONSES OF ATHLETES AND SEDENTARY SUBJECTS TO EXERCISE

A. LYMPHOCYTES

At any given absolute work rate, the leukocytosis tends to be less in athletes than in sedentary subjects (Table 3). Nevertheless, one factor that has contributed to apparently discordant results has been a difference in the relative intensity and duration of the test exercise between investigations. If sedentary and athletic groups are each stressed at maximum or at an equivalent percentage of maximal effort, the leukocytosis may become comparable in the two groups.[34,53] Dorner et al.[19] attributed the leukocytosis in athletic individuals to neutrophilia rather than lymphocytosis, but Masuhara et al.[73] found that the exercise-induced lymphocytosis was also greater in subjects with a large aerobic power.

Brahmi et al.[6] and Deuster et al.[18] found no essential differences in overall T cell or subset responses to exercise between trained and untrained human subjects. Oshida et al.[91] further noted that while exercise invariably decreased the percentage of lymphocytes that were T cells and T helper cells, an acute bout of exercise markedly increased the percentage of T suppressor cells in trained subjects.

Mahan and Young[71] compared responses to a single exhausting bout of swimming in trained and untrained rats. They noted a greater suppression of the Con A response in untrained (55%) than in trained (26%) animals. However, in human studies (where the intensity of training has probably been

Table 3 Comparisons of Immune Response to Exercise Between Trained (T) and Untrained (UT) Subjects

Variable	Subject Numbers	Findings	Ref.
NK activity against K562 tumor cells	—	No differences	6
Granulocyte response	6 Marathoners, 7 UT	Exercise depresses lysozyme response in UT but not T	9
CD25 cells %	16 T, 8 UT	Increase of CD25% with exercise greater in UT	14
NK activity	7 T, 7 UT elderly F	Greater increase in T	15
Lymphocyte subsets	20 Young men	No difference with fitness	18
Granulocyte, lymphocyte	37 F, 179 M	Granulocytes + in fit, lymphocytes in those with low peak power (w/kg)	19
IL-1 activity	5 T, 4 UT	Greater increase of IL-1 in UT	24
Leukocyte, lymphocyte counts	16 T, 13 UT	No difference in response to maximum exercise	34
CD25 %	10 Cyclists, 6 UT	CD25% decreased 6 h postexercise, less decrease in UT	37
CD4, CD8, NK cells	30 Men, varying fitness	Fitness has no marked effect on lymphocyte enumerative response to exercise	53
Neutrophil, monocyte adherence, phagocytosis	20 T, 19 UT	Exercise decreased adherence in T, increased neutrophil phagocytosis in UT	59
Lymphocyte proliferation	32 Men, varying fitness	Exercise reduces proliferation most in UT	70
Lymphocyte %	—	Increase in lymphocyte % related to aerobic power	73
Lymphocytes, NK cells, neutrophils, subsets	6 Athletes, 5 UT	NK% increased more in athletes	91
Lymphocyte proliferation	10 T, 10 UT	Exercise suppresses in T	126

higher), the opposite response has been seen. Telgenhoff and Renk[126] found that 15 min of cycle ergometer exercise suppressed mitogen responses in conditioned but not in sedentary subjects. Likewise, Oshida et al.[91] noted that relative to trained individuals, untrained subjects showed a smaller fall in PHA response immediately after an acute bout of exercise, and a larger overshoot during the following 3 d.

B. NATURAL KILLER CELLS

Oshida et al.[91] found a much larger increase of NK percentage in trained than in untrained subjects at the immediate end of an acute bout of exercise. The IL-2α (CD25) receptors showed a smaller increase in trained than in untrained individuals at the end of exercise,[14] and the untrained individuals also showed a smaller decrease postexercise.[37]

C. NEUTROPHILS

Lewicki et al.[59] found that whereas untrained subjects showed increased phagocytic activity, trained individuals showed decreased adherence and bactericidal activity in response to exercise. Dorner et al.[19] commented that whereas subjects with a low aerobic power output (W/kg) showed lymphocytosis during exercise, well-trained subjects showed granulocytosis. They further observed a differential increase of plasma catecholamine receptors on the neutrophils of trained subjects. The ability of the neutrophils of trained subjects to produce reactive oxygen species was also depressed relative to untrained subjects during exercise.[120] Busse et al.[9] observed that a 13-km run did not change the lysozyme response of granulocytes to isoproterenol in trained subjects, but in untrained individuals a maximal treadmill run was enough to reduce this response.

D. MONOCYTES AND MACROPHAGES

Lewicki et al.[59] found that exercise decreased the adherence of macrophages in trained but not in untrained subjects.

E. SOLUBLE FACTORS

Evans et al.[24] found a greater increase of IL-1-like activity in untrained than in trained subjects during an acute bout of exercise; however, the untrained individuals commenced from a lower baseline.

Most authors have found either no differences or even an increase of immunoglobulin readings with moderate training, particularly if care has been taken to allow for training-induced changes of plasma volume.[85, 92]

Nieman and Nehlsen-Cannarella[85] reported that complement levels during and following exercise were lower in marathoners than in age-matched controls. They speculated that repeated distance running may have overloaded the liver's ability to synthesize complement, although alterations of blood volume, catabolism, and immune reactions could have contributed to the observed differences.

V. DELIBERATE TRAINING OF ANIMALS AND HUMANS

Deliberate training experiments can be conducted in either animals or in humans. There are several advantages to animal experiments. It is not necessary to restrict cell analysis to the peripheral blood, as is done in most human studies; specimens can be collected from such sites as the spleen and the liver. Further, animals can be exercised to more severe exhaustion than is possible in most human studies. The food intake of animals can be rigorously controlled, and the impact of immune changes on resistance to experimental infections and neoplasms can be examined directly. On the other hand, only small volumes of blood can be collected from small mammals; and given differences from the human life span, it is difficult to equate the duration of training between animal and human experiments. There are also problems in determining maximal oxygen intake in animals, leading in turn to problems in rating the intensity of training. Some types of exercise are stressful for animals, and this may modify their immune responses. Finally, the importance of the spleen as a storage reservoir seems to differ between humans and many animal species.

The response to deliberate training depends on the intensity, frequency, and duration of the applied regimen, and on the initial condition of the individual. There seems to be a J-shaped response, moderate training having a positive effect and excessive training leading to a depression of immune function. It is thus necessary to distinguish carefully between experiments that have used a moderate training stimulus and those that have demanded very heavy training. Moreover, well-trained athletes are able to undertake a much larger volume of training than sedentary individuals before this becomes an excessive stress for them. Finally, in some studies, changes that have been reported a result of training may in fact reflect incomplete recovery from the most recent training session.[25,26] A minimum of 24 h of recovery is needed following exercise, and with very vigorous effort recovery may be incomplete for much longer.[113]

A. LYMPHOCYTES

Training typically reduces overall leukocyte counts,[74] and attenuates the overall lymphocytosis that accompanies exhausting exercise in a sedentary individual.[123] Surkina and Kozlovskaya[125] found an increase in the proportion of B cells after intensive training of figure skaters, but others have suggested that T cells account for a larger percentage of total lymphocytes after conditioning.[123,134]

Table 4   Effect of Training on Resting Immune Function

Variables	Subjects	Findings	Ref.
NK activity	18 Rheumatoid arthritis patients	No change over 8 weeks training	2
Lymphocyte subsets	20 Runners	Increase of monocytes, sIL2-R, ICAM1, and CD4CD45RO+ as training peaks	3
T cell function	Beagle dogs: 8T, 8 UT	No change with training	11
T cell function	Young rats: 11T, 6 UT	Impaired by training	25
IL-2 release in rat splenocytes	5 T, 5 controls	Increased in T	26
CD56, CD25, HLA-DR	5 Men, overtrained	Decreased CD56 Increased CD25 and HLA-DR	31
NK (CD57) %	9 T, 9 UT males	Increase in NK%	45
T cell function	Pigs	No change with training	48
Lymphocyte subsets	12 Runners	High-intensity T more immunosuppressant than high volume T	50
IgM and IgG production	18 T, 9 controls	Enhanced IgM, IgG output in T	52
Lymphocyte subsets	7 T, 7 controls	Increase of CD2, CD4, CD45RACD4, CD8, and CD20 cells with training	57
Splenocyte proliferation	4 T, 4 UT rats	Training decreased proliferation to Con A and *Staph. ent. B*, IL-2 production decreased	61
Salivary IgA, IgM	12 Males	Levels unchanged by 8 weeks interval training	66
Salivary IgA	8 F field hockey players	Decrease over 5 d intense training	68
Splenic NK activity and cytotoxicity	Mice- wheel run or treadmill	Training increased *in vitro* splenic NK activity and *in vivo* cytotoxicity	69

Table 4 (continued)   Effect of Training on Resting Immune Function

Variables	Subjects	Findings	Ref.
Leukocyte count	Track and field athletes	Decreased with overtraining	74
Ig production, lymphocyte proliferation	11 T, 10 controls	No change of lymphocyte proliferation or Ig production over 12 weeks moderate T	80
T cell function	Rats	Impaired by T in young but not old rats	82
Ig production	18 T, 18 UT	Enhanced by brisk walking	83
Lymphocyte subsets	17 Male swimmers	Decreased CD4, increased CD8, NK and B cell counts over training season	84
Activity, NK count	18T, 18UT	Increased NK activity at 6 weeks but not 15 weeks no effect on NK count	88
IL-2 relase by rat splenocytes	Rats: 17T, 17 UT	Increased by T	93
Lymphocyte proliferation	Hamsters	Enhanced by T	99
Neutrophil phagocytosis	91 Athletes	Decreased ingestion of bacteria with heavier training	101
Thymus size	Mice: 25T, 25 UT	Decreased thymus size in T	103
NK count, NK activity		Increased resting NK count, NK activity	105
Lymphocyte subsets	Athletes	Decreased CD4, increased CD8 count	108
Coxsackie virus antibodies	68 Track and field athletes	No relation to training status	109
Lymphocyte count	17 T, 12 controls	Training reduces exercise lymphocytosis	123
Leukocyte subsets	Young figure skaters	Increased B cell, decreased T cell, neutrophil and eosinophil count	125

Table 4 (continued) Effect of Training on Resting Immune Function

Variables	Subjects	Findings	Ref.
Salivary IgA	50 boys	Increase over basketball season	127
Lymphocyte subsets and proliferation	16 Volunteers	Back muscle training no effect	130
Lymphocyte counts Mitogen stimulated cell proliferation and Ig synthesis	10 Runners	Decreased IgG synthesis with heavy training	133
T cell mitogenesis, NK activity	Men	Training increased T cell mitogenesis, NK activity	134
Leukocyte subsets	11 Men	No change of lymphocyte, neutrophil, or monocyte counts	136
IgA, IgG, IgM	217 Athletes	Decrease with peak T	137
Macrophage response to thioglycollate	Mice: 6 exhaustive T vs. 6 moderate T	Reduced inflammatory response	138
Neutrophil number and function	7 Men	Training no effect	139

LaPerriere et al.[57] noted that 10 weeks of moderate training led to increased B and T cell counts, with increases in CD4, CD8, and CD45RACD4 (CD4-inducer) cell subsets. However, heavy training generally leads to a decrease in the ratio of helper:suppressor cells.[125,132,133] High-intensity training exerts a greater suppressant effect than high-volume training.[50] Baum et al.[3] commented that the CD4CD45RO+ subset of cells increased as the training of a group of 20 runners peaked. This finding was associated with increased blood levels of sIL-2r. Fry et al.[31] found an increase of IL-2α (CD25) and human leukocyte antigen (HLA) receptors over 10 d of very heavy training.

Data on the proliferation of lymphocytes are complicated by the effects of recent training, and sometimes (in the case of athletes) by steroid abuse, which can increase proliferation rates.[10] Studies subjecting average individuals to 6[123] or 15 weeks[134] of aerobic training, and of distance runners to 3 weeks of much increased training[132,133] have all shown a tendency for resting mitogen-induced lymphocyte proliferation to be increased; however, because of a variable response, quite large average changes (up to a 64% increment) have sometimes been statistically nonsignificant. Other authors have found an unchanged or an insignificantly depressed resting response to both Con A and PHA; it is unclear how far these differences reflect the length of the recovery interval after the final bout of training. Verde et al.[132,133] further reported that a combination of very heavy training and an acute bout of submaximal exercise decreased the response to mitogens.

Animal training studies have reached conflicting conclusions, but offer some evidence that exercise-induced changes can extend beyond the circulating blood. Thus Reyes et al.[103] observed that nine consecutive days of swimming to exhaustion induced a decrease in the mass of the rat thymus. No changes of lymphocyte function were seen in dogs[11] or pigs.[48] Others reported a decreased responsiveness of lymphocytes to mitogen stimulation in young but not in older rats.[25,61,82,93] Hoffman-Goetz[43] noted that after 6 weeks of treadmill exercise, mouse splenic lymphocytes showed a decreased responsiveness to mitogen stimulation, perhaps due to an alteration in the relative proportions of T and B cells and perhaps due also to the action of T suppressor cells[71] or macrophage-secreted prostaglandin E_2.[98] The responsiveness of the mice splenic lymphocytes was not restored by 2 d of subsequent rest. In keeping with the comments on human studies, Hoffman-Goetz et al.[45] observed a decreased response to mitogens at the immediate end of training, but an increased response after 72 h of recovery. In elderly rats[82] and hamsters,[99] training enhanced lymphocyte responsiveness.

B. NATURAL KILLER CELLS

Using the E-rosetting technique, Watson et al.[134] found a decrease in the number of NK cells with heavy aerobic training. This was attributed to either a redistribution of cells between the peripheral blood and reservoir sites, or to a conversion of the NK cells into rosetting T cells. Fry et al.[31] also described a decrease of NK cell (CD56) counts with very heavy training. In contrast, Crist et al.[15] found that basal NK cell activity was increased in a geriatric population after the participants had completed a low-level aerobic training program. Nieman et al.[88] also saw little change in the NK cell counts of 36 obese women assigned to a controlled study of light aerobic training; the NK cell activity of the experimental group was increased at 6 weeks of training, but not at 15 weeks.

Blank et al.[5] observed that mice had reduced NK cell activity after 10 weeks of training on a motorized treadmill. Hoffman-Goetz et al.[46] found no effect of 8 weeks running–wheel training on the resting NK cell activity of mice splenocytes. However, other experiments with mice demonstrated increased *in vitro* splenic NK cell activity and a greater *in vivo* cytotoxicity after 9 weeks of treadmill training or voluntary wheel running.[44,69,119] The increased activity was not accompanied by any increase in serine esterase, leaving the mechanism of the augmented cytolysis uncertain.

C. NEUTROPHILS

Current information suggests a dose-dependent suppression of neutrophil activity. Wilkinson et al.[136] did not see any change in neutrophil counts over a 6-week high-intensity interval cycle training program. However, Surkina and

Kozlovskaya[125] reported a decrease in segmented neutrophils in young figure skaters when they were engaged in intensive training. Petrova et al.[101] tested three training regimens of differing intensity, finding a progressive decrease in the ability of neutrophils to ingest bacilli as the training dose was increased.

D. EOSINOPHILS

Surkina and Kozlovskaya[125] commented on a decrease in the eosinophil count during intensive training.

E. MONOCYTES AND MACROPHAGES

Wilkinson et al.[136] found no change of monocyte count in response to 6 weeks of high-intensity interval training. However, Baum et al.[3] observed a rise in monocyte count, but a decrease of oxidative capacity in 20 runners as their training peaked. This was associated with an increase of the adhesion molecule ICAM1.

As with other leukocytes, the effect of training appears dose dependent. Soman et al.[122] found that the density of monocyte insulin receptors (and presumably their metabolic activity) was increased by moderate training, but Michel et al.[77] found a decrease with very intensive training. Animal data present a similar picture. Michna[78] reported that 3 weeks of daily treadmill exercise enhanced macrocyte migration, chemotaxis, enzyme content, and phagocytosis in mice. However, Woods and Davis[138] found that exhausting training reduced the macrophage response of small mammals to thioglycolate inflammation.

F. SOLUBLE FACTORS

Both swim training[93] and treadmill training[26] enhance the IL-2 release from rat splenocytes. Swim training also enhances IgM and IgG production in rats.[52] In humans, Tharp[127] also observed that moderate basketball training increased IgA levels. Likewise, Nehlsen-Cannarella et al.[83] found enhanced serum levels of IgA, IgG, and IgM in response to a brisk walking program. Roberts et al.[109] studied antibodies to Coxsackie viruses 1 through 5 in a group of 68 elite track and field athletes; after controlling for past infections, there was no evidence of a link between antibody titers and training. On the other hand, the response to heavy training has been less favorable. Tharp and Barnes[128] saw a decrease of salivary IgA levels in swimmers as they approached the peak of their training. B. H. Sabiston (personal communication, 1988) found that postexercise levels of IgG and IgM fell progressively during 6 d of repeated 35 km/d marches. The abnormal findings still prevailed after 24 h of subsequent rest. Wit[137] noted low levels of IgG, IgA, and IgM when subjects were tested at times of heavy training, particularly immediately before and during major competitions. Likewise, Verde et al.[133] noted a decrease of mitogen-stimulated IgG synthesis following 3 weeks of increased training.

Exercise Training and Immune Function **113**

VI. CONCLUSIONS

The evidence reviewed here shows that moderate training has a beneficial effect on many aspects of immune function, both under resting conditions and during an acute exercise challenge. However, periods of intense and highly competitive training commonly have adverse effects. There is growing evidence that intensive training has a negative impact on health, temporarily lowering the resistance of the individual to viral infections, although there remains a need to confirm that clinical effects are linked directly to immune suppression rather than operating through some associated factor. By implication, moderate exercise should reduce the risk of cancer, and there may be an increased risk of carcinogenesis in the person who is overtrained; however, these concepts have yet to be demonstrated convincingly in human subjects.[115]

The threshold for adverse immunological reactions to any given bout of exercise appears to depend on the relative intensity of effort. Regular moderate training can thus shift the threshold for adverse reactions upward. As with most issues relating to training, there remains a need for a clearer delineation of the relative effects of program intensity, frequency, and duration relative to the initial fitness of the individual.

ACKNOWLEDGMENTS

This research is supported in part by research contracts from the Defense and Civil Institute of Environmental Medicine, Downsview, Ontario. One of us (R.J.S.) also receives support as Canadian Tire Acceptance Ltd. Resident Scholar in Health Studies at Brock University.

REFERENCES

1. Ardawi, M. S. and Newsholme, E. A., Metabolism in lymphocytes and its importance in the immune response, *Essays Biochem.*, 21, 1, 1985.
2. Baslund, B., Lyngberg, K., Andersen, V., Dristensen, J. H., Hansen, M., Klokker, N., and Pedersen, B. K., Effect of 8 wk of bicycle training on the immune system of patients with rheumatoid arthritis, *J. Appl. Physiol.*, 75, 1691, 1993.
3. Baum, M., Liesen, H., and Enneper, J., Leucocytes, lymphocytes, activation parameters and cell adhesion molecules in middle-distance runners under different training conditions, *Int. J. Sports Med.*, 15, S122, 1994.
4. Berglund, B. and Hemmingson, P., Infectious disease in elite cross-country skiers: a one year incidence study, *Clin. Sports Med.*, 2, 19, 1990.
5. Blank, S. E., Johansson, J. O., Origines, M. M., and Meadows, G. G., Modulation of NK activity by moderate intensity endurance training and chronic ethanol consumption, *J. Appl. Physiol.*, 72, 8, 1992.
6. Brahmi, Z., Thomas, J. E., Park, M., and Dowdeswell, I. R. G., The effects of acute exercise on natural killer cell activity of trained and sedentary human subjects, *J. Clin. Immunol.*, 5, 321, 1985.

7. Brenner, I., Shek, P. N., and Shephard, R. J., Infection in athletes, *Sports Med.*, 17, 86, 1994.
8. Budgett, R. G. and Fuller, G. N., Illness and injury in international oarsmen, *Clin. Sports Med.*, 1, 57, 1989.
9. Busse, W. W., Anderson, C. L., Hanson, P. G., and Folts, J. D., The effects of exercise on the granulocyte response to isoproterenol in the trained athlete and the unconditioned individual, *J. Allergy Clin. Immunol.*, 65, 358, 1980.
10. Calabrese, J. R., Kling M. A., and Gold, P. W., Alterations in immunocompetence during stress, bereavement, and depression: focus on neuroendocrine regulation, *Am. J. Psychiatry*, 144, 1123, 1987.
11. Campbell, S. A., Hughes, H. C., Griffin, H. E., Landi, M. S., and Mallon, F. M., Some effects of limited exercise on purpose-bred beagles, *Am. J. Vet. Res.*, 49, 1298, 1988.
12. Cannon, G., Exercise and resistance to infection, *J. Appl. Physiol.*, 74, 873, 1993.
13. Cannon, J. G. and Kluger, M. J., Exercise enhances survival rate in mice infected with *Salmonella typhimurium*, *Proc. Soc. Exp. Biol. Med.*, 175, 518, 1984.
14. Ciusani, E., Grazzi, L., Salmaggi, A., Eoli, M., Ariano, C., Vascovi, A., Parati, E., and Nespolo, A., Role of physical training on immune function: preliminary data, *Int. J. Neurosci.*, 51, 249, 1990.
15. Crist, D. M., Mackinnon, L. T., Thompson, R. F., Atterbom, H. A., and Egan, P. A., Physical exercise increases natural cellular-mediated tumor cytotoxicity in elderly women, *Gerontology*, 35, 66, 1989.
16. Davidson, R. J. L., Robertson, J. D., Galea, G., and Maughan, R. J., Hematological changes associated with marathon running, *Int. J. Spts. Med.*, 8, 19, 1987.
17. De la Fuente, M., Martin, M. I., and Ortega, E., Changes in the phagocytic function of peritoneal macrophages from old mice after strenuous physical exercise, *Comp. Immunol. Microbiol. Inf. Dis.*, 13, 189, 1990.
18. Deuster, P. A., Curiale, A. M., Cowan, M. L., and Finkelman, F. D., Exercise-induced changes in populations of peripheral blood mononuclear cells, *Med. Sci. Sports Exerc.*, 20, 276, 1988.
19. Dorner, H., Heinhold, D., and Hilmer, W., Exercise-induced leukocytosis — its dependence on physical capability, *Int. J. Sports Med.*, 8, 152, 1987, (Abstr.).
20. Douglas, D. J. and Hanssen, P. G., Upper respiratory infections in the conditioned athlete, *Med. Sci. Sports Exerc.*, 10, 55, 1978, (Abstr.).
21. Dufaux, B., Order, U., Geyer, H., and Hollmann, W., C-reactive protein concentration in well-trained athletes, *Int. J. Sports Med.*, 5, 102, 1984.
22. Elson, S. H. and Abelmann, W. H., Effects of muscular activity upon the acute myocarditis of C3H mice infected with *Trypsonoma cruzi*, *Am. Heart J.*, 69, 629, 1965.
23. Espersen, G. T., Elback, A., Ernst, E., Toft, E., Kaalund, S., Jersild, C., and Grunnet, N., Effect of physical exercise on cytokines and lymphocyte subpopulations in human peripheral blood, *APMIS*, 98, 395, 1990.
24. Evans, W. J., Meredith, C. N., Cannon, D. J., Dinarello, C. A., Frontera, W. R., Hughes, V. A., Jones, B. H., and Knuttgen, H. G., Metabolic changes following eccentric exercise in trained and untrained men, *J. Appl. Physiol.*, 61, 1864, 1986.
25. Ferry, A., Rieu, P., Laziri, F., Guezennec, C. Y., Elhabazi, A., LePage, C., and Rieu, M., Immunomodulations of thymocytes and splenocytes in trained rats, *J. Appl. Physiol.*, 71, 815, 1991.
26. Ferry, A., Rieu, P., Laziri, F., Elhabazi, A., and Rieu, M., Effect of moderate exercise on rat T cells, *Eur. J. Appl. Physiol.*, 65, 464, 1992.
27. Fitzgerald, L., Exercise and the immune system, *Immunol. Today*, 9, 337, 1988.
28. Folinsbee, L. J., Ambient air pollution and endurance performance, in *Endurance in Sports*, Shephard, R. J. and Åstrand, P. O., Eds., Blackwell Scientific, Oxford, 1992, 479.
29. Frenkl, R., Hatfaludy, Z., and Petrekanits, M., Serum protein changes during exhaustive training and competition, *Hung. Rev. Sports Med.*, 32, 85, 1991.

30. Fry, R. W., Morton, A. R., and Keast, D., Overtraining in athletes: an update, *Sports Med.*, 12, 32, 1991.
31. Fry, R. W., Morton, A. R., Garcia-Webb, P., Crawford, G. P. M., and Keast, D., Biological responses to overload training in endurance sport, *Eur. J. Appl. Physiol.*, 64, 335, 1992.
32. Gabriel, L., Schwarz, L., Urhausen, A., and Kindermann, W., Leukocyten- und Lymphozytensubpopulationen im peripheren Blut von Sportlerinnen und Sportlern unter Ruhebedingungen, *Dtsch. Z. Sportmed.*, 43, 196, 1992.
33. Gemsa, D., Leser, F. G., Deimann, W., and Resch, K., Suppression of T lymphocyte proliferation during lymphoma growth in mice: role of PGE_2-producing macrophages, *Immunobiolology*, 161, 385, 1982.
34. Gimenez, M., Mohan-Kumar, T., Humbert, J. C., de Talance, N., Teboul, M., and Arino-Belenguer, F. J., Training and leucocyte, lymphocyte and platelet response to dynamic exercise, *J. Sports Med. Phys. Fitness*, 27, 172, 1987.
35. Goodwin, J. S., Messner, R., and Peake, G. L., Prostaglandin suppression of mitogen-stimulated lymphocytes *in vitro*: changes with mitogen dose and preincubation, *J. Clin. Invest.*, 62, 753, 1978.
36. Gordon, D., Henderson, D. C., and Westwick, J., Effects of prostaglandins E_2 and I_2 on human lymphocyte transformation 144 in the presence and the absence of inhibitors of prostaglandin synthesis, *Br. J. Pharmacol.*, 67, 17, 1979.
37. Gray, A. B., Smart, Y. C., Telford, R. D., Weidmann, M. J., and Roberts, T. K., Anaerobic exercise causes transient changes in leukocyte subsets and IL-2R expression, *Med. Sci. Sports Exerc.*, 24, 1332, 1992.
38. Green, R. L., Kaplan, S. S., Rabin, B. S., Stanitski, C. L., and Zdziarski, U., Immune function in marathon runners, *Ann. Allergy*, 47, 73, 1981.
39. Griffiths, M. and Keast, D., The effect of glutamine on murine splenic leukocyte responses to T- and B-cell mitogens, *Cell Biol.*, 68, 405, 1990.
40. Hack, V., Strobel, G., Rau, J. P., and Weicker, H., The effect of maximal exercise on the activity of neutrophil granulocytes in highly trained athletes in a moderate training period, *Eur. J. Appl. Physiol.*, 65, 520, 1992.
41. Hanson, P. G. and Flaherty, D. K., Immunological responses to training in conditioned runners, *Clin. Sci.*, 60, 225, 1981.
42. Heath, G. W., Ford, E. S., Craven, T. E., Macera, C. A., Jackson, K. L., and Pate, R. R., Exercise and incidence of upper respiratory tract infections, *Med. Sci. Sports Exerc.*, 23, 152, 1991.
43. Hoffman-Goetz, L., Exercise, natural immunity, and tumor metastasis, *Med. Sci. Sports Exerc.*, 26, 157, 1994.
44. Hoffman-Goetz, L., Serine esterase (BLT esterase) activity in murine splenocytes is increased with exercise but not with training, *Int. J. Sports Sci.*, 2, 94, 1995.
45. Hoffman-Goetz, L., Simpson, R. J., and Houston, M. E., Lymphocyte subset response to repeated submaximal exercise in men, *J. Appl. Physiol.*, 68, 1069, 1990.
46. Hoffman-Goetz, L., Arumugam, Y., and Sweeny, L., Lymphokine activated killer cell activity following voluntary physical activity in mice, *J. Sports Med. Phys. Fitness*, 34, 83, 1994.
47. Horstmann, D. M., Acute poliomyelitis; relation of physical fitness at time of onset to course of disease, *JAMA*, 142, 236, 1950.
48. Jensen, M., The influence of regular physical activity on the cell-mediated immunity in pigs, *Acta Vet. Scand.*, 30, 19, 1989.
49. Joseph, S. W., Conway, J. B., and Kalichman, S. G., Aquatic and terrestrial bacteria in diving environments: monitoring and significance, *Undersea Biomed. Res.*, 18, 187, 1991.
50. Kajiura, J. S., Ernst, O. E., and MacDougall, J. D., Immune system response to changes in training intensity and volume in runners, *Med. Sci. Sports Exerc.*, 25(Abstr.), S122, 1993.
51. Karper, W. B. and Borschen, M. B., Effects of exercise on acute respiratory tract infections and related symptoms, *Geriatr. Nurs.*, 14, 15, 1993.

52. Kaufman, J. C., Harris, T. J., Higgins, J., and Maisel, A. S., Exercise-induced enhancement of immune function in the rat, *Circulation*, 90, 525, 1994.
53. Kendall, A., Hoffman-Goetz, L., Houston, M., MacNeil, B., and Arumugam, Y., Exercise and blood lymphocyte subset responses: intensity, duration, and subject fitness effects, *J. Appl. Physiol.*, 69, 251, 1990.
54. Kono, I., Matsuda, H. K. M., Haga, S., Fukushima, H., and Kashiwagi, H., Weight reduction in athletes may adversely affect the phagocytic function of monocytes, *Physician Sports Med.*, 16(7), 56, 1988.
55. Kuipers, H. and Keizer, H. A., Overtraining in elite athletes, *Sports Med.*, 6, 79, 1988.
56. Kusaka, Y., Kondou, H., and Morimoto, K., Healthy lifestyles are associated with higher natural killer cell activity, *Prev. Med.*, 21, 602, 1992.
57. LaPerriere, A., Antoni, M. H., Ironson, G., Perry, A., McCabe, P., Klimas, N., Helder, L., Schneiderman, N., and Fletcher, M. A., Effects of aerobic exercise training on lymphocyte subpopulations, *Int. J. Spts. Med.*, 5, S127, 1994.
58. Lee, D. J., Meehan, R. T., Robinson, C., Mabry, T. R., and Smith, M. L., Immune responsiveness and risk of illness in US Air Force Academy cadets during basic cadet training, *Aviat. Space Environ. Med.*, 63, 517, 1992.
59. Lewicki, R., Tchorzewski, H., Denys, A., Kowalska, M., and Golinska, A., Effect of physical exercise on some parameters of immunity in conditioned sportsmen, *Int. J. Sports Med.*, 8, 309, 1987.
60. Liesen, H., Reidel, H., Order, U., Mücke, S., and Widenmayer, W., Zellülarer Immunität bei Hochleistungssportlern, *Dtsch. Z. Sportmed.*, 40(11), 4, 1990.
61. Lin, Y. S., Jan, M. S., and Chen, H. I., The effect of chronic and acute exercise on immunity in rats, *Int. J. Sports Med.*, 14, 86, 1993.
62. Linde, F., Running and upper respiratory tract infections, *Scand. J. Sports Sci.,* 9, 21, 1987.
63. Linenger, J.M., Flink, S., Thomas, B., and Johnson, C.W. Musculo-skeletal and medical morbidity associated with rigorous physical training, *Clin. J. Sports Med.*, 3, 229, 1993.
64. Lötzerich, H., Fehr, H. G., and Appell, H. J., Potentiation of cytostatic but not cytolytic activity of murine macrophages after running stress, *Int. J. Sports Med.,*. 11, 61, 1990.
65. Mackinnon, L., *Exercise and Immunology*, Human Kinetics Publishers, Champaign, IL, 1992.
66. MacKinnon, L. T. and Jenkins, D. G., Decreased salivary immunoglobulins after intense interval exercise before and after training, *Med. Sci. Sports Exerc.*, 25, 678, 1993.
67. MacKinnon, L. T., Chick, T. W., van As, A., and Tomasi, T. B., Effects of prolonged intense exercise on natural killer cell number and function, in *Exercise Physiology: Current Selected Research*, Dotson, C. O. and Humphrey, J. H., Eds., AMS Press, New York, 1988, 77.
68. MacKinnon, L. T., Ginn, E., and Seymour, G., Comparison of the effects of training and competition on secretory IgA levels, *Med. Sci. Sports Exerc.*, 22, S125, 1990, (Abstr.).
69. MacNeil, B. and Hoffman-Goetz, L., Effects of exercise on natural cytotoxicity and pulmonary tumor metastases in mice, *Med. Sci. Sports Exerc.*, 25, 922, 1993.
70. MacNeil, B., Hoffman-Goetz, L., Kendall, A., Houston, M., and Arumugam, Y., Lymphocyte proliferation response after exercise in men: fitness, intensity and duration effects, *J. Appl. Physiol.*, 70, 179, 1991.
71. Mahan, M. P. and Young, M. R., Immune parameters of untrained or exercise-trained rates after exhaustive exercise, *J. Appl. Physiol.*, 66, 282, 1989.
72. Martin, B. J., Limitations imposed by respiratory muscle fatigue, *Can. J. Sports Sci.*, Suppl. 12, 61S, 1987.
73. Masuhara, M., Kami, K., Umobayasi, K., and Tatsumi, N., Influences of exercise on leucocyte count and size, *J. Sports Med. Phys. Fitness*, 27, 285, 1987.
74. Matvienko, L. A., A study of peripheral blood in track and field athletes, *Teor. Prakt. Fizicheskoi Kult.*, 2, 31, 1979 (translated in *Soviet Sports Rev.*, 16, 50, 1980).
75. McCarthy, D. A. and Dale, M. M., The leukocytosis of exercise, *Sports Med.*, 6, 333, 1988.

76. McCarthy, D. A., Perry, J. D., Melsom, R. D., and Dale, M. M., Leukocytosis induced by exercise, *Br. Med. J.*, 295, 636, 1987.

77. Michel, G., Vocke, T., Fiehn, W., Weicker, H., Schwarz, W., and Bieger, W. P., Bidirectional alteration of insulin receptor affinity by different forms of physical exercise, *Am. J. Physiol.*, 246, E153, 1984.

78. Michna, H., The human macrophage system: activity and functional morphology, *Biblio. Anat.*, 31, 1, 1988.

79. Midtvedt, T. and Midtvedt, K., Sport and infection, *Scand. J. Soc. Med.*, Suppl. 29, 241, 1982.

80. Mitchell, J. B., Paquet, A. J., Pizza, F. X., Starling, R. O., Holtz, R. W., and Grandjean, P. W., Effect of aerobic training on immune function, *Med. Sci. Sports Exerc.*, 25, S78, 1993, (Abstr.).

81. Nakachi, K. and Imai, K., Environmental and physiological influences on human natural killer cell activity in relation to good health practices, *Jpn. J. Cancer Res.*, 83, 798, 1992.

82. Nasrullah, I. and Mazzeo, R. S., Age-related immunosenescence in Fischer 344 rats: influence of exercise training, *J. Appl. Physiol.*, 73, 1932, 1992.

83. Nehlsen-Cannarella, S. L., Nieman, D. C., Balk-Lamberton, A. J., Markoff, P. A., Chritton, D. B. W., Gusewitch, G., and Lee, J. W., The effects of moderate exercise training on immune response, *Med. Sci. Sports Exerc.*, 23, 64, 1991.

84. Neisler, H. M., Bean, M. H., Thompson, W. R., and Hall, M., Alterations of lymphocyte subsets during a competitive swim training session, in *Biomechanics and Medicine in Swimming*, MacLaren, D., Reilly, T., and Lees, A., Eds., E. & F.N. Spon., London, 1992, 333.

85. Nieman, D. C. and Nehlsen-Cannarella, S. L., Exercise and infection, in *Exercise and Disease*, Watson, R. R. and Eisinger, M., Eds., CRC Press, Boca Raton, FL, 1992, 121.

86. Nieman, D. C., Johanssen, L. M., and Lee, J. W., Infectious episodes in runners before and after a road race, *J. Sports Med. Phys. Fitness*, 29, 289, 1989.

87. Nieman, D. C., Johanssen, L. M., Lee, J. W., and Arabatzis, K., Infectious episodes in runners before and after the Los Angeles marathon, *J. Sports Med. Phys. Fitness*, 30, 316, 1990.

88. Nieman, D. C., Nehlsen-Cannarella, S. L., Markoff, P. A., Balk-Lamberton, A. J., Yang, H., Chritton, D. B. W., Lee, J. W., and Arabatzis, K., The effects of moderate exercise training on natural killer cells and acute upper respiratory tract infections, *Int. J. Sports Med. Phys. Fitness*, 11, 467, 1990.

89. Nieman, D. C., Henson, D. A., Sampson, C., Herring, J. L., Suttles, J., Conley, M., and Stone, M. H., Natural killer cell cytotoxic activity in weight lifters and sedentary controls, *J. Strength Cond. Res.*, in press.

90. Niinimaa, V., Cole, P., Mintz S., and Shephard, R. J., The switching point from nasal to oronasal breathing, *Resp. Physiol.*, 42, 61, 1981.

91. Oshida, Y., Yamanouchi, K., Hayamizu, S., and Sato, Y., Effect of acute physical exercise on subpopulations in trained and untrained subjects, *Int. J. Sports Med.*, 9, 137, 1988.

92. Osterback, L. and Qvarnberg, Y., A prospective study of respiratory infections in 12-year old children, *Acta Pediatr. Scand.*, 76, 944, 1987.

93. Pahlavani, M., Cheung, T. H., Chesky, J. A., and Richardson, A., Influence of exercise on immune function of rats of various ages, *J. Appl. Physiol.*, 64, 1997, 1988.

94. Papa, S., Vitale, M., Mazzotti, G., Neri, L. M., Monti, G., and Manzoli, F. A., Impaired lymphocyte stimulation induced by the long-term training, *Immunol. Lett.*, 22, 29, 1989.

95. Parry-Billings, M., Budgett, R., Koutedakis, V., Blomstad, E., Brooks, S., Williams, C., Calder, P. C., Pilling, S., Baigrie, R., and Newsholme, E. A., Plasma amino acid concentrations in the overtraining syndrome: possible effects on the immune system, *Med. Sci. Sports Exerc.*, 24, 1353, 1992.

96. Pedersen, B. K., Tvede, N., Hansen, F. R., Andersen, V., Bendix, T., Bendixen, G., Bendtzen, K., Galbo, H., Haahr, P. M., Klarlund, K., Sylvest, J., Thomsen, B. S., and Halkjaer-Kristensen, J., Modulation of natural killer cell activity in peripheral blood by physical exercise, *Scand. J. Immunol.*, 27, 673, 1988.

97. Pedersen, B. K., Tvede, N., Christensen, L. D., Klarlund, K., Kragbak, S., and Halkjaer-Kristensen, J., Natural killer cell activity in peripheral blood of highly trained and untrained persons, *Int. J. Sports Med.*, 10, 129, 1989.

98. Pedersen, B. K., Tvede, N., Klarlund, K., Christensen, L. D., Hansen, F. R., Galbo, H., Kharamazi, A., and Halkjaer-Kristensen, J., Indomethacin in vitro and in vivo abolishes post-exercise suppression of natural killer cell activity in peripheral blood, *Int. J. Sports Med.*, 11, 127, 1990.

99. Peters, B. A., Sothmann, M., and Wehrenberg, W. B., Blood leukocyte and spleen lymphocyte immune responses in chronically physically active hamsters, *Life Sci.*, 45, 2239, 1989.

100. Peters, E. M. and Bateman, E. D., Ultramarathon running and upper respiratory infections, *S. Afr. Med. J.*, 64, 582, 1983.

101. Petrova, I. V., Kuz'min, S. N., Kurshakova, T. S., Suzdal'nitskii, R. S., Levando, V. A., and Moshiashavili, I. Y., Phagocytic activity of neutrophils and humoral factors of systemic and local immunity during intensive physical loads, *Zh. Mikrobiol. Epidemiol. Immunobiol.*, 12, 53, 1983.

102. Reyes, M. P. and Lerner, A. M., Interferon and neutralizing antibody in sera of exercised mice with coxsackie virus B-3 myocarditis, *Proc. Soc. Exp. Biol. Med.*, 151, 333, 1976.

103. Reyes, M. P., Lerner, A. M., and Ho, K. L., Diminution in the size of the thymus in mice during forced swimming, *J. Infect. Dis.*, 143, 292, 1981.

104. Rhind, S. G., Shek, P. N., Shinkai, S., and Shephard, R. J., Differential expression of interleukin-2 receptor alpha and beta chains in relation to natural killer cell subsets and aerobic fitness, *Int. J. Sports Med.*, 15, 311, 1994.

105. Rhind, S., Shek, P. N., and Shephard, R. J., Effects of moderate endurance exercise and training on lymphocyte activation: in vitro lymphocyte proliferative response, IL-2 production, and IL-2 receptor expression, *Eur. J. Appl. Physiol.*, submitted.

106. Ricken, K. H. and Kindermann, W., Der Immunstatus des Leistungssportlers-Ursachen der Infektanfälligkeit, *Dtsch. Z. Sportmed.*, 37, 38, 1986.

107. Ricken, K. H. and Kindermann, W., Cell-mediated immunity of male and female athletes, *Int. J. Sports Med.*, 8, 157, 1987.

108. Ricken, K. H., Rieder, T., Hauck, G., and Kindermann, W., Changes in lymphocyte subpopulations in after prolonged exercise, *Int. J. Sports Med.*, 11, 132, 1990.

109. Roberts, J. A., Wilson, J. A., and Clements, G. B., Virus infections and sports performance: a prospective study, *Br. J. Sports Med.*, 22, 161, 1990.

110. Rylander, R., Pulmonary defence mechanisms to airborne bacteria, *Acta Physiol. Scand.*, Suppl. 306, 6, 1968.

111. Schouten, W. J., Verschuur, R., and Kemper, H. C. G., Physical activity and upper respiratory infection in a population of young men and women: the Amsterdam growth and health study, *Int. J. Sports Med.*, 9, 451, 1988.

112. Seyfried, P. L., Tobin, R. S., Brown, N. E., and Ness, P. F., A prospective study of swimming-related illness. I. Swimming associated health risk, *Am. J. Public Health*, 75, 1068, 1985.

113. Shek, P. N., Sabiston, B. H., Vidal, D., Paucod, J. C., Bourdon, M. L., Melin, B., Buguet, A. C., and Radomski, M. W., Immunological changes induced by exhaustive exercise in conditioned athletes, *Proc. Int. Congr. Immunol.*, 8, 706, 1992.

114. Shephard, R. J., Exercise and lifestyle change, *Br. J. Sports Med.*, 23, 11, 1989.

115. Shephard, R. J., Exercise in the prevention and treatment of cancer, *Sports Med.*, 15, 258, 1993.

116. Shephard, R. J., Verde, T. J., Thomas, S. G., and Shek, P. N., Physical activity and the immune system, *Can. J. Sports Sci.*, 16, 163, 1991.

117. Shephard, R. J., Kavanagh, T., Mertens, D. J., and Qureshi, S., Personal health benefits of Masters athletics competition, *Br. J. Sports Med.*, 29, 35, 1995.

118. Simon, H. B., Immune mechanisms and infectious disease in exercise and sports, in *Sports Medicine*, Strauss, R., Eds., W. B. Saunders, Philadelphia, 1991, 95.

119. Simpson, J. A. R. and Hoffman-Goetz, L., Exercise, serum zinc, and interleukin-1 concentrations in man: some methodological considerations, *Nutr. Res.*, 11, 309, 1991.

120. Smith, J. A., Telford, R. D., Mason, I. B., and Weidemann, M. J., Exercise, training and neutrophil microbicidal activity, *Int. J. Sports Med.*, 11, 179, 1990.

121. Smith, J., Telford, R. D., Baker, M. S., Hapel, A. J., and Weidemann, M. J., Cytokine immunoreactivity in plasma does not change after moderate endurance exercise, *J. Appl. Physiol.*, 73, 1396, 1992.

122. Soman, V. R., Koivisto, V. A., Deibert, D., Felig, P., and de Fronzo, R. A., Increased insulin sensitivity and insulin binding to monocytes after physical training, *N. Engl. J. Med.*, 301, 1200, 1979.

123. Soppi, E., Varjo, P., Eskola, J., and Laitinen, L. A., Effect of strenuous physical stress on circulating lymphocyte number and function before and after training, *J. Lab. Clin. Immunol.*, 8, 43, 1982.

124. Strauss, R. H., Lanese, R. R., and Leizman, D. J., Illness and absence among wrestlers, swimmers and gymnasts at a large university, *Am. J. Sports Med.*, 16, 653, 1988.

125. Surkina, L. D. and Kozlovskaya, L. V., Blood leucocytes in sportsmen during adaptation to exercise, *Lab. Delo*, 10, 597, 1980.

126. Telgenhoff, G. and Renk, C., Effect of acute exercise on lymphocyte mitogenic responses in conditioned and non-conditioned male subjects, *Med. Sci. Sports Exerc.*, 21, S110, 1989, (Abstr.).

127. Tharp, G. D., Basketball exercise and secretory immunoglobulin A, *Eur. J. Appl. Physiol.*, 63, 312, 1991.

128. Tharp, G. D. and Barnes, M. V., Reduction of salivary immunoglobulin levels by swim training, *Eur. J. Appl. Physiol.*, 60, 61, 1990.

129. Tomasi, T. B., Trudeau, F. B., Czerwinski, D., and Erredge, S., Immune parameters in athletes before and after strenuous exercise, *J. Clin. Immunol.*, 2, 173, 1982.

130. Tvede, N., Pedersen, B. K., Hansen, F. R., Bendix, T., Christensen, L. D., Galbo, H., and Halkjaer-Kristensen, J., Effect of physical exercise on blood mononuclear subpopulations and in vitro proliferative responses, *Scand. J. Immunol.*, 29, 383, 1989.

131. Tvede, N., Steensberg, J., Baslund, B., Halkjaer-Kristensen, J., and Pedersen, B. K., Cellular immunity in highly trained racing cyclists and controls during periods of training with high and low intensity, *Scand. J. Sports Med.*, 1, 163, 1991.

132. Verde, T. J., Thomas, S., and Shephard, R. J., Potential markers of heavy training in highly trained distance runners, *Br. J. Sports Med.*, 26, 167, 1992.

133. Verde, T., Thomas, S., Shek, P. N., and Shephard, R. J., The effects of heavy training on two in-vitro assessments of cell-mediated immunity, *Clin. J. Sports Med.*, 3, 211, 1993.

134. Watson, R. R., Moriguchi, S., Jackson, J. C., Werner, L., Wilmore, J. H., and Freund, B. J., Modifications of cellular immune functions in humans by endurance training during β-adrenergic blockade with atenolol or propranolol, *Med. Sci. Sports Exerc.*, 18, 95, 1986.

135. von Weiss, M. J., Fuhrmansky, J., Lulay, R., and Weicker, H., Häufigkeit und Ursache von Immunoglobulinmangel bei Sportlern, *Dtsch. Z. Sportmed.*, 35, 146, 1985.

136. Wilkinson, J. G., Biskup, B. G., and Martin, D. T., High intensity interval training does not result in chronic leucocytosis, *Med. Sci. Sports Exerc.*, 25, S123, 1993, (Abstr.).

137. Wit, B., Immunological responses to physical effort, in *International Perspectives in Exercise Physiology*, Nazar, K., Terjung, R. L., Kaciuba-Uscilko, H., and Budohoski, L., Eds., Human Kinetics Publishers, Champaign, IL, 1990, 220.

138. Woods, J. A. and Davis, J. M., Exercise, monocyte/macrophage function, and cancer, *Med. Sci. Sports Exerc.*, 26, 147, 1994.

139. Woolley, K. L., Kajiura, J., MacDougall, D., and Jones, N., Effects of exercise and training on neutrophil number and function, *Med. Sci. Sports Exerc.*, 25, S78, 1993, (Abstr.).

Chapter 7

IMMUNE RESPONSES TO OVERTRAINING AND FATIGUE

David Keast

CONTENTS

I. INTRODUCTION

    Anecdotal evidence has accumulated over the last 20 to 30 years, suggesting that a significant proportion of athletes enjoy increased feelings of health and have fewer infectious illnesses than untrained individuals. On the other hand, a significant number of athletes eventually consistently underperform; some appear to suffer increased episodes of infectious illness which occur more often than in untrained individuals and may eventually lead to serious and sustained illness. Scientists are now attempting to verify these observations scientifically and to look for reasons why the illnesses occur. Research in this field is now established in at least five major areas:

1. Epidemiological studies are aimed at verification of the incidence of infectious illness in the athlete, along with its association with training load and any temporal effects with respect to training programs and performance at major athletic events. Presumably both maximal physical and mental stress prevail in the athlete in order to produce the best performance possible at the time.
2. Physiological studies are conducted on the outcome of performance techniques and on the ways training may be improved to reduce training stress on the athlete.
3. Biochemical studies elucidate the adaptations which the body has to undergo in order for the athlete not only to increase performance, but also to both sustain that increased performance and to improve on it without detriment to the athlete through, for example, increased susceptibility to infection.
4. Psychological stress studies are done to determine the role in performance and the ways this may influence training, performance of the day, and recovery from exercise stress. More recently studies have begun to establish a role for psychological stress in the function of the immune system.
5. Immunological studies have probably become the keystone area of research attempting to link exercise-induced infection with suppression or some other abnormality induced in the immune system by training programs.

There is no doubt that all these areas interact as athletes proceed through training programs, and one of the pressing requirements at the present time is to pinpoint where normal homeostasis begins to become compromised and whether this eventually leads to increased incidences of infection and other more serious syndromes.

II. THE TRAINING SPECTRUM

Modern elite athletic performance is now so refined that long-term training programs designed to increase both skills and cardiorespiratory endurance energy systems are obligatory to any expectation of top-level performance.

However, it has become clear that these training programs must be carefully structured to provide both a training stress and more importantly a substantial recovery period between exercise bouts.[2,10] During the recovery period the body adjusts to the training stress and establishes an adaptive homeostasis capable of sustained performance at the new level. Short-term fatigue is a natural outcome of training and, in association with balanced-increased workloads, provides the environment for development of endurance needed by any athlete to perform at any level of sport. Development of the modern training program therefore is through what has been termed overload training.[66] Only when inadequate rest and/or too great an exercise stress has been undertaken during a training program may the athlete reach a state of failing adaptation. This is associated with increased fatigue and the requirement for longer recovery times between exercise bouts. Should the athlete fail to recognize this and/or continue to increase the training load, then chronic fatigue will develop. Chronic fatigue is characterized by a serious deterioration in performance which may be associated with increased physical injury and increased susceptibility to infection. This situation is probably the most critical one with which the athlete has to contend; if chronic fatigue is ignored, there is a very high probability that the athlete will develop what is now being recognized as a serious long-term clinical illness, the overtraining syndrome.[11,36,75,76,81,141]

The transition from one of the above stages to another is through ill-defined zones where some characteristics of both states coexist (Table 1). Part of the adaptive process involves the acceptance of the new level of training stress into the normal homeostatic mechanisms in order that the athlete can perform more work for the same homeostatic displacement. This is called super compensation and occurs mainly over the rest periods when the athlete is in the natural state of a fatigue valley.[66] If the athlete is not allowed to fully recover before the next exercise bout, then the athlete progresses to a more highly trained state, provided that the process is applied sensibly.

There is now ample evidence that biochemical and physiological supercompensation occur in several sports such as running[1] and swimming[18] and in arm strength and power sports.[19] There is little doubt that sport-induced changes can occur in other body systems not directly associated with improved physical performance. It has been recognized for a considerable time that the homeostatic mechanisms of the immune system can be influenced by exercise, and it was proposed sometime ago that in heavily trained individuals increased susceptibility to infection could occur due to the adverse effects of training on the immune system.[133] Understanding of the effects of training, both in the short term and in the long term, on the immune system therefore provides an opportunity to study mechanisms which might be involved in the fine-tuning of immunity to combat infection, on the one hand, and to recognize factors which can lead to a breakdown in immunity and increase susceptibility to infection, on the other hand.[66,67,95,143]

TABLE 1   The Training Continuum and Its Properties

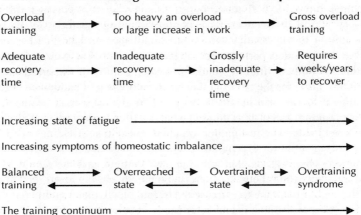

Overload → Too heavy an overload → Gross overload
training   or large increase in work   training

Adequate → Inadequate → Grossly → Requires
recovery   recovery   inadequate   weeks/years
time   time   recovery   to recover
                                 time

Increasing state of fatigue ────────────────→

Increasing symptoms of homeostatic imbalance ────────→

Balanced → Overreached → Overtrained → Overtraining
training ←   state ←   state ←   syndrome

The training continuum ─────────────────→

III. FATIGUE

It is clear from the literature that there is still a need for the sports scientist to come to grips with the role of energetics on the immune system.[16,40,66] There exists a plethora of information on both the acute and the longer term effects of exercise on the immune system. However, much of the discussion has been based on the nonreproducibility of results between groups, when the researchers have used experimental systems where the exercise protocols have induced significantly different short-term biochemical changes in the subjects. The results have suggested that the internal environment of the subjects might in fact have been quite different and could have exerted substantially different metabolic stresses on all systems of the body, not only that of the immune system. In addition, much of the work has been with *in vitro* systems with no acknowledgment of likely hormonal influences on the results obtained. Research designed to stress adenosine 5′-triphosphate (ATP)/creatine metabolism, anaerobic metabolism, or aerobic metabolism provided substantial evidence on how in the short term effects on the immune system were quite different.[67] These studies also suggested that the fatigue valley into which the subjects progressed after their exercise could be controlled by quite different mechanisms.

A. SHORT-TERM FATIGUE: NATURAL

As stated above fatigue is a normal expectation of exercise. Following acute bouts of exercise, on the whole this fatigue probably lasts from a few hours to less than 24 h. Fatigue results from the cumulative metabolic and physical stress of the exercise bout. The components making up short-term fatigue are likely to vary considerably in their relative importance depending on the design of the exercise and the subsequent physical, hormonal, physiological, and biochemical factors stressed. It may well be that the *in vitro* changes associated with the immune system, which appear to occur in the acute exercise situation, are a reflection of population shifts of the cellular component of the immune system rather than exercise-induced metabolism within the cells.[41,63] These population shifts may well be induced as a result of blood volume changes and/or hormonal changes such as those associated with the mobilization of cells of the immune system by catecholamines.[13,46,47,61,63,129,139,146]

More recent studies employing acute exercise have shown that only in situations where subjects exercise at greater than 75 to 80% of their $\dot{V}O_2$max do major changes in biochemical and cellular distributions become evident.[41,42,48,99] At these levels of exercise major biochemical and physiological changes occur in the athlete and acute fatigue is most pronounced. Evidence is being accumulated that in these circumstances the majority of biochemical parameters return to normal well within 24 h. Any significant population changes that occur in cells of the immune system also return to normal. Many of the *in vitro* responses seen can be explained by these subpopulation shifts.[42,99]

One intriguing aspect of these studies, which has yet to be resolved, is whether these subpopulation changes of short duration are sufficient to open a window of opportunity for infection to occur in some instances. On the other hand, the fact that a very large proportion of the subpopulation changes can be accounted for in circulation, at least initially, by increased numbers of natural killer (NK) cells and phagocytic cells, may provide the clue to the proposed decreased susceptibility to infection that well-trained athletes indicate they experience.[35,40,41,46,66,110,130]

B. LONG-TERM FATIGUE: EXTREME

It follows that we need to establish whether the biochemical, physiological, hormonal, and immunological changes which are seen in short-term fatigue are also seen after longer and more sustained exercise programs. There are two elements for discussion in this area. First, the athlete under a sustained training schedule often has to respond, through his/her training routines, to an additional acute bout of exercise. Second, there is the long-term effect on the athlete of the training program that may persist for weeks, months, or even years. Endurance athletes would fall into this category. The running of a marathon or the performance of a biathlon or triathlon might be considered to represent an extension of an acute bout of exercise for these athletes. For biathletes and the triathletes, participation in different sports concurrently at competition level requires that the training programs be multifocal and long in duration. Therefore, within any one day these athletes may be severely stressed both biochemically and physiologically, as well as physically.

At the present time it appears that the athlete in a well-structured long-term training program will respond to an acute bout of exercise with the traditional valley of fatigue that probably varies little from that outlined above. However, the training program is likely designed to gradually increase many of the parameters to fit within an increased homeostasis.[36,66] Therefore, more effort will be required by these athletes to move parameters beyond normal as the program develops. This must be considered to be a normal course of events.

A second possibility is that significant changes may occur in biochemical, physiological, and immunological parameters over the course of a longer term exercise program. In order to explore this, any range of parameters will need to be studied after the effects of the last exercise have been dissipated. Most acute exercise effects on the above parameters appear to return to baseline within about 12 to 18 h. Therefore, samples taken early in the morning prior to exercise of the day and after an overnight fast will probably yield the most consistent results. It has been reported in the literature that both increases and decreases occur in many of the biochemical, physiological, and immunological parameters measured (see References 37, 43, 44, 49, 50, 102, 105, 107, 114, 120, 129, 135, and 144). However, once training programs have become routine the feelings of the normal fatigue valley appear to dominate in well-trained individuals. Only when athletes begin to overexercise do both prolonged feelings of fatigue persist and some, but not all, biochemical and immunological parameters fail to return to baseline levels. In our own studies, where we induced short-term overtraining in extremely fit subjects, other than creatine phosphokinase, only glutamine, cortisol, NK cell numbers, and the two lymphocyte activation markers CD-25 and HLA-DR remained significantly reduced in peripheral blood 18 h after each daily set of weight-bearing (running) exercises.[42,68] While creatine phosphokinase and cortisol returned to baseline levels after 5 d of recovery time, glutamine and immunological parameters often remained significantly reduced. Plasma ferritin also became significantly reduced.[42] Even after the recovery period of 5 d, subjects still reported chronic feelings of fatigue which suggested the persistence of a central psychological component to the fatigue process.

C. EXTENDED FATIGUE: OVERTRAINING

A proportion of athletes seriously overtrain as a result of their own motivation or of coaches providing them with ill-conceived training programs. These athletes do not have to be elite athletes, but can come from all levels of sports. However, such individuals typically have very high levels of achievement as their drive to take on the very heavy training programs. This type of training program appears to be obligatory to the development of what has now become known as the overtraining syndrome (see References 8, 11, 21, 23, 30, 36, 66, 75, 76, 81, 115, and 124). Apart from the overtraining syndrome (which develops as a response to severe overtraining), there are two other categories that merit mention. First, some athletes relate the development of the overtraining syndrome directly to the effects of an episode of acute viral infection. The syndrome in this case may develop as an acute or a persistent lethargy following any of a series of common viruses, and has become known as the postviral syndrome. Second, there is a clinical condition known as the chronic fatigue syndrome which can also be linked in some instances to viral infection.[38,39,74,148] In our studies on the chronic fatigue syndrome, a high proportion of the cases have been elite or highly motivated athletes immediately prior to developing the syndrome. We have attempted to relate the features of the overtraining syndrome to the chronic fatigue syndrome.[38,39]

While clinical criteria have been developed which allow for a more consistent diagnosis of these syndromes,[11,57,148] the overriding feature has been extended chronic fatigue persisting from 3 to 6 months to several years.[4,38,39] In these circumstances fatigue persists in the absence of any form of exercise. In fact, exercise exacerbates the fatigue to the extent that often the individual can no longer remain employed and is actually or nearly bedridden.

There have been numerous studies in this area with little to no success in the understanding or alleviation of the syndrome. In the case of the chronic fatigue syndrome in athletes, published material has yielded little consistent information.[3-8] Views on the cause of the syndrome range from it being a chronic breakdown of physical capacity with associated immunological anergy, to a syndrome associated with central nervous incapacitation or a combination of both.[8,11,30,66,75,76,81,115,124,126,127] Often an acute loss of performance has been the only indicator of the onset of the syndrome; by this time it is too late to prevent a complete breakdown of the individual's capacity to perform at any but the basic physiological levels. However, because this syndrome develops in individuals under extreme training stress, there is no reason to believe that there will be a common mechanism for the development of the overtraining syndrome. It may well reflect the individual's weakest link in the biological training chain. In support of this possibility are anecdotal and epidemiological reports suggesting that individuals with the overtraining syndrome and chronic fatigue syndrome are more susceptible to and experience higher than expected frequencies of infection.[14,30,36,66,67,97]

There has also been the interesting observation that circulating levels of the amino acid glutamine are significantly reduced in the overtraining syndrome and they remain low as the syndrome persists.[95,106,107,122,123] In our studies, we have shown that in short-term overtraining circulating glutamine levels fall rapidly before the onset of the overtraining.[68] Glutamine levels remain low for several days of a recovery period, with the return to normal levels appearing to match the recovery from fatigue.[68] In another study in which we surveyed a large range of biochemical, physiological, and immunological parameters, glutamine was the only parameter which was consistently significantly reduced in the ten athletes from a wide variety of sports who suffered from the overtraining syndrome.[122] It is tempting, therefore, to suggest that the reduced level of glutamine in circulation is a reliable predictor of the overtraining syndrome.[68,95,106,107,123,124] However, results do not provide evidence that the reduced levels of glutamine are causal in the overtraining syndrome and may only represent fortuitous observations. Nevertheless, there is an increasing body of information which indicates that the immune system may well rely on circulating glutamine to function optimally, and a glutamine debt may explain some of the observations of increased levels of infections claimed to occur in overtrained athletes.[36,95] Further work is required not only to verify the results presented so far, but also to determine the mechanisms for the reduction in circulating glutamine. A recent study with chronic fatigue subjects did not reveal any significant changes in immunological cytokines within this group, but the results suggested that gentle exercise could relieve some of the feelings of fatigue and improve their sense of well-being.[78]

D. CONCLUSIONS

Fatigue is a normal and expected consequence of exercise. When training programs are successful, there are two components to fatigue. First, an acute bout of exercise must stress the athlete sufficiently to induce a valley of fatigue. This valley of fatigue is likely to last not much longer than 18 to 24 h for some but not all parameters. During the recovery period the biological components of homeostasis adjust to the new levels of stress. Ideally the next training bout should occur over the latter part of this recovery period or shortly thereafter. Through these mechanisms the training process occurs, is sustainable, and can be built on for long periods of time. There is both a general component to this training process and sport specific processes: the latter requires a great amount of attention to provide for top sport-specific performances. The development of chronic fatigue provides a physical and physiological indication that inadequate adjustment occurs to the exercise loads. Should the athlete and/or the coach ignore these warning signs, then it is likely that performance will deteriorate. In some instances an athlete will develop a serious and often long-term debilitating overtraining syndrome.

IV. IMMUNITY

While it is still largely unproved, there is a large pool of data that can be interpreted as supporting the notion that balanced exercise, on the one hand, can improve health and reduce the incidence of infectious disease in athletes; on the other hand, overtraining or possibly imbalanced training programs can lead to increased infections in athletes (Figure 1; see also References 2, 11, 14, 36, 55, 66, 72, 75, 96, 111, 118, 131, and 133). Many of the earlier observations were based on anecdotal information, and only relatively recently have epidemiological studies begun to support these observations scientifically.[14,97]

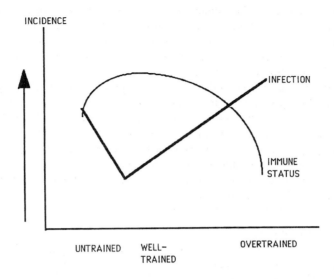

FIGURE 1 The proposed relationship between levels of infection, immune status, and training spectrum in man. (Adapted from Nieman, D. C., et al., Int. *J. Sports. Med.*, 15, 199, 1994.)

A. IMPLICATIONS FOR THE CELLULAR IMMUNE SYSTEM

The majority of information now available suggests that single exercise bouts can lead to major shifts in the populations of leukocytes in circulation, with the subpopulations of lymphocytes including NK cells being grossly affected. Many of the variations in published information may result from differences in intensity and specific nature of the exercise undertaken. It has often been interpreted that these shifts may provide a window of opportunity for infections to occur.[38,66] However, this is by no means proof.[63] Soluble communication molecules for and from the immune system can be activated in situations where tissue damage has occurred.[23,24,53,66,67,101,141] These soluble factors may have been stimulated into production by injury, which does not imply any early indications of infection. There is also evidence that hormonal changes, in particular the catecholamines and growth hormone, may contribute to the mobilization of cells from peripheral pools, including the spleen[36,60,66,112,159] There is also evidence that NK cells, mobilized into circulation following acute exercise, are metabolically activated.[35] It is likely that similar immediate effects on the immune system will occur in overtrained individuals. However, these changes will be influenced to some degree, by any long-term effects already in existence due to the overtraining.[36,66,80,83,109,140]

NK cells are known to play a significant role in an innate mechanism of immunity known as immune surveillance. Immune surveillance is involved in the early recognition of infectious agents, and as a result initiates their removal from the body through the recognition of the first cells replicating the virus.[35,66] Any involvement of lymphocytes occurs later if there is a requirement to develop specific immunity to the infection. Alternatively, immunogenic products arising from the cytotoxic activities of immune surveillance, mediated mainly through NK cell and/or LAK cytotoxicity, would also provide the drive for the development of specific adaptive immunity. Some studies have indicated that the longer the hours of training and/or performance, the greater the likelihood of infection days or weeks after a competition.[14,96,97,118] At these times, specific adaptive immunity directed through the lymphocytes may be involved.[14] There are several instances when increased numbers of infections have been reported in athletes where the athletes have come together from many areas of the world to compete.[14,98,111] These examples and others, on the one hand, may be examples of classical herd immunity; on the other hand, they may indicate that the athletes were already compromised immunologically by their training programs and the contact with other athletes (and their assorted microorganisms) was sufficient to set up the conditions for infection to occur, i.e., provided the window of opportunity.[6,8,33,66,79,90,147] Notably the requirement for the compromised immune system and the infectious agent to be brought together, by whatever means, must occur before fulminated infection can appear.[66]

The early morning preexercise status of overtrained individuals appears to become modified by exercise in many cases.[73,85,86,108,133,142] However, at the present time the variations of these changes suggest that at the level of overtraining each individual may respond differently, due in part to heredity, rather than to specific effects of the long periods of sustained exercise which have led to the state of overtraining.[11,36,66,75,76,81] Furthermore, there is still some doubt as to whether the cellular immune system has been seriously compromised.[63,66,122]

B. IMPLICATIONS FOR THE HUMORAL SYSTEM
1. Antibody Production

The main classes of antibodies, IgM, IgG, IgA, and IgE, and the circulating levels of IgM, IgG, or IgA are apparently uncompromised with extended bouts of exercise, such as marathon running.[51] Furthermore, the immunization of marathon runners with tetanus toxoid after a race led to normal antibody production.[22] There is also evidence that long-term moderate exercise can increase the levels of circulating immunoglobulins.[84] However, because high proportions of the infections recorded by athletes are those of the upper respiratory tract, it may be that local immunity — cell-mediated and/or involving IgA antibody levels in the bronchial tract, nares, and saliva — may be important in the initial stages.[77,82,84,91,136,137] The secretory IgA antibody has been reported to be compromised in endurance sports. It has also been suggested that the breathing of cold air may play a role in the reduction of this antibody in saliva.[137]

Recent studies with elite swimmers undertaking long-term intensive training indicate that IgA production may become compromised, especially if the athlete is progressing toward the overtraining syndrome.[82] However, in our studies the levels of all the classes of antibodies in circulation appear to be normal, even in subjects with the overtraining syndrome.

2. The Cytokines

The cytokines form a series of soluble communication molecules without which the immune system is unable to function.[66] Part of the cytokine network for cooperation between populations and subpopulations of cells within the immune system is made up of interleukins, interferons, tumor necrosis factors, and prostaglandins. Many of the functions and interactions of these factors are now being investigated, but the full impact of these substances, which can be both stimulatory or inhibitory to the immune system, is as yet not understood.[66] There are sources of these cytokines in cells and organs ranging far from that of the immune system. Several properties of the cytokines have now been associated with hormonal control centers and cachectic-type reactions.[121] Chronic exercise is known to induce both tissue and muscle damage; and some of the interleukins, in particular interleukin-6[71] and interleukin-1,[21] can originate from these damaged tissues per se and thus increase in circulation as a direct result of this damage.[34,54,57,66] These interleukins are immediately available to initiate stimulation of both phagocytic cells and lymphocytes or may be able to pass to the brain where it is thought that they may be involved in central nervous (CN) suppression.[66] Currently this area forms one of the interesting developments on the effects of exercise on central control areas and immunity because the cytokines have the potential to cause major modification to immune responses.[41,66,128] Long-term exercise programs suggest that interleukin levels may become chronically increased, probably as a reflection of continuing tissue damage. However, little is known about their effects or contribution to the overtraining syndrome. Our unpublished data suggest that there is little change of the interleukins in circulation, but we have not studied the wider range of cytokines.

V. THE OVERTRAINING SYNDROME

There is no doubt that while athletes can undertake prodigious amounts of work through their training programs, this may also lead to overtraining. As stated earlier, this overtraining may result from the competition between the time required for exercise and the necessity for recovery when homeostasis is adjusting to new levels. Apart from extended feelings of fatigue, loss of performance is probably the first indicator of overtraining. Experienced athletes learn to recognize these early symptoms of overtraining and take extended rest and/or lighten their exercise programs temporarily in order to give their bodies time to readjust. Should the indicators be ignored, a proportion of athletes will deteriorate, sometimes in a very short time, into what has become known as the overtraining syndrome.[8,11,30,36,66,76,81,124,126,127]

There have been detailed a large array of symptoms which accompany the overtraining syndrome.[66] This, in itself, indicates that the likelihood of an individual's final response to serious overtraining may be closely associated with heredity and makes a classical diagnosis of the condition virtually impossible. Athletes at all levels of performance can be at risk to the overtraining syndrome, with high motivation as an important risk factor in its development in many cases.[20,25,62,100,103,132,138] In addition, there is increasing evidence that psychological stress, a common situation for athletes, can exert immunosuppressive effects on the immune system.[69,89] Indeed, immunological and associated factors have been reported as becoming compromised with the development of the overtraining syndrome.[8,11,30,36,66,76,81,124,126,127] There have also been reports of increased susceptibility to infections, in particular those associated with the upper respiratory tract.[66,82] Increases in allergies to environmental allergens and to food allergens at the gut level have also been reported. At the cellular level decreased numbers of lymphocytes, NK cells, neutrophils, and eosinophils have also been reported which have been associated with significant variations in the CD4:CD8 lymphocyte ratio and reduced mitogen responses *in vitro*. There have been reports of various stages of lymphoid cell activation, as determined by increases in the number of lymphoid cells in circulation exhibiting CD69, CD25, and HLA-DR receptors, although this has not been a universal observation.[122]

Animal models have indicated that phagocytic activity of the Kupffer cells of the liver can be depressed while that of the alveolar spaces can be increased by long-term training.[85] In our own studies, while some of the above features were recorded in ten athletes with the long-term overtraining syndrome, they were randomly spread through this small population.[122] The only consistent feature found was that of a significant reduction in circulating levels of glutamine.[122] This amino acid has been implicated in the function of the immune system.[68,95,107,122,123]

A. HORMONES AND OVERTRAINING

There is now substantial evidence that some hormones can play a significant role as immunoregulators and that exercise can vary the levels of these hormones in circulation.[17,19,22,26,27,66,100,117.] There is no doubt that overtraining can be associated with increased levels of cortisol and thyroid hormones and tends to decrease testosterone. Cortisol can be inhibitory to cells of the immune system, and the thyroid hormones are also metabolically active within the immune system. A reduced ratio of free testosterone to cortisol has been suggested as an indicator of overtraining.[9,31] Although these hormones vary with overtraining, the changes recorded are, once again, not universal.[7,9,12,17,25,31,149]

The catecholamines, in particular epinephrine, have been shown to aid in the short-term the mobilization of cells of the immune system following exercise.[46,59,112,135,139] It has been suggested that the levels of circulating epinephrine can be reduced in overtraining;[70] however, one would still expect the concentration to rise, in the short term, when an overtrained individual was subjected to further stress. Undoubtedly other hormones are also involved.[66]

More importantly, hormonal and neuroendocrine communication networks, rather than individual hormones, may determine the final immunological status of the overtrained individual.[28,29,45,87,104,119] Exercise induces significant changes in the hypothalamic-pituitary-adrenal (H-P-A) axis and as a result induces immunomodulation. In addition, the overtraining syndrome is often associated with anxiety, depression, loss of appetite, weight loss, decreased libido, and lack of self-esteem.[29,45,88,89,116] All of these observations suggest that in the overtraining syndrome major modification to hormone networks may have occurred, but is not necessarily accompanied by large changes in absolute levels of individual hormones. These changes could conceivably be responsible for major shifts in metabolism, immunological status, behavior, and extended recovery timescales associated with the overtraining syndrome. It is also tempting to suggest that long-term aberrations in hormonal synthesis may contribute to the significantly lowered levels of circulating glutamine experienced by the chronically overtrained athlete.[122,123]

VI. GLUTAMINE, IMMUNITY, AND THE OVERTRAINING SYNDROME

It was first reported in the early 1980s that cells of the immune system could not synthesize glutamine and rely on the amino acid for both energy and nucleic acid metabolism.[3-5] It followed that glutamine was required by lymphoid cells *in vitro* in order to respond to a mitogen[5] and that this requirement was equally important for both B and T cell mitogens.[52,64,65] Furthermore, the production of the two major interleukins associated with lymphocyte proliferation in response to mitogens or antigen, interleukin-1 and interleukin-2, was shown to be proportional *in vitro* to the amount of available glutamine.[15,52] It has also been shown *in vitro* that the phagocytic capacity of both unopsonized and opsonized macrophages[15,145] and the amount of antibody synthesized[125] were governed by the availability of glutamine. Gutamine is required late in the activation cycle by lymphocytes previously stimulated by the mitogen anti-CD3 monoclonal antibody.[58] Furthermore, the original hypothesis that lymphocytes have an absolute requirement for glutamine has now been modified by the fact that nucleobases or nucleotides can replace a significant portion of the glutamine requirement in the lymphocytic response to the T cell mitogen, phytohemagglutinin.[134] However, the replication of lymphocytes is strongly in favor of the utilization of glutamine as a substrate.

Following the recognition that a major source for glutamine found in circulation was the skeletal muscle, a supply and demand network between muscle and the immune system was proposed; and this network has been extended to incorporate the brain.[58,94] Following short-term acute exercise, glutamine levels in circulation can be temporarily raised.[134] Although when tested over a wide range of exercise intensities, however, this rapidly becomes a glutamine deficit[68] which can last for up to 12 to 18 h.[61] It has been shown that in both short-term overtraining[68] and the overtraining syndrome[32,59,60] a significant and persistent reduction in glutamine levels in peripheral blood occurs.[122,123] These observations, taken together, have led to the proposal that the deficit in circulating glutamine may be responsible for the increased susceptibility to infection seen in some overtrained athletes.[55,69,89,113] It is unlikely that the reduced levels of glutamine in circulation are the prime cause for the development of the overtraining syndrome. However, changes in blood glutamine may well provide a pointer to some more critical aspect of metabolism which is at fault. This now represents a major challenge to sports biochemists.[123]

Work to date suggests that a prolonged deficit in circulatory glutamine may be an excellent indicator that serious overtraining is present.[68,122,123] This may provide the first parameter, which if found to be consistently significantly reduced from normal levels of around 1 M, will indicate that serious overtraining is present in an athlete. In this context, an early morning blood sample, taken under fasting conditions, would provide for the most consistent results.

A. CONCLUSIONS

There are two important aspects to the immune response in the overtrained athlete. First, there is still the need to understand the details of the athlete's immediate response to a single bout of exercise. Second, there remains the fundamental underlying change in the immune system which may have occurred as a result of the overtraining process. Accepting that there are still degrees of overtraining that remain poorly defined,[66] it appears that the distribution of circulating cells has been modified from normal in the long term and numbers are often depleted. Functionally, three of the important populations of cells appear to be compromised: NK cells can be both metabolically activated and yet show suppressed cytotoxicity; phagocytic cells can be severely compromised; and lymphocyte responses, both cell mediated in origin and in the production of antibodies, can be significantly affected by overtraining. Hormonal variation is almost certainly involved, but wide-ranging differences are again prevalent observations. An understanding of the influences of cytokines on these systems is developing rapidly, but whether the greatest influence on the immune system comes from nonspecific cytokinesis due to tissue damage or some more direct immunological mechanism is still uncertain. The role of the amino acid glutamine in the development and possible maintenance of overtraining currently presents an interesting challenge. It may well be that glutamine can be used in the short term as an indicator of overtraining despite the lack of understanding for why glutamine has been reduced.[123] The use of glutamine supplementation or the development of a diet(s) capable of releasing large amounts of glutamine, and how these may help recovery of the overtrained athlete have yet to be explored.

REFERENCES

1. Adams, W. C., The effects of selective pace variations on the O_2 requirements of running a 4.37 mile, *Natl. Coll. Phys. Educ. Assoc. Men,* 1966.
2. Anderson, O., A run a day keeps the doctor at bay, *Runners World*, January, 54, 1989.
3. Ardawi, M. S. M. and Newsholme, E. A., Maximum activities of some enzymes of glycolysis, the tricarboxcylic acid cycle and ketone-body and glutamine utilisation pathways in lymphocytes of the rat, *Biochem. J.*, 208, 743, 1982.
4. Ardawi, M. S. M. and Newsholme, E. A., Glutamine metabolism in lymphocytes in the rat, *Biochem. J.*, 212, 835, 1983.
5. Ardawi, M. S. M. and Newsholme, E. A., Metabolism in lymphocytes and its importance in the immune response, *Essays Biochem.*, 21, 1, 1985.
6. Baron, R. C., Hatch, M. H., Kleeman, K., and MacCormack, J. N., Aseptic meningitis among members of a high school football team, *J. Am. Med. Assoc.*, 248, 1724, 1982.
7. Barron, J. L., Noakes, T. D., Levy, W., et al., Hypothalamic dysfunction in overtrained athletes, *J. Clin. Endocrinol. Metab.*, 60, 803, 1985.
8. Becker, T. M., Kodsi, R., Bailey, P., et al., Grappling with herpes: herpes gladiatorum, *Am. J. Sports Med.*, 16, 665, 1988.
9. Belcastro, A. N., Dallaire, J., McKenzie, D. C., et al., CASS overstress study: blood monitoring, *Med. Sci. Sports Exerc.*, 22, S131, 1990.
10. Bompa, T. O., *Theory and methodology of training*, Kendall/Hunt Publishing, Dubuque, IA, 1983.
11. Budgett, R., Overtraining syndrome, *Br. J. Sports Med.*, 24, 231, 1990.
12. Budgett, R., Koutedakis, Y., Walker, R., et al., The overtraining syndrome/staleness, *Proc. IOC Conf.*, Colorado Springs, 1989.
13. Bunt, J. C., Hormonal alterations during exercise, *Sports Med.*, 3, 331, 1986.
14. Cabinian, A. E., Kiel, R. J., Smith, F., Ho, K. L., Khatib, R., and Reyes, M. P., Modification of exercise-aggravated Coxsackie B3 virus murine myocarditis by T lymphocyte suppression in an inbred model, *J. Lab. Clin. Med.*, 115, 454, 1990.
15. Calder, P. C. and Newsholme, E. A., Glutamine promotes interleukin-2 production by concanavalin A-stimulated lymphocytes, *Proc. Nutr. Soc.*, 51, 105A, 1992.
16. Cameron, K. R., Morton, A. R., and Keast, D., T-cell sub-populations and polyclonal lymphocyte function in continuous and intermittent exercise, *Aust. J. Sci. Med. Sports*, 21, 15, 1989.
17. Carli, G., Martelli, G., Viti, A., et al., Modulation of hormone levels in male swimmers during training, *Biochmech. Med. Swimming: Int. Ser. Sports Sci.*, 14, 33, 1983.
18. Costill, D. L., Flynn, M. G., Kirwan, J. P., et al., Effects of repeated days of intensified training on muscle glycogen and swimming performance, *Med. Sci. Sports Exerc.*, 20, 249, 1988.
19. Costill, D. L., King, D. S., Thomas, R., and Hargreaves, M., Effects of reduced training on muscle power in swimmers, *Physician Sports Med.*, 13, 94, 1985.
20. Costill, D. L., *Inside Running — Basics of Sports Physiology*, Benchmark Press, Indianapolis, IN, 1986.
21. di Giovine, F. S. and Duff, G. W., Interleukin 1: the first interleukin, *Immunol. Today*, 11, 13, 1992.

22. Eskola, J., Ruuskanen, O., Soppi, E., Viljanen, M., Jarvinen., H., and Toivonen, K., Effect of sport stress on lymphocyte transformation and antibody formation, *Clin. Exp. Immunol.*, 32, 339, 1978.

23. Espersen, G. T., Elback, A., Ernst, E., Toft, E., Kaalund, S., Jersild, C., and Grunnet, N., Effect of physical exercise on cytokines and lymphocyte subpopulations in human peripheral blood, *APMIS*, 98, 395, 1990.

24. Evans, W. J., Meredith, C. N., and Cannon, J. G., Metabolic changes following eccentric exercise in trained and untrained men, *J. Appl. Physiol.*, 61, 1864, 1986.

25. Falsetti, H. L., Overtraining in athletes — a round table, *Physician Sports Med.*, 11, 93, 1983.

26. Fauci, A. S., Mechanisms of corticosteriods on lymphocyte subpopulations. I. Redistribution of circulating T- and B-lymphocytes to the bone marrow, *Immunology*, 28, 669, 1975.

27. Fauci, A. S., Mechanisms of corticosteriods on lymphocyte subpopulations. II. Differential effect of *in vivo* hydrocortisone, predisone and dexamethasone on *in vitro* expression of lymphocyte function, *Clin. Exp. Immunol.*, 24, 54, 1976.

28. Fauman, F. A., The central nervous system and the immune system, *Biol. Psychiatry*, 17, 1459, 1982.

29. Feigley, D. A., Psychological burn out in high level athletes, *Physician Sports Med.*, 12, 109, 1984.

30. Fitzgerald, L., Overtraining increases the susceptibility to infection, *Int. J. of Sports Med.*, 12, S5, 1991.

31. Flynn, M. G., Pizza, F. X., Boone, J. B., et al., Indices of overtraining syndrome during a running season, *Med. Sci. Sports Exerc.*, 22, S131, 1990.

32. Fox, G. N., Revisiting the revisited football team hepatitis outbreak, correspondence, *J. Am. Med. Assoc.*, 254, 317, 1985.

33. Freidman, L. S., O'Brien, T. F., and Morse, L. J., Revisiting the Holy Cross football team outbreak (1969) by serological analysis, *J. Am. Med. Assoc.*, 254, 774, 1985.

34. Friden, J., Muscle soreness after exercise: implications of morphological change, *Int. J. Spots Med.*, 5, 57, 1984.

35. Frisina, J. P., Gaudieri, S., Cable, T., Keast, D., and Palmer, T. N., Effects of acute exercise on lymphocyte subsets and metabolic activity, *Int. J. Sports Med.*, 15, 36, 1994.

36. Fry, R., Morton, A. R., and Keast, D., Overtraining syndrome: an update, *Sports Med.*, 12, 32, 1991.

37. Fry, R. W., Morton, A. R., Garcia-Webb, P., and Keast, D., Monitoring exercise stress by changes in metabolic and hormonal responses over a 24 hour period, *Eur. J. Appl. Physiol.*, 63, 228, 1991.

38. Fry, R. W., Morton, A. R., and Keast, D., Overtraining syndrome and the chronic fatigue syndrome, I. *N. Z. J. Sports Med.*, 19, 48, 1991.

39. Fry, R. W., Morton, A. R., and Keast, D., Overtraining and the chronic fatigue syndrome, II. *N. Z. J. Sports Med.*, 19, 76, 1991.

40. Fry, R. W., Morton, A. R., and Keast, D., Periodisation of training stress — a review, *Can. J. Sports Sci.*, 17, 234, 1992.

41. Fry, R. W., Morton, A. R., Crawford, G. P. M., and Keast, D., Cell numbers and in vitro responses of leucocytes and lymphocyte subpopulations following maximal exercise and interval training sessions of different intensities, *Eur. J. Appl. Physiol.*, 64, 218, 1992.

42. Fry, R. W., Morton, A. R., and Keast, D., Acute intense interval training and T-lymphocyte function, *Med. Sci. Sports Exerc.*, 24, 339, 1992.

43. Fry, R. W., Morton, A. R., Garcia-Webb, P., Crawford, G. P. M., and Keast, D., Biological responses to overload in endurance sports, *Eur. J. Appl. Physiol.*, 64, 335, 1992.

44. Fry, R. W., Lawrence, S. R., Morton, A. R., Schreiner, A. B., Polglaze, T. D., and Keast, D., Monitoring training stress in endurance sports using biological parameters, *Clin. J. Sports Med.*, 3, 6, 1993.

45. Fry, R. W., Grove, J. R., Morton, A. R., Zeroni, P. M., Gaudeiri, S., and Keast, D., Psychological and immunological correlates of acute overtraining, *Br. J. Sports Med.*, 28, 241, 1994.

46. Gabriel, H., Scwarz, L., Born, P., and Kindermann, W., Differential mobilization of leucocyte and lymphocyte subpopulations into the circulation during endurance exercise, *Eur. J. Appl. Physiol.*, 65, 529, 1992.

47. Galbo, H., in *Hormonal and Metabolic Adaptation to Exercise*, Georg Thieme, Stuttgart/Springer-Verlag, Austria, 1983.

48. Goodman, C., Rogers, G. G., Vermaak, H., and Goodman, M. P., Biochemical responses during recovery from maximal and sub maximal swimming exercise, *Eur. J. Physiol.*, 54, 436, 1985.

49. Graham, T. E. and MacLean, D. D., Ammonia and amino acid metabolism in human skeletal muscle during exercise, *Can. J. Physiol. Pharmacol.*, 70, 132, 1992.

50. Grazzi, L., Salmaggi, A., Dufour, A., Gritti, A., et al., Short and medium term influence of physical activity on immune parameters, *Int. J. Neurosci.*, 71, 267, 1993.

51. Green, R. L., Kaplan, S. S., Rabin, B. S., Stanitski, C. L., and Zdziarski, U., Immune function in marathon runners, *Am. Allergy*, 47, 73, 1981.

52. Griffiths, M. and Keast, D., The effect of glutamine on murine splenic leukocyte responses to T- and B- cell mitogens, *Immunol. Cell Biol.*, 68, 405, 1990.

53. Haahr, P. M., Pedersen, B. K., Formsgaard, A., Tvede, N., Diamant, M., Klarlund, K., Hakjaer-Kristensen, J., and Bendtzen, K., Effect of physical execise on the in vitro production of IL-1, IL-6, TNF alpha, IL-2 and IFN, *Int. J. Sports Med.*, 12, 223, 1991.

54. Hagerman, F. C., Hikida, R. S., Staron, R. S., et al., Muscle damage in marathon runners, *Physician Sports Med.*, 12, 39, 1984.

55. Heath, G. W., Ford, E. S., Craven, T. E., Macera, C. A., Jackson, K. L., and Pate, R. R., Exercise and the incidence of upper respiratory tract infections, *Med. Sci. Sports Exerc.*, 23, 152, 1991.

56. Hikida, R. S., Staron, R. S., Hagerman, F. C. et al., Muscle fibre necrosis associated with human marathon runners, *J. Neurol. Sci.*, 59, 185, 1983.

57. Horig, H., Spagnoli, G. C., Filgueira, L., Babst, R., Gallati, H., Harder, F., Juretic, A., and Heberer, M., Exogenous glutamine requirement is confined to late events of T cell activation, *J. Cell. Biochem.*, 53, 343, 1993.

58. Holmes, G. P., Kaplan, J. E., Ganyz, N. M., et al., Chronic fatigue syndrome: a working case definition, *Ann. Intern. Med.*, 108, 387, 1988.

59. Iversen, P. O., Arvesen, B. L., and Benestad, H. B., No mandatory role for the spleen in the exercise induced leucocytosis in man, *Clin. Sci.*, 86, 505, 1994.

60. Kappel, M., Hansen, M. B., Diamant, M., Jorgensen, J. O., Gyhrs, A., and Pedersen, B. K., Effects of an acute bolus growth hormone infusion on the human immune system, *Hormone Metab. Res.*, 25, 579, 1993.

61. Kargotich, S., Keast, D., Fry, R. W., and Goodman, C., Plasma volume changes following acute interval training varying intensity in weight bearing and non-weight bearing exercise, submitted.

62. Karpovitch, P. V., *Physiology of Muscular Activity*, W. B. Saunders, Philadelphia, 1965.

63. Katz, P., Exercise and the immune response, *Baillieres Clin. Rheum.*, 8, 53, 1994.

64. Keast, D. and Newsholme, E. A., Effects of mitogens on the maximal activities of hexokinase, lactate dehydrogenase, citrate synthase and glutaminase in rat mesenteric lymph node lymphocytes and splenocytes during the early period of culture, *Int. J. Biochem.*, 22, 133, 1990.

65. Keast, D. and Newsholme, E. A., Effect of B and T cell mitogens on the maximum activities of hexokinase, lactate dehydrogenase, citrate syhtase and glutaminase in bone marrow cells and thymocytes of the rat during four hours of culture, *Int. J. Biochem.*, 23, 823, 1991.

66. Keast, D. and Morton, A. R., Long-term exercise and immune functions, in *Exercise and Disease*, Watson, R. R. and Eisinger, M., Eds., CRC Press, Boca Raton, FL, 1992, chap. 7.

67. Keast, D., Cameron, K., and Morton, A. R., Exercise and the immune response, *Sports Med.*, 5, 248, 1988.

68. Keast, D., Arstein, D., Harper, W. M., Fry, R. W., and Morton, A. R., Depression of plasma glutamine concentration after exercise and its possible influence on the immune system, *Med. J. Aust.*, 162, 15, 1995.

69. Khansari, D. N., Murgo, A. J., and Faith, R. E., Effects of stress on the immune system, *Immunol. Today*, 11, 170, 1990.

70. Kindermann, W., Overtraining — an expression of faulty regulated development *Dtsch. Z. Sportmed.*, 37, 238, 1986.

71. Kishimoto, T., The biology of interleukin-6, *Blood*, 74, 1, 1989.

72. Koch, C., Cold protection, *Triathlon Mag.*, January, 16, 1988.

73. Kokot, K., Schaefer, R. M., Teschner, M., Gilge, U., Plass, R., and Heidland, A., Activation of leucocytes during prolonged physical exercise, *Adv. Exp. Med. Biol.*, 240, 57, 1988.

74. Klonoff, D. C., Chronic fatigue syndrome, *Clin. Inf. Dis.*, 15, 812, 1992.

75. Kuipers, H. and Keizer, H. A., Overtraining in elite athletes. Reviews and direction for the future, *Sports Med.*, 6, 79, 1988.

76. Lehmann, M., Foster, C., and Keul, J., Overtraining in endurance athletes: a brief review, *Med. Sci. Sports Exerc.*, 25, 854, 1993.

77. Liew, F. Y., Russell, S. M., Appleyard, G., Brand, G. M., and Beale, J., Cross protection of mice infected with influenza A virus by the respiratory route is correlated with local IgA antibody rather than serum antibody or cytotoxic T cell reactivity, *Eur. J. Immunol.*, 14, 350, 1984.

78. Lloyd, A., Gandevia, S., Brockman, A., Hales, J., and Wakefield, D., Cytokine production and fatigue in patients with chronic fatigue syndrome and healthy control subjects in response to exercise, *Clin. Infect. Dis.*, 18, S142, 1994.

79. Ludlam, H. and Cookson, B., Scrum kidney: pyoderma caused by a nephrotogenic strep-tococcus pyogenes in a rugby team, *Lancet*, 9, 331, 1986.

80. MacKinnon, L. T., Exercise and natural killer cells. What is the relationship?, *Sports Med.*, 7, 141, 1989.

81. MacKinnon, L. T., and Hooper, S., Overtraining: state of the art review, *Excel*, 8, 3, 1992.

82. MacKinnon, L. T. and Hooper, S., Mucosal secretory immune system responses to exercise of varying intensity and during overtraining, *Int. J. Sports Med.*, 15, S179, 1994.

83. MacKinnon, L. T., Chick, T. W., van As, A., and Tomasi, T. B., Effects of prolonged intense exercise on natural killer cells, *Med. Sci. Sports Exerc.*, 19, S10, 1987.

84. MacKinnon, L. T., Chick, A., van As, A., and Tomasi, T. B., The effect of exercise on secretory and natural immunity, *Adv. Exp. Med. Biol.*, 216A, 869, 1987.

85. Maianskii, D. N. and Voronina, N. P., Changes of macrophage function after graded physical loading, *Patol. Fitziol. Eksp.*, 3, 56, 1989.

86. Matvienko, L. A., A study of peripheral blood in track and field athletes, *Teor. Prakita Fiz. Kultury*, 2, 31, 1979; translation in *Soviet Sports Rev.*, 16, 50, 1981.

87. Miller, T. W., Vaughn, M. P., and Miller, J. M., Clinical issues and treatment strategies in stress-orientated athletes, *Sports Med.*, 9, 370, 1990.

88. Morgan, W. P., Selected psychological factors limiting performance: a mental health model, in *Units of Human Performance,* Clarke, D. H. and Eckert, H. M., Eds., Human Kinetics Publishers, Champaign, IL, 1985.

89. Morgan, W. P., Brown, D. R., Raglin, J. S., et al., Psychological monitoring of overtraining and staleness, *Br. J. Sports Med.*, 21, 107, 1987.

90. Morse, L. J., Bryan, J. A., Murle, J. P., Thommasen, H., Belzberg, A., and Hogg, J. C., Holy Cross football team hepatitis outbreak, *J. Med. Med. Assoc.*, 219, 706, 1972.

91. Muns, G., Liesen, H., Riedel, H., and Bergman, K. C., Influence of long distance running on IgA in nasal secretion and salvia, *Dtsch. Z. Sportsmed.*, 40, 63, 1989.

92. Nehlsen-Cannarella, S. L., Nieman, D. C., Balk-Lamberton, A. J., Markoff, P. A., Chritton, D. B., Gusewitch, G., and Lee, J. W., The effects of moderate exercise training in immune response, *Med. Sci. Sports Exerc.*, 23, 64, 1991.

93. Newsholme, E. A., Biochemical mechanism to explain immunosuppression in well-trained and overtrained athletes, *Int. J. Sports Med.*, 15, S142, 1994.

94. Newsholme, E. A. and Parry-Billings, M., Properties of glutamine release from muscle and its importance for the immune system, *J. Parent. Enterol. Nutr.*, 14, 63, 1990.

95. Nieman, D. C., Exercise, infection, and immunity, *Int. J. Sports Med.*, 15, S131, 1994.

96. Nieman, D. C., Johanssen, L. M., and Lee, J. W., Infectious episodes in runners before and after a road race, *J. Sports Med. Phys. Fitness*, 29, 289, 1989.

97. Nieman, D. C. and Nehlsen-Cannerella, S. L., Exercise and infection, in *Exercise and Disease*, Watson, R. R. and Eisinger, M., Eds., CRC Press, Boca Raton, FL, 1992, chap. 7.

98. Nieman, D. C., Johanssen, L. M., Lee, J. W., and Arabatzis, K., Risk of infectious episodes in runners before and after the Los Angeles Marathon, *J. Sports Med. Phys. Fitness*, *30*, 316, 1990.

99. Nieman, D. C., Miller, A. R., Henson, D. A., Warren, B. J., Gusewitch, G., Johnson, R. L., Davis, J. M., Butterworth, D. E., Herring, J. L., and Nehlsen-Cannarella, S. L., Effect of high-versus moderate-intensity exercise on lymphocyte subpopulations and proliferative response, *Int. J. Sports Med.*, 15, 199, 1994.

100. Noakes, T., *Lore of Running*, Oxford University Press, Cape Town, 1989.

101. Northoff, H. and Berg, A., Immunologic mediators as parameters of the reaction to strenuous exercise, *Int. J. Sports Med.*, 12, S9, 1991.

102. Northoff, H., Weinstock, C., and Berg, A., The cytokine response to strenuous exercise, *Int. J. Sports Med.*, 15, S167, 1994.

103. O'Brien, T. F., Overtraining and Sports Psychology, in *The Olympic Book of Sports Medicine*, Vol. 1, Dirix, A. et al., Eds., Blackwell Scientific, Cambridge, MA, 1988, 635.

104. Ottaway, C. A. and Husband, A. J., Central nervous system influences on lymphocyte migration, *Brain, Behav. Immunity*, 6, 97, 1992.

105. Ortega, R. E., Physiology and biochemistry: influence of exercise on phagocytosis, *Int. J. Sports Med.*, 15, S172, 1994.

106. Parry-Billings, M., Blomstrand, E., McAndrew, N., and Newsholme, E. A., A communicational link between skeletal muscle, brain and cells of the immune system, *Int. J. Sports Med.*, 11, S1, 1990.

107. Parry-Billings, M., Budgett, R., Koutedakis, Y., et al., Plasma amino acid concentrations in the overtraining syndrome: possible effects on the immune system, *Med. Sci. Sports Exerc.*, 24, 1353, 1992.

108. Papa, S., Vitale, M., Mazzotti, G., et al., Impaired lymphocyte stimulation induced by long term training, *Immunol. Lett.*, 22, 29, 1989.

109. Pedersen, B. K., Tvede, N., Hansen, F. R., Andersen, V., Bendix, T., Bendixen, G., Bendtzen, K., Galbo, H., Haahr, P. M., Karlund, K., Sylvest, J., Thomsen, B., and Halkjaer-Kristensen, J., Modulation of natural killer cell activity in peripheral blood by physical exercise, *Scand. J. Immunol.*, 26, 673, 1988.

110. Pedersen, B. K., Tvede, N., Karlund, K., Christensen, L. D., Hansen, F. F., Galbo, H., Kharazmi, A., and Halkjaer-Kristensen, J., Indomethacin in vitro and in vivo abolishes post-execise suppression of natural killer cell activity in peripheral blood, *Int. J. Sports Med.*, 11, 127, 1990.

111. Peters, E. M. and Bateman, E. D., Ultramarathon running and upper respiratory tract infections — an epidemiological survey, *S. Afr. Med. J.*, 64, 582, 1983.

112. Peters, A. M., Allsop, P., Stuttle, A. W. J., Arnot, R. N., Gwilliam, M., and Hall, G. M., Granulocyte margination in the human lung and its response to strenuous exercise, *Clin. Sci.*, 82, 237, 1992.

113. Petrova, I. V., Kuzmin, S. N., Kurshakova, T. S., et al., Neutrophil phagocytic activity and the humoral factors of general and local immunity under intensive physical loading, *Zh. Microbiol. Epidemiol. Immunobiol.*, 12, 53, 1983.

114. Pyne, D. B., Uric acid as an indicator of training stress, *Sports Health*, 11, 26, 1993.

115. Pyne, D. B., Reglation of neutrophil function during exercise, *Sports Med.*, 17, 245, 1994.

116. Raglin, J. S., Exercise and mental health beneficial and detrimental effects, *Sports Med.*, 9, 323, 1990.

117. Ricter, E. A., Kiens, B., Raben, A., Tvede, N., and Pedersen, B. F., Immune parameters in male athletes after a lacto-ovo vegetarian diet and a mixed Western Diet, *Med. Sci. Sports Exerc.*, 23, 517, 1991.

118. Roberts, J. A., Wilson, J. A., and Clements, G. B., Virus infections and sports performance: a prospective study, *Br. J. Sports Med.*, 22, 161, 1988.

119. Rogers, M. P., Dubey, D., and Reich, P., The influence of the psyche and the brain on immunity and disease susceptbility: a critical review, *Psychosom. Med.*, 41, 147, 1979.

120. Rogers, G., Goodman, C., Mitchell, D., and Hattingh, J., The response of runners to arduous triathlon competition, *Eur. J. Appl. Physiol.*, 55, 405, 1986.

121. Roitt, I., *Essential Immunology*, Blackwell Scientific, Oxford, 1994.

122. Rowbottom, D., Keast, D., Goodman, C., and Morton, A. R., Glutamine and the overtraining syndrome, *Eur. J. Physiol.*, 70, 502, 1995.

123. Rowbottom, D., Keast, D., and Morton, A. R., The emerging role of glutamine as an indicator of exercise stress and overtraining, *Sports Med.*, in press.

124. Ryan, A. J., Brown, R. L., Frelerick, E. C., et al., Overtraining in athletes, *Phys. Sports. Med.*, 11, 93, 1983.

125. Schneider, Y. J. and Lavoix, A., Monoclonal antibody production in semi-continuous serum- and protein-free culture, *J. Immunol. Methods*, 129, 251, 1990.

126. Sharp, N. C. C. and Koutedes, Y., Sport and the overtraining syndrome — immunological aspects, *Br. Med. Bull.*, 48, 518, 1992.

127. Sharp, C. and Parry-Billings, M., Can exercise damage your health?, *New Sci.*, 135, 33, 1992.

128. Shepard, R. J., Rhind, S., and Shek, P. N., Exercise and training: influences on cytotoxicity, interleukin-1, interleukin-2, and receptor structures, *Int. J. Sports Med.*, 15, S154, 1994.

129. Shepard, R. J., Verde, T. J., Thomas, S. G., and Shek, P., Physical activity and the immune system, *Can. J. Sports Sci.*, 16, 169, 1991.

130. Shinkai, S., Shore, S., Shek, P. N., and Shephard, R. J., Acute exercise and immune function. Relationship between lymphocyte activity and changes in subset counts, *Int. J. Sports Med.*, 13, 452, 1992.

131. Schouten, W. J., Verschuur, R., and Kemper, H. C., Physical activity and upper respiratory tract infections in a normal population of young men and women: the Amsterdam growth and health study, *Int. J. Sports Med.*, 9, 451, 1988.

132. Stray-Gundersen, J., Videman, T., and Snall, P. G., Changes in selected objective parameters during overtraining, *Med. Sci. Sports Exerc.*, 18 (Abstr.), 268, 1986.

133. Surkina, D. L., Stress and immunity among athletes, *Teor. Pratika Fiz. Kultury*, 3, 18, 1981; translation in *Soviet Sports Rev.*, 17, 198, 1982.

134. Szondy, Z. and Newsholme, E. A., The effects of various concentrations of nucleobases and nucleotides or glutamine on the incorporation of [3H] thymidine into DNA in rat mesenteric-lymph-node lymphocytes stimulated by phytohaemagglutinin, *Biochem. J.*, 270, 437, 1990.

135. Taylor, C., Rogers, G., Goodman, C., Baynes., et al., Hematologic, iron related, and acute-phase protein response to sustained strenuous exercise, *J. Appl. Physiol.*, 62, 464, 1987.

136. Tharp, G. D. and Barnes, M. W., Reduction of salivary immunoglobulin levels by swim training, *Eur. J. Appl. Physiol.*, 60, 61, 1990.

137. Tomasi, T. B., Trudeau, F. B., Czerwinski, D., and Erredge, S., Immune parameters in athletes before and after strenuous exercise, *J. Clin. Immunol.*, 2, 173, 1982.

138. Town, G. P., *Science of Triathlon Training and Competition*, Human Kinetics, Champaign, IL, 1985.

139. Tvede, N., Kappel, M., Karlund, K., Duhn, S., Halkjaer-Kristensen, J., Kjaer, M., Galbo, H., and Pedersen, B. K., Evidence that the effect of bicycle exercise on blood mononuclear cell proliferative responses and subsets is mediated by epinephrine, *Int. J. Sports Med.*, 15, 100, 1994.

140. Tvede, N., Pedersen, B. K., Hansen, F. R., Bendix, T., Christensen, L. D., Galbo, H., and Halkjaer-Kristensen, J., Effects of physical exercise on blood mononuclear cell subpopulations in vitro proliferative reponses, *Scand. J. Immunol.*, 29, 383, 1989.

141. Ullum, H., Haahr, P. M., Diamont, M., Palmo, J., Halkaer-Kristensen, J., and Pedersen, B. K., Bicycle exercises enhances plasma IL-6, but do not change pre-mRNA for IL-1alpha, IL-beta, IL-6 or TNF alpha in blood mononuclear cells, *J. Appl. Physiol.*, 74, 93, 1994.

142. Umarova, L. S., The state of natural immunity in athletes of different ages, *Teor. Prakita Fiz. Kultury*, 8, 26, 1981; translation in *Soviet Sports Rev.*, 17, 104, 1982.

143. Verde, T. J., Short-term exercise and immune function, in *Exercise and Disease*, Watson, R. R. and Eisinger, M., Eds., CRC Press, Boca Raton, FL, 1992, chap. 6.

144. Verde, T., Thomas, S., and Shepherd, R. J., Potential markers of heavy training in highly trained distance runners, *Br. J. Sports Med.*, 26, 167, 1992.

145. Wallace, C. and Keast, D., Glutamine and macrophage function, *Metabolism*, 41, 1016, 1992.

146. Weicker, H. and Werle, E., Interaction between the hormones and the immune system, *Int. J. Sports Med.*, 12, S30, 1991.

147. Weinstein, L., Poliomyelitis — a persistent problem, *N. Eng. J. Med.*, 288, 370, 1973.

148. Wessely, S., Chronic fatigue syndrome: current issues, *Rev. Med. Microbiol.*, 3, 211, 1992.

149. Wishnitzer, R., Berribi, A., Hurwitz, N., et al., Decreased cellularity and hemosiderin of the bone marrow in healthy overtrained competitive distance runners, *Physician Sports Med.*, 14, 86, 1986.

Chapter 8

PROLONGED AEROBIC EXERCISE, IMMUNE RESPONSE, AND RISK OF INFECTION

_____ David C. Nieman

CONTENTS

I. INTRODUCTION

Among elite athletes and their coaches, a common perception is that heavy exertion lowers resistance and is a predisposing factor to upper respiratory tract infections.[28,42] During the winter and summer Olympic Games, it has been regularly reported by clinicians that "upper respiratory infections abound"[21] and that "the most irksome troubles with the athletes were infections."[28] Many elite athletes including Sebastian Coe, Uta Pippig, Liz McColgan, Darren Baker, Michelle Akers-Stahl, Alberto Salazar, and Steve Spence have reported significant bouts with infections that have interfered with their ability to compete and train.[42]

In this chapter, emphasis will be placed on the relationship between prolonged aerobic endurance exercise, chronic and acute alterations in immunity, and risk of upper respiratory tract infections (URTI). Research on the potential for skin infections and other infections in athletes (e.g., hepatitis B and human immunodeficiency viruses) has been reviewed elsewhere.[5,43] It has been proposed that the relationship between aerobic exercise and URTI may be modeled in the form of a "J" curve.[42,43] This model suggests that although the risk of URTI may decrease below that of a sedentary individual when one engages in moderate exercise training, risk may rise above average during periods of excessive amounts of high-intensity exercise. At present, there is more evidence characterizing the relationship between heavy exertion and infection, and these data will be emphasized here.

II. RESTING IMMUNITY IN ENDURANCE ATHLETES VS. NONATHLETES

Relatively few researchers have published cross-sectional comparisons of immune function in aerobic endurance athletes and nonathletes. In this type of study design is a logical starting point when considering the question of prolonged aerobic endurance exercise and immunity. If a significant contrast between athletes and nonathletes could be established for a certain component of the immune system, additional studies, both cross sectional and prospective in design, could be conducted to determine the exercise training and workload thresholds associated with the alteration in immune function. Table 1 summarizes the data currently available on cross-sectional comparisons of human endurance athletes and nonathletes for natural killer cell activity (NKCA),[4,46,47,49,60,78] neutrophil function,[2,18-20,32,66,73] and lymphocyte proliferative response.[2,46,47,49,58,59]

A. NATURAL KILLER CELL ACTIVITY

Natural killer (NK) cells are large granular lymphocytes that can mediate non-MHC restricted cytolytic reactions against a variety of neoplastic and viral-infected cells.[33] NK cells also exhibit key noncytolytic functions, and can inhibit microbial colonization and growth of certain viruses, bacteria, fungi, and parasites.

Of the six studies listed for NKCA, four support the finding of enhanced NKCA in athletes when compared to nonathletes, in both younger and older groups (Table 1). The weighted average elevation in NKCA for the 124 athletes in these four studies is 43.5%. Of interest are the data of Tvede et al.[78] which support a higher NKCA in cyclists during the summer (intensive training period) than during the winter (low training period). Several prospective studies utilizing moderate endurance training regimens have reported no significant elevation in NKCA relative to sedentary controls.[42,48] Together, these data imply that endurance exercise may have to be intensive and prolonged (i.e., at athletic levels) before NKCA is chronically elevated. Researchers disagree on whether the higher NKCA is due to a greater concentration of circulating NK cells or an enhanced cytotoxic capacity of these cells.[47,60,62,78] Data by Tvede et al.[78] suggest that the answer to this question may vary according to the time of the year and the training intensity.

B. NEUTROPHIL FUNCTION

The cross-sectional NKCA data are in contrast to those for neutrophil function (another component of the innate immune system). As summarized in Table 1, no researcher has reported an elevation in neutrophil function (both phagocytic and oxidative burst) among athletes when compared to nonathletes. Instead, during periods of high-intensity training, neutrophil function has been reported to be suppressed in athletes. This is especially apparent in the studies by Hack et al.[20] and Baj et al. [2] where neutrophil function in athletes was similar to controls during periods of low training workloads, but then was significantly suppressed during the summer months of intensive training. Pyne[66] reported that elite swimmers undertaking intensive training have a significantly lower neutrophil oxidative activity at rest than do age- and sex-matched sedentary individuals, and that function is further suppressed during periods of strenuous training prior to national-level competition.

Neutrophils are an important component of the innate immune system, aiding in the phagocytosis of many bacterial and viral pathogens, and the release of immunomodulatory cytokines. Acute exercise bouts have a large effect on the demargination of neutrophils from endothelial tissues and bone marrow, and their function. In general, moderate exercise tends to enhance neutrophil activity while intensive exercise may suppress it.[2,73] In one study, immediately following a 20-km race, neutrophils in a nasal lavage taken from 12 male runners were less able to ingest bacteria, an effect which lasted for 3 d.[41]

Pyne[66] in a recent review on the regulation of neutrophil function during exercise has proposed that repetitive high-intensity training sessions by elite athletes "may leave a significant proportion of their circulating neutrophils in a chronically refractory state. This may be one explanation for the observation that elite athletes, as a group, are more prone to upper respiratory tract illnesses than their sedentary counterparts."

C. LYMPHOCYTE PROLIFERATIVE RESPONSE

Determination of the proliferative response of human lymphocytes upon stimulation with various mitogens *in vitro* is a well-established test to evaluate the functional capacity of T and B lymphocytes. Mitogen stimulation of lymphocytes *in vitro* using optimal and suboptimal doses is believed to mimic events which occur after antigen stimulation of lymphocytes *in vivo*.

Data on the lymphocyte proliferative response to athletic endeavor are less clear than for NK cells and neutrophils, but generally support no significant difference between athletes and nonathletes (Table 1). Only one study by Papa et al.[59] using a limited number of athletes and nonathletes reported a decrease in the resting mitogen-induced lymphocyte proliferative response of the athletes.

Table 1   Resting Immune Function in Human Endurance Athletes and Nonathletes

Subjects	Major Results	Ref.
Natural Killer Cell Activity		
5 Trained male athletes 10 Untrained males and females	↔ No significant difference	4
27 Elite male cyclists 15 Untrained males	↑ 26% Higher in athletes	60
29 Elite male cyclists (low training) 15 Untrained males	↑ 27% Higher in athletes	78
14 Elite male cyclists (high training) 10 Untrained males	↑ 64% Higher in athletes	
12 Elderly female athletes 32 Sedentary elderly females	↑ 55% Higher in athletes	49
18 Male endurance athletes 11 Untrained males	↔ No significant difference	46
22 Male marathon runners 18 Untrained males	↑ 57% Higher in athletes	47
Neutrophil Function		
20 Male marathon runners Pool of untrained males	↔ No significant difference	18
20 Elite male cyclists 19 Untrained males	↓ 90% Lower in athletes	32
11 Elite male cyclists 9 Untrained males	↓ 50% Lower in athletes	73

Table 1 (continued)   Resting Immune Function in Human Endurance Athletes and Nonathletes

Subjects	Major Results	Ref.
20 Elite male runners/triathletes 10 Untrained males	↔ No significant difference during low training period	19
12 Elite male and female swimmers 11 Untrained females and males	↓ 50% Lower in athletes before and after 16 weeks of intensive training	66
7 Elite male runners 10 Untrained males	↔ No significant difference during low training period; ↓ lower in athletes during high training period	20
15 Elite male cyclists 16 Untrained males	↔ No significant difference during low training period; ↓ 33% lower in athletes during high training period (PMA stimulated)	2

Lymphocyte Proliferative Response

Subjects	Major Results	Ref.
6 Elite male runners 5 Untrained males	↔ No significant difference	58
7 Elite water polo players 7 Untrained males	↓ PHA 28% lower in athletes; PWM 60% lower in athletes	59
29 Elite male cyclists (low training) 15 Untrained males	↔ No significant difference	78
14 Elite male cyclists (high training) 10 Untrained males	↔ No significant difference	
12 Elderly female athletes 32 Sedentary elderly females	↑ PHA 56% higher in athletes	49
15 Elite male cyclists 16 Untrained males	↔ No significant difference during low training period; ↑ PHA 35%, anti-CD3 mAb 50% higher in athletes, during high training period (no effect on Con A, PWM)	2
18 Male endurance athletes 11 Untrained males	↔ No significant difference	46
22 Male marathon runners 18 Untrained males	↔ No significant difference	47

Baj et al.[2] reported no difference between elite cyclists and nonathletes during low training periods (March), but increased levels in the athletes for phyto-hemagglutinin (PHA) and anti-CD3 mAb (but not concanavalin A [Con A] or pokeweed mitogen [PWM]) during intensive training. Interleukin-2 generation, however, was suppressed in the athletes vs. controls during intensive training. These data contrast with that of Tvede et al.[78] who found no difference between athletes and nonathletes during both low- or high-training periods.

Among highly conditioned elderly women, PHA-induced lymphocyte proliferative response was 56% higher than among sedentary controls.[49] These data are interesting because T cell function tends to diminish with age. However, moderate exercise training for 12 weeks failed to alter T cell function in elderly women, indicating that an unusual committment to vigorous exercise may be necessary before an effect on T cell function can be measured in the elderly population.

D. OTHER MEASURES OF IMMUNITY

Other components of immunity have been less well studied among human athletes and nonathletes. Tomasi et al.[74] reported that resting salivary IgA levels were lower in elite cross-country skiers than in age-matched controls, but this was not confirmed in a follow-up study of elite cyclists.[36] As reviewed by MacKinnon and Hooper,[37] the secretory immune system of the mucosal tissues of the upper respiratory tract is considered the first barrier to colonization by pathogens, with IgA the major effector of host defense. Secretory IgA inhibits attachment and replication of pathogens, preventing their entry into the body. While several studies have shown that salivary IgA concentration decreases after a single bout of intense endurance exercise, further research is needed to determine the overall chronic effect.[36-38]

Complement but not serum immunoglobulins (especially when adjusted for the higher plasma volumes of athletes) has been reported to be lower in marathon runners vs. sedentary controls.[55,57] Production of tumor necrosis factor in lipopolysaccharide-stimulated blood has been described as significantly depressed in elite cross-country skiers relative to controls.[31] Most studies have failed to demonstrate any important effects of regular exercise training on concentrations of circulating total leukocytes or lymphocytes or their various subpopulations.[18,46,47,49,54]

Together these data support the concept that the innate immune system responds differentially to the chronic stress of intensive exercise, with NKCA tending to be enhanced while neutrophil function is suppressed. The adaptive immune system in general seems to be largely unaffected, although the research data at present are mixed. Further research is needed with larger groups of athletes and nonathletes to allow a more definitive comparison.

III. THE ACUTE IMMUNE RESPONSE TO PROLONGED AEROBIC EXERCISE

As will be discussed in the next section, epidemiological studies suggest that marathon and ultramarathon race events are associated with a significant increase in risk of upper respiratory tract infections during the 1 to 2 week recovery period.[42,51,63-65] In light of the mixed results regarding the effect of chronic, intensive training on resting immune function (previous section), several authors have posited that prolonged cardiorespiratory endurance exercise (defined in this chapter as ≥ 2 h) leads to transient but significant perturbations in immunity and host defense, providing a possible physiological rationale for the epidemiological data.[37,42,62]

For example, mitogen-induced lymphocyte proliferation,[12,17,58,56,71] neutrophil phagocytic function,[41,66] salivary IgA concentration,[36-38,74] and NKCA[3,35,44,54,71] have all been reported to be suppressed for several hours during recovery from prolonged, intense endurance exercise. During this "window of decreased host protection," viruses and bacteria may gain a foothold, increasing the risk of subclinical and clinical infection. This may be especially apparent when the athlete goes through repeated cycles of heavy exertion.[66]

There are no convincing data at this time, however, that exercise-induced changes in immune function explain the increased risk of URTI suggested by epidemiological data.[42] Researchers disagree on the mechanistic interpretation of their findings, and none have provided follow-up data of large numbers of subjects to determine whether various changes in immunity translate to altered host protection. Further research is needed to settle these issues, and to determine whether the large but transient perturbations in leukocyte cell concentrations in both blood and peripheral lymphoid tissue (which often underlie reported *in vitro* functional alterations) are important from a clinical viewpoint.

A. NATURAL KILLER CELL ACTIVITY

To illustrate the problems involved in the interpretation of results from a host protection perspective, consider the effect of endurance exercise on NKCA. Of the three major lymphocyte subpopulations (T, B, and NK cells), NK cells are by far most responsive to acute aerobic exercise.[44,45,52,53,61,72,76,77] Figure 1 summarizes the results of a recent study by Nieman et al.,[44] where the effect of 2.5 h of treadmill running at $75.6 \pm 0.9\%$ VO_2max on NKCA was investigated in 22 experienced marathon runners (VO_2max 57.9 ± 1.1 ml/kg/min, age 38.7 ± 1.5 years). Ten sedentary controls (34.7 ± 1.0 ml/kg/min, 45.3 ± 2.3 years) sat in the laboratory during testing and had their blood sampled at the same time points. The pattern of change in NKCA over time was significantly different between groups [$F(4,27) = 6.53$, $p = 0.001$], with the runner's NKCA dropping 51 to 61% below preexercise levels throughout 6 h of recovery.

As depicted in Figure 1, resting NKCA was elevated in the runners compared to controls. Subsequent to 2.5 h of running, and despite a reduction of more than 50%, NKCA was merely lowered to sedentary control levels. In other words, during the 6-h recovery time period, the runners appeared to lose their normal training-induced advantage in NKCA. How this translates to actual host protection in the athletes is difficult to determine at this time.

Although some reason that the drop in NKCA can be ascribed to numerical shifts in NK cells,[13,44,53,72] others report that prostaglandins from activated monocytes and neutrophils[61,62,76] or elevated stress hormone levels[3] suppress the ability of NK cells to function appropriately. Preincubation of blood mononuclear cells *in vitro* with indomethacin (an inhibitor of prostaglandin) had no effect on the difference in pattern of change in NKCA between marathoners and controls, and did not attenuate the postexercise reduction in the runners.[44] When NKCA was adjusted on a per NK cell basis, group differences were removed, and the postexercise decline in NKCA was eliminated. NKCA data from this study and others suggest that even though the per

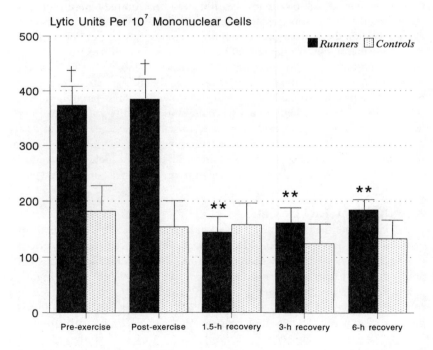

FIGURE 1   The pattern of change in natural killer cell activity (NKCA, expressed in total lytic units) over time between runners (2.5 h at 76% VO_2max) and sitting controls was significantly different [$F(4, 27) = 6.53$, $p = 0.001$]. NKCA was significantly higher in the runners vs. controls both immediately before and after the 2.5-h run. † $p < 0.0125$, difference between groups at time point. ** $p < 0.0125$, difference in change from baseline between groups.

NK cell function is not impaired following exercise, the loss of NK cells from the circulation means that the blood compartment as a whole suffers a transient decrease in NKCA capacity.[13,53] Whether this is important for total body host protection is unknown.

Serum cortisol concentrations were significantly elevated above control levels for several hours following the 2.5-h run (Figure 2). Cortisol has been related to many of the immunosuppressive changes experienced during recovery.[10,16,22,40,75] Glucocorticoids administered *in vivo* have been reported to cause neutrophilia, eosinopenia, lymphocytopenia, and suppression of both NK and T cell function. However, although long-term incubation (>20 h) of BMNC with cortisol *in vitro* or administration *in vivo* of long-acting glucocorticoids has been shown to suppress NKCA,[16,24] short-term (<5 h) infusion of cortisol into human volunteers has been shown to have no effect on NKCA.[24,75] Also, when cortisol is added to the 4-h NKCA assay, no effect can be measured.[16,24,75] This suggests that the transient elevation of cortisol above control levels following 2.5 h of running is of insufficient duration to have a major direct influence on NKCA. It is plausible, however, that cortisol may induce an

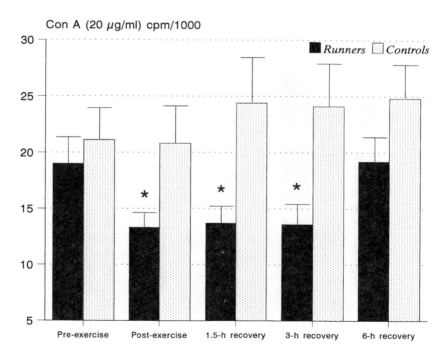

FIGURE 2 Serum cortisol response to 2.5 h of running at ~76% VO_2max in marathon runners compared to values obtained from resting, sedentary controls. The pattern of change was significantly different between groups (F[4, 27] = 9.39, $p < 0.001$). * = $p < 0.0125$, between groups at given time point.

indirect effect on NKCA through its effect on removing NK cells from the circulation in excess of other types of lymphocytes.[10,53]

B. LYMPHOCYTE PROLIFERATIVE RESPONSE

In this same study (2.5-h run), the Con A-induced lymphocyte proliferative response was decreased relative to controls for more than 3 h postexercise, and except for the immediate postexercise time point, tended to parallel the decrease in T cell (CD3+) concentrations (Figure 3).[56] Eskola et al.,[12] Gmünder et al.,[17] and Shinkai et al.[71] have also reported significant decreases in mitogen-induced lymphocyte proliferation immediately following prolonged, intense aerobic exercise; however, the mechanisms (e.g., numerical redistribution of cells, direct hormonal influences, or down-regulation by other substances released during exercise) underlying the decrease are not clear at present. Thus the same sort of interpretation problems associated with the NKCA data are found with the lymphocye proliferative response to prolonged endurance exercise.

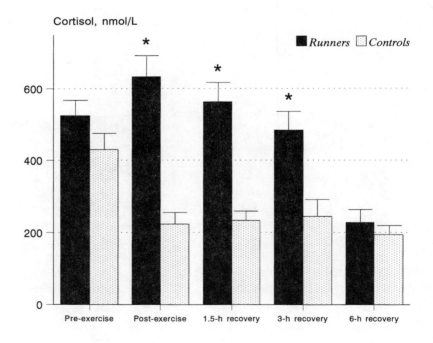

FIGURE 3   Whole blood, Con A-induced lymphocyte proliferative response to 2.5 h of running at ~76% VO$_2$max in marathon runners compared to values obtained from resting, sedentary control subjects. The pattern of change was significantly different between groups (F[4, 116] = 2.51, p = 0.045). * = p < 0.0125, between groups at given time point.

IV. RISK OF UPPER RESPIRATORY TRACT INFECTION IN ENDURANCE ATHLETES

Several epidemiological reports suggest that athletes engaging in marathon-type events and/or very heavy training are at increased risk of URTI.[23,34,51,63-65] Several reviews of this information are available;[5,42,43,54,70] and in this chapter, emphasis will be placed on studies of endurance athletes. (Table 2).

Peters and Bateman[64] were the first to report an increased risk of URTI among athletes following heavy exertion. They studied the incidence of URTI in 150 randomly selected runners who took part in a 56-km Cape Town race in comparison to matched controls who did not run. Symptoms of URTI occurred in 33.3% of runners compared with 15.3% of controls during the 2-week period following the race, and were most common in those who achieved the faster race times.

Two subsequent studies from this group of researchers have confirmed this finding.[63,65] During the 2-week period following the 56-km Milo Korkie Ultramarathon in Pretoria, South Africa, 28.7% of the 108 subjects who completed the race reported nonallergy derived URTI symptoms as compared to 12.9% of controls.[63] In the most recent report from Peters et al.,[65] 68% of runners reported the development of symptoms of URTI within 2 weeks after the 90-km Comrades Ultramarathon. Using a double-blind placebo research design, it was determined that only 33% of runners taking a 600-mg vitamin C supplement daily for 3 weeks prior to the race developed URTI symptoms. The incidence of URTI symptoms was greatest among the runners who trained the hardest (85%) compared to those training more moderately (46%) prior to the race. Duration of URTI symptoms was shortest in the vitamin C-supplemented runners and their matched controls. The authors suggested that because heavy exertion enhances the production of free oxygen radicals, vitamin C, which has antioxidant properties, may be required in increased quantities.

Nieman et al.[51] researched the incidence of URTI in a group of 2311 marathon runners who varied widely in running ability and training habits. Runners retrospectively self-reported demographic, training, and URTI episode and symptom data for the 2-month period (January, February) prior to and the 1-week period immediately following the 1987 Los Angeles Marathon race. During the week following the race, 12.9% of the marathoners reported an URTI compared to only 2.2% of control runners who did not participate (odds ratio, 5.9). Of the runners 40% reported at least one URTI episode during the 2-month winter period prior to the marathon race. Controlling for various confounders, it was determined that runners training more than 96 km/week doubled their odds for sickness compared to those training less than 32 km/week.

Other epidemiological data support these findings. Linde[34] studied URTI in a group of 44 elite orienteers and 44 nonathletes of the same age, sex, and occupational distribution during a 1-year period. The orienteers experienced

Table 2   Epidemiological Research on the Relationship Between Prolonged Endurance Exercise and Upper Respiratory Tract Infection (URTI)

Subjects	Method of Determining URTI	Major Finding	Ref.
141 South African marathon runners vs. 124 live-in controls	2-week recall of URTI incidence and duration after 56 km race	URTI incidence twice as high in runners after 56-km race vs. controls (33.3 vs 15.3%)	64
44 Danish elite orienteers vs. 44 matched nonathletes	URTI symptoms self-recorded in daily log for 1 year	Orienteers vs. controls had 2.5 vs. 1.7 URTIs during year	34
294 California runners	2-Month recall of URTI incidence training for race; 1-week recall after March 5,10, 21 km races	Training 42 vs. 12 km/week associated with lower URTI; no effect of race participation on URTI	50
108 South African marathon runners vs. 108 live-in controls	2-Week recall of URTI incidence and duration after 56-km race	URTI incidence 28.7% in runners vs. 12.9% in controls after 56-km race	63
2311 Los Angeles marathon runners	2-Month recall of URTI incidence during training for marathon; 1-week recall after March race	Runners training ≥97 vs. <32 km/week at higher URTI risk; odds ratio 5.9 for partcipants vs. nonparticipants 1 week after 42.2-km race	51
530 Runners, South Carolina	1-Year daily log using self-reported, precoded, symptoms	Increase in running distance positively related to increased URTI risk	23
84 South African marathon runners vs. 73 nonrunner controls	2-Week recall of URTI incidence and duration after 90-km race	URTI incidence 68% in runners vs. 45% in controls after 56-km race; 33% in runners using vitamin C vs. 53% of controls	65
170 North Carolina marathon runners	1-Week recall of URTI incidence after July marathon race	URTI reported by only 3% of marathoners during week after summer race	Nieman (unpubl. data)

significantly more URTI episodes during the year in comparison to the control group (2.5 vs. 1.7 episodes, respectively). Heath et al.[23] followed a cohort of 530 runners who self-reported URTI symptoms daily for 1 year, and found that total running distance for a year was a significant risk factor for URTI among recreational runners, with risk increasing as the running distance rises.

URTI risk following a race event may depend on the distance, with an increased incidence conspicuous only following marathon or ultramarathon events. For example, Nieman et al.[50] were unable to establish any increase in prevalence of URTI in 273 runners during the week following 5-, 10-, and 21.1-km events as compared to the week before. URTI incidence was also measured during the two-winter-month period prior to the three races; and in this group of recreational runners, 25% of those running 25 or more kilometers per week (average of 42 km/week) reported at least one URTI episode, as opposed to 34% training less than 25 km/week (average of 12 km/week) ($p = 0.09$). These findings suggest that, in recreational running, an average weekly distance of 42 vs. 12 km is associated with either no change in or even a slight reduction of URTI incidence. Further, they suggest that racing 5 to 21.1 km is not related to an increased risk of sickness during the ensuing week.

The time of year may also play a role. As shown in Table 2, studies (D. C. Nieman, unpublished observations) were made on 170 marathon runners who ran the July 1993 Grandfather Mountain Marathon in North Carolina. Only 3% of runners reported URTI symptoms during the week after the race, which is less than one fourth the incidence reported in marathoners following the March 1987 Los Angeles Marathon.[51] In other words, incidence of URTI may be higher following marathons run during the cold/flu season than during the summer.

Together, these epidemiological studies imply that heavy acute or chronic exercise is associated with an increased risk of URTI.[42,54] The risk appears to be especially high during the 1- or 2-week period following marathon-type race events. Among runners varying widely in training habits, the risk for URTI is slightly elevated for the highest distance runners, but only when several confounding factors are controlled.

V. MANAGEMENT OF THE ATHLETE DURING AN INFECTIOUS EPISODE

Endurance athletes are often uncertain of whether they should exercise or rest during an infectious episode. There are few data available in humans to provide definitive answers. Most clinical authorities in this area recommend that if the athlete has symptoms of a common cold with no constitutional involvement, then regular training may be safely resumed a few days after the resolution of symptoms.[6,67-69] Mild exercise during sickness with a common cold does not appear to be contraindicated, but there is insufficient evidence at present to say one way or the other. However, if there are symptoms or signs of systemic involvement (fever, extreme tiredness, muscle aches, swollen lymph glands, etc.), then 2 to 4 weeks should probably be allowed before resumption of intensive training.

For example, Burch[6] has urged that there is no method available to predict in advance which individual with an URTI will develop viral myocarditis, cardiomyopathy, pericarditis, or valvulitis; and that the best course of action is to avoid strenuous physical stress for at least 2 weeks postinfection. Sharp[69] cautions that attempting to "sweat it out" can be dangerous if the individual is febrile because it can lead to permanent damage of the myocardium.

These recommendations are speculative, however, and are primarily based on animal studies and some case reports among humans who died following bouts of vigorous exercise during an acute viral illness.[42] Depending on the pathogen (with some more affected by exercise than others), animal studies generally support the finding that one or two periods of exhaustive exercise following inoculation of the animal leads to a more frequent appearance of infection and a higher fatality rate.[8] For example, there are many reports that the virulence of the Coxsackie virus B3 is markedly augmented by intense exercise in mice, including increased replication of the virus in heart muscle cells leading to necrosis and death.[42]

If an athlete experiences sudden and unexplained deterioration in performance during training or competition, viral infection should be suspected.[69] In some athletes, a viral infection may lead to a severely debilitating state known as postviral fatigue syndrome (PVFS).[39] The symptoms can persist for several months, and include lethargy, easy fatiguability, and myalgia. Maffulli et al.[39] followed eight varsity endurance runners who developed PVFS. The aerobic and anaerobic capacities of the runners were seriously affected by PVFS for over a year.

It is well established that various measures of physical performance capability are reduced during an infectious episode.[11,14,25,67] Several case histories have been published demonstrating that sudden and unexplained deterioration in athletic performance can in some individuals be traced to either recent URTI or subclinical viral infections that run a protracted course.[67-69]

For elite athletes who may be undergoing heavy exercise stress in preparation for competition, several precautions may help them reduce their risk of URTI. Considerable evidence indicates that two other environmental factors, improper nutrition[7] and psychological stress,[9,29] can compound the negative influence that heavy exertion has on the immune system. Based on current understanding, the athlete is urged to eat a well-balanced diet, keep other life stresses to a minimum, avoid overtraining and chronic fatigue, obtain adequate sleep, and space vigorous workouts and race events as far apart as possible.[42,43] Immune system function appears to be suppressed during periods of low caloric intake and weight reduction;[30] therefore when necessary, the athlete is advised to lose weight slowly during noncompetitive training phases. Cold viruses are spread by both personal contact and breathing the air near sick people.[1,26,27] Therefore, if at all possible, athletes should avoid being around sick people before and after important events. If the athlete is competing during the winter months, a flu shot is recommended.

VI. SUMMARY

The epidemiological data suggest that endurance athletes are at increased risk for URTI during periods of heavy training and the 1 to 2 week period following marathon-type race events. At present, there is no clear indication that either acute or chronic alterations in immune function explain the increased risk. For example, while several researchers have reported a diminished neutrophil function in athletes during periods of intense and heavy training, others have shown an enhanced NKCA.

Following acute bouts of prolonged heavy endurance exercise, several components of the immune system demonstrate suppressed function for several hours. This has led to the concept of the "open window" theory described as the 1-9 hour time period following prolonged endurance exercise when host defense is decreased and risk of URTI is elevated. However, researchers disagree on the mechanisms underlying the suppression of immune function (i.e., numerical redistribution vs. direct per cell suppression by various factors). Further research is needed to provide a better understanding of these mechanisms before clinical applications can be formulated. Nonetheless, there is sufficient evidence to caution athletes to practice various hygienic measures to lower their risk of URTI and to avoid heavy exertion during systemic illness.

REFERENCES

1. Ansari, S. A., Springthorpe, V. S., Sattar, S. A., Rivard S., and Rahman, M., Potential role of hands in the spread of respiratory viral infections: studies with human parainfluenza virus 3 and rhinovirus 14, *J. Clin. Microbiol.*, 29, 2115, 1991.
2. Baj, Z., Kantorski, J., Majewska, E., Zeman, K., Pokoca, L., Fornalczyk, E., Tchórzewski, H., Sulowka, Z., and Lewicki, R., Immunological status of competitive cyclists before and after the training season, *Int. J. Sports Med.*, 15, 319, 1994.
3. Berk, L. S., Nieman, D. C., Youngberg, W. S., Arabatzis, K., Simpson-Westerberg, M., Lee, J. W., Tan, S. A., and Eby, W. C., The effect of long endurance running on natural killer cells in marathoners, *Med. Sci. Sports Exerc.*, 22, 207, 1990.
4. Brahmi, Z., Thomas, J. E., Park, M., Park, M., and Dowdeswell, I. A. G., The effect of acute exercise on natural killer-cell activity of trained and sedentary human subjects, *J. Clin. Immunol.*, 5, 321, 1985.
5. Brenner, I. K. M., Shek, P. N., and Shephard, R. J., Infection in athletes, *Sports Med.*, 17, 86, 1994.
6. Burch, G. E., Viral diseases of the heart, *Acta Cardiol.*, 34(1), 5, 1979.
7. Chandra, R. K., 1990 McCollum award lecture. Nutrition and immunity: lessons from the past and new insights into the future, *Am. J. Clin. Nutr.*, 53, 1087, 1991.

8. Chao, C. C., Strgar, F., Tsang, M., and Peterson, P. K., Effects of swimming exercise on the pathogenesis of acute murine *Toxoplasma gondii* Me49 infection, *Clin. Immunol. Immunopathol.*, 62, 220, 1992.

9. Cohen, S., Tyrrell, D. A., and Smith, A. P., Psychological stress and susceptibility to the common cold, *N. Engl. J. Med.*, 325, 606, 1991.

10. Cupps, T. R. and Fauci, A. S., Corticosteroid-mediated immunoregulation in man, *Immunol. Rev.*, 65, 133, 1982.

11. Daniels, W. L., Sharp, D. S., Wright, J. E., Vogel, J. A., Friman, G., Beisel, W. R., and Knapik, J. J., Effects of virus infection on physical performance in man, *Mil. Med.*, 150, 8, 1985.

12. Eskola, J., Ruuskanen, O., Soppi, E., Viljanen, M. K., Järvinen, M., Toivonen, H., and Kouvalainen, K., Effect of sport stress on lymphocyte transformation and antibody formation, *Clin. Exp. Immunol.*, 32, 339, 1978.

13. Field, C. J., Gougeon, R., and Marliss, E. B., Circulating mononuclear cell numbers and function during intense exercise and recovery, *J. Appl. Physiol.*, 71, 1089, 1991.

14. Friman, G., Ilbäck, N. G., Crawford, D. J., and Neufeld, H. A., Metabolic responses to swimming exercise in *Streptococcus pneumoniae* infected rats, *Med. Sci. Sports Exerc.*, 23, 415, 1991.

15. Gabriel, H., Müller, H. J., Urhausen, A., and Kinderman, W., Suppressed PMA-induced oxidative burst and unimpaired phagocytosis of circulating granulocytes one week after a long endurance exercise, *Int. J. Sports Med.*, 15, 441, 1994.

16. Gatti, G., Cavallo, R., Sartori, M. L., del Ponte, D., Masera, R., Salvadori, A., Carignola, R., and Angeli, A., Inhibition by cortisol of human natural killer (NK) cell activity, *J. Steroid Biochem.*, 26, 49, 1987.

17. Gmünder, F. K., Lorenzi, G., Bechler, B., Joller, P., Müller, J., Ziegler, W. H., and Cogoli, A., Effect of long-term physical exercise on lymphocyte reactivity: similarity to spaceflight reactions, *Aviat. Space Environ. Med.*, 59, 146, 1988.

18. Green, R. L., Kaplan, S. S., Rabin, B. S., Stanitski, C. L., and Zdziarski, U., Immune function in marathon runners, *Ann. Allergy*, 47, 73, 1981.

19. Hack, V., Strobel, G., Rau, J. P., and Weicker, H., The effect of maximal exercise on the activity of neutrophil granulocytes in highly trained athletes in a moderate training period, *Eur. J. Appl. Physiol.*, 65, 520, 1992.

20. Hack, V., Strobel, G., Weiss, M., and Weicker, H., PMN cell counts and phagocytic activity of highly trained athletes depend on training period, *J. Appl. Physiol.*, 77, 1731, 1994.

21. Hanley, D. F., Medical care of the US Olympic team, *JAMA*, 12(236), 147, 1976.

22. Haq, A., Al-Hussein, K., Lee, J., Al-Sedairy, S., Changes in peripheral blood lymphocyte subsets associated with marathon running, *Med. Sci. Sports Exerc.*, 25, 186, 1993.

23. Heath, G. W., Ford, E. S., Craven, T. E., Macera, C. A., Jackson, K. L., and Pate, R. R., Exercise and the incidence of upper respiratory tract infections, *Med. Sci. Sports Exerc.*, 23, 152, 1991.

24. Holbrook, N. J., Cox, W. I., and Horner, H. C., Direct suppression of natural killer activity in human peripheral blood leukocyte cultures by glucocorticoids and its modulation by interferon, *Cancer Res.*, 43, 4019, 1983.

25. Ilbäck, N. G., Friman, G., Crawford, D. J., and Neufeld, H. A., Effects of training on metabolic responses and performance capacity in *Streptococcus pneumoniae* infected rats, *Med. Sci. Sports Exerc.*, 23, 422, 1991.

26. Jackson, G. G., Dowling, H. G., Anderson, T. O., Riff, L., Saporta, J., and Turck, M., Susceptibility and immunity to common upper respiratory viral infections-the common cold, *Ann. Intern. Med.*, 53, 719, 1960.

27. Jennings, L. C. and Dick, E. C., Transmission and control of rhinovirus colds, *Eur. J. Epidemiol.*, 3, 327, 1987.

28. Jokl, E., The immunological status of athletes, *J. Sports Med.*, 14, 165, 1974.
29. Khansari, D. N., Murgo, A. J., and Faith, R. E., Effects of stress on the immune system, *Immunol. Today*, 11(5), 170, 1990.
30. Kono I., Kitao, H., Matsuda, M., Haga, S., Fukushima, H., and Kashiwagi, H., Weight reduction in athletes may adversely affect the phagocytic function of monocytes, *Physician Sports Med.*, 16(7), 56, 1988.
31. Kvernmo, H., Olsen, J. O., and Osterud, B., Changes in blood cell response following strenuous physical exercise, *Eur. J. Appl. Physiol.*, 64, 318, 1992.
32. Lewicki, R., Tchórzewski, H., Denys, A., Kowalska, M., and Golinska, A., Effect of physical exercise on some parameters of immunity in conditioned sportsmen, *Int. J. Sports Med.*, 8, 309, 1987.
33. Lewis, C. E. and McGee, J. O. D., *The Natural Killer Cell*, Oxford University Press, New York, 1992, 175.
34. Linde, F., Running and upper respiratory tract infections, *Scand. J. Sport Sci.*, 9, 21, 1987.
35. MacKinnon, L. T., Chick, T. W., van As, A., and Tomasi, T. B., Effects of prolonged intense exercise on natural killer cell number and function, *Exerc. Physiol.: Cur. Selected Res.*, 3, 77, 1988.
36. MacKinnon, L. T., Chick, T. W., van As, A., and Tomasi, T. B., The effect of exercise on secretory and natural immunity, *Adv. Exp. Med. Biol.*, 216A, 869, 1987.
37. MacKinnon, L. T. and Hooper, S., Mucosal (secretory) immune system responses to exercise of varying intensity and during overtraining, *Int. J. Sports Med.*, 15, S179, 1994.
38. MacKinnon, L. T. and Jenkins, D. G., Decreased salivary immunoglobulins after intense interval exercise before and after training, *Med. Sci. Sports Exerc.*, 25, 678, 1993.
39. Maffulli, N., Testa, V., and Capasso, G., Post-viral fatigue syndrome. A longitudinal assessment in varsity athletes, *J. Sports Med. Phys. Fitness*, 33, 392, 1993.
40. Munck, A., Guyre, P. M., and Holbrook, N. J., Physiological functions of glucocorticoids in stress and their relation to pharmacological actions, *Endocr. Rev.*, 5, 25, 1984.
41. Müns, G., Effect of long-distance running on polymorphonuclear neutrophil phagocytic function of the upper airways, *Int. J. Sports Med.*, 15, 96, 1993.
42. Nieman, D. C., Exercise, infection, and immunity, *Int. J. Sports Med.*, 15, S131, 1994.
43. Nieman, D. C., Physical activity, fitness and infection, in *Exercise, Fitness, and Health: A Consensus of Current Knowledge,* Bouchard, C., Ed., Human Kinetics Books, Champaign, IL, 1993.
44. Nieman, D. C., Ahle, J. C., Henson, D. A., Warren, B. J., Suttles, J., Davis, J. M., Buckley, K. S., Simandle, S., Butterworth, D. E., Fagoaga, O. R., and Nehlsen-Cannarella, S. L., Indomethacin does not alter the natural killer cell response to 2.5 hours of running, *J. Appl. Physiol.* 79, 748, 1995.
45. Nieman, D. C., Berk, L. S., Simpson-Westerberg, M., Arabatzis, K., Youngberg, W., Tan, S. A., and Eby, W. C., Effects of long endurance running on immune system parameters and lymphocyte function in experienced marathoners, *Int. J. Sports Med.*, 10, 317, 1989.
46. Nieman, D. C., Brendle, D., Henson, D. A., Suttles, J., Cook, V. D., Warren, B. J., Butterworth, D. E., Fagoaga, O. R., and Nehlsen-Cannarella, S. L., Immune function in athletes versus nonathletes, *Int. J. Sports Med.*, 16, 329, 1995.
47. Nieman, D. C., Buckley, K. S., Henson, D. A., Warren, B. J., Suttles, J., Ahle, J. C., Simandle, S., Fagoaga, O. R., and Nehlsen-Cannarella, S. L., Immune function in marathon runners versus sedentary controls, *Med. Sci. Sports Exerc.*, 27, 986, 1995.
48. Nieman, D. C., Cook, V. D., Henson, D. A., Suttles, J., Rejeski, W. J., Ribisl, P. M., Fagoaga, O. R., and Nehlsen-Cannarella, S. L., Moderate exercise training and natural killer cell cytotoxic activity in breast cancer patients, *Int. J. Sports Med.*, 16, 334, 1995.
49. Nieman, D. C., Henson, D. A., Gusewitch, G., Johnson, R. L., Davis, J. M., Butterworth, D. E., and Nehlsen-Cannarella, S. L., Physical activity and immune function in elderly women, *Med. Sci. Sports Exerc.*, 25, 823, 1993.

50. Nieman, D. C., Johanssen, L. M., and Lee, J. W., Infectious episodes in runners before and after a roadrace, *J. Sports Med. Phys. Fitness*, 29, 289, 1989.
51. Nieman, D. C., Johanssen, L. M., Lee, J. W., and Arabatzis, K., Infectious episodes in runners before and after the Los Angeles Marathon. *J. Sports Med. Phys. Fitness*, 30, 316, 1990.
52. Nieman, D. C., Miller, A. R., Henson, D. A., Warren, B. J., Gusewitch, G., Johnson, R. L., Davis, J. M., Butterworth, D. E., Herring, J. L., and Nehlsen-Cannarella, S. L., Effects of high-versus moderate-intensity exercise on circulating lymphocyte subpopulations and proliferative response, *Int. J. Sports Med.*, 15, 199, 1994.
53. Nieman, D. C., Miller, A. R., Henson, D. A., Warren, B. J., Gusewitch, G., Johnson, R. L., Davis, J. M., Butterworth, D. E., and Nehlsen-Cannarella, S. L., The effects of high- versus moderate-intensity exercise on natural killer cell cytotoxic activity, *Med. Sci. Sports Exerc.*, 25, 1126, 1993.
54. Nieman, D. C. and Nehlsen-Cannarella, S. L., Effects of endurance exercise on immune response, in *Endurance in Sport*, Shephard, R. J. and Astrand, P. O., Eds., Blackwell Scientific, Oxford, England, 1992, 487.
55. Nieman, D. C. and Nehlsen-Cannarella, S. L., The effects of acute and chronic exercise on immunoglobulins, *Sports Med.*, 11, 183, 1991.
56. Nieman, D. C., Simandle, S., Henson, D. A., Warren, B. J., Suttles, J., Davis J. M., Buckley, K. S., Ahle, J. C., Butterworth, D. E., Fagoaga, O. R., and Nehlsen-Cannarella, S. L., Lymphocyte proliferation response to 2.5 hours of running, *Int. J. Sports Med.*, 16, 404, 1995.
57. Nieman, D. C., Tan, S. A., Lee, J. W., and Berk, L. S., Complement and immunoglobulin levels in athletes and sedentary controls, *Int. J. Sports Med.*, 10, 124, 1989.
58. Oshida, Y., Yamanouchi, K., Hayamizu, S., and Sato, Y., Effect of acute physical exercise on lymphocyte subpopulations in trained and untrained subjects, *Int. J. Sports Med.*, 9, 137, 1988.
59. Papa, S., Vitale, M., Mazzotti, G., Neri, L. M., Monti, G., and Manzoli, F. A., Impaired lymphocyte stimulation induced by long-term training, *Immunol. Lett.*, 22, 29, 1989.
60. Pedersen, B. K., Tvede, N., Christensen, L. D., Klarlund, K., Kragbak, S., and Halkjaer-Kristensen, J., Natural killer cell activity in peripheral blood of highly trained and untrained persons, *Int. J. Sports Med.*, 10, 129, 1989.
61. Pedersen, B. K., Tvede, N., Klarlund, K., Christensen, L. D., Hansen, F. R., Galbo, H., Kharazmi, A., and Halkjaer-Kristensen, J., Indomethacin in vitro and in vivo abolishes post-exercise suppression of natural killer cell activity in peripheral blood, *Int. J. Sports Med.*, 11, 127, 1990.
62. Pedersen, B. K. and Ullum, H., NK cell response to physical activity: possible mechanisms of action, *Med. Sci. Sports Exerc.*, 26, 140, 1994.
63. Peters, E. M., Altitude fails to increase susceptibility of ultramarathon runners to post-race upper respiratory tract infections, *S. Afr. J. Sports Med.*, 5, 4, 1990.
64. Peters, E. M. and Bateman, E. D., Respiratory tract infections: an epidemiological survey, *S. Afr. Med. J.*, 64, 582, 1983.
65. Peters, E. M., Goetzsche, J. M., Grobbelaar, B., and Noakes, T. D., Vitamin C supplementation reduces the incidence of postrace symptoms of upper-respiratory-tract infection in ultramarathon runners, *Am. J. Clin. Nutr.*, 57, 170, 1993.
66. Pyne, D. B., Regulation of neutrophil function during exercise, *Sports Med.*, 17, 245, 1994.
67. Roberts, J. A., Loss of form in young athletes due to viral infection, *Br. J. Med.*, 290, 357, 1985.
68. Roberts, J. A., Viral illnesses and sports performance, *Sports Med.*, 3, 296, 1986.
69. Sharp, J. C. M., Viruses and the athlete, *Br. J. Sports Med.*, 23, 47, 1989.
70. Shephard, R. J. and Shek, P. N., Infectious diseases in athletes: new interest for an old problem, *J. Sports Med. Phys. Fitness*, 34, 11, 1994.

71. Shinkai, S., Kurokawa, Y., Hino, S., Hirose, M., Torii, J., Watanabe, S., Watanabe, S., Shiraishi, S., Oka, K., and Watanabe, T., Triathlon competition induced a transient immunosuppressive change in the peripheral blood of athletes, *J. Sports Med. Phys. Fitness*, 33, 70, 1993.

72. Shinkai, S., Shore, S., Shek, P. N., and Shephard, R. J., Acute exercise and immune function: relationship between lymphocyte activity and changes in subset counts, *Int. J. Sports Med.*, 13, 452, 1992.

73. Smith, J. A., Telford, R. D., Mason, I. B., and Weidemann, M. J., Exercise, training and neutrophil microbicidal activity, *Int. J. Sports Med.*, 11, 179, 1990.

74. Tomasi, T. B., Trudeau, F. B., Czerwinski, D., and Erredge, S., Immune parameters in athletes before and after strenuous exercise, *J. Clin. Immunol.*, 2, 173, 1982.

75. Tonnesen, E., Christensen, N. J., and Brinklov, M. M., Natural killer cell activity during cortisol and adrenaline infusion in healthy volunteers, *Eur. J. Clin. Invest.*, 17, 497, 1987.

76. Tvede, N., Kappel, M., Halkjaer-Kristensen, J., Galbo, H., and Pedersen, B. K., The effect of light, moderate, and severe bicycle exercise on lymphocyte subsets, natural and lymphokine activated killer cells, lymphocyte proliferative response and interleukin 2 production, *Int. J. Sports Med.*, 14, 275, 1993.

77. Tvede, N., Kappel, M., Klarlund, K., Duhn, S., Halkjaer-Kristensen, J., Kjaer, M., Galbo, H., and Pedersen, B. K., Evidence that the effect of bicycle exercise on blood mononuclear cell proliferative responses and subsets is mediated by epinephrine, *Int. J. Sports Med.*, 15, 100, 1994.

78. Tvede, N., Steensberg, J., Baslund, B., Kristensen, J. H., and Pedersen, B. K., Cellular immunity in highly-trained elite racing cyclists and controls during periods of training with high and low intensity, *Scand. J. Sports Med.*, 1, 163, 1991.

Chapter 9

EXERCISE AND AUTOIMMUNE DISEASES

Arnaud Ferry

CONTENTS

I. INTRODUCTION

The capacity of the immune system (IS) to keep the *milieu intérieur* compatible with living processes is first linked to its own ability to discriminate self and nonself. However, in some cases self-recognition or self-tolerance induction does not operate leading to autoimmune diseases (AID). Disturbance of the primary function of the IS is not uncommon; approximately 1 to 2% of the human population is affected by AID characterized by a destruction of various tissues/organs by cells of the body's own IS.[27]

Removal of the antigen introduced in the body acts to down-regulate the immune response. The IS also includes paracrine or autocrine fine regulation by the production from specialized immunocytes of various immunotransmitters (e.g., cytokines, putative immunologically derived classical hormones and neurotransmitters, thymic hormones). Moreover, as with other physiological systems the immune response is highly integrated. Numerous experiments have demonstrated the existence of hormone and neurotransmitter receptors on immunocytes, the innervation of lymphoid organs, and the effects of hormones and neurotransmitter administration or blockade; these results suggest a complex regulation of the IS by neuroendocrine and nervous systems.[13,26,43] Finally, the immunotransmitters coordinate and regulate not only immune but also nervous and neuroendocrine functions. Blalock[13] and Besedowsky and del Rey[11] proposed that the IS may sense stimuli (such as antigens, bacteria, or tumor cells) and transmit message via immunotransmitters to the central and peripheral nervous system. This interaction allows adapted neuroendocrine and autonomic nervous responses that regulate a set of coordinated physiological functions (e.g., thermoregulation, carbohydrate metabolism) at the level of the whole body during antigen challenge.[11] With regard to the introduction of foreign macromolecules, the modification of self-antigens, and the appearance of neoantigens, the immune response belongs perfectly to the category of homeostatic mechanisms that reestablish the *milieu intérieur* with the help of the other homeostatic mechanisms. However, disturbances in immune-neuroendocrine-central nervous (CN) system interactions could lead to nonhomeostatic or even antihomeostatic responses, including AID.[11] It is also possible that stressors, such as exercise, may affect these interactions.

II. BIOLOGICAL FACTORS OF AUTOIMMUNITY

A. IMMUNE STIMULUS AS A STRESSOR

It has been suggested that antigen challenge is a stressor and that the immune response is a stress response. This idea has been articulated because neuroendocrine and autonomic responses occur during the activation of IS by antigen, inoculation of virus and bacterial endotoxins, and transplantation of tumor.[11] These responses are only detected in susceptible animals, i.e., those who are able to mount an immune response directed against the antigen.

Adjuvant arthritis (AA) and streptococcal cell wall arthritis (SCWA), two animal models of rheumatoid arthritis (RA), provoke a chronic activation of the hypothalamic-pituitary-adrenal axis (H-P-A). Neidhart et al.[75] demonstrated activation of the central nervous system and the release of pituitary hormones during the development of AA. Morning levels of blood glucocorticoids (GC) were elevated just before the appearance of the clinical signs of AA in rats.[83,95] Moreover, corticotropin-releasing hormone (CRH) was markedly increased in the inflammed joints with AA or SCWA.[102] In the case of experimental autoimmune encephalomyelitis (EAE), a model of multiple sclerosis (MS), animals also exhibited increasing serum GC immediately before and during the disease,[47,97] similar to patients with MS.[72] Local production of adrenocorticotrophic hormone (ACTH) by activated lymphocytes is unlikely sufficient to be considered as the significant signal leading to H-P-A axis activation. IL-1 has the capacity to induce rapid CRH responses (far more potent than IL-6 and TNFα) and is thought to act via a central mode of action on CRH hypothalamic neurons.[6,100,101] IL-1 also exerts direct effects on pituitary cells in regulating the release of POMC-derived peptides or adrenal medulla cells.[6,13,43,101]

In addition changes in the blood levels of thyroid hormones, insulin, testosterone, and prolactin are known to occur after antigen challenge or tumor cell inoculation.[11] Decreased serum testosterone levels in AA rats were not due to an inhibition of the release of LH since LH concentration in serum was elevated during the course of the disease.[16] In contrast, rats with EAE experience a threefold rise in blood prolactin levels on days 4 to 10 before the appearance of the clinical signs.[79] Of interest here is the finding that lymphocytes may be able to produce prolactin or growth hormone-like molecule.[13]

Autonomic nervous system changes also occur during the immune response. In animals with acute symptoms of EAE, splenic noradrenaline levels rise above control values.[68] Elevated concentrations of local catecholamines in tissues are also detected in rats in which EAE is induced by transfer of encephalitogenic lymphocytes.[59] However, soon after antigen challenge sympathic activity in the spleen decreases.[11] Similar results are observed in rats with EAE, 3 to 7 d postimmunization.[68]

These peripheral nervous and neuroendocrine responses are likely mediated by immune system-central nervous system (CNS) communication since the firing of individual hypothalamic neurons are detected soon after injection of antigen. Moreover, changes in electrical activity in the CNS are associated with a modified turnover rate of catecholamines (i.e., norepinephrine) in the hypothalamus.[6,11]

B. PHYSIOLOGICAL INTERPRETATION OF NEUROENDOCRINE CHANGES INDUCED BY ANTIGEN CHALLENGE

1. Negative Feedback

Given the well-known immunosuppressive potential of GC,[43,74] and the finding that elevated GC levels are detected only after the development of the immune response, activation of the H-P-A axis is thought to exert a negative feedback to prevent excessive activation of the IS.[74] The same hypothesis may be applied to the activation of the autonomic nervous system several days after antigen challenge.[8,68] It has been hypothesized that activation of the H-P-A axis contributes to maintenance of immunological specificity.[11] As the immune response proceeds, the higher GC release prevents the excessive expansion of lymphocytes with low affinity for antigen (e.g., autoreactive cells) that are recruited under the influence of cytokines. These lymphocytes are vulnerable to GC suppression.

Evidence for this hypothesis comes from numerous experimental results concerning the control of EAE by GC. First, administration of GC before the onset of disease inhibited the appearance of clinical signs; this effect was blocked by RU 38486, a GC receptor antagonist.[15] Second, adrenalectomy or RU 38486 administration after the first episode of chronic relapsing EAE increased the frequency of relapses.[63,64,70]

The negative feedback exerted by GC characterizes other AID. Adrenalectomy before and during the onset of AA has a detrimental effect both in terms of the severity and the survival of rodents.[38] Animals that normally do not develop SCWA become susceptible when pretreated with RU 38486.[89] Futhermore, GC administration reduces insulin-dependent diabetes mellitus (IDDM) and autoimmune thyroidis.[43] The development of an autoimmune thyroid dysfunction has been observed after adrenalectomy in humans.[93]

2. Permissive Influence

Neuroendocrine and nervous responses occurring immediately after antigen challenge may be permissive or facilitate immune responses. Prolactin and growth hormone (GH) responses to antigen challenge appear to be a one of the signals necessary to the progression of the cell cycle.[10] Several results support this theory: (1) GH or prolactin deficiency lead to lymphocyte unresponsiveness;[10,43] (2) hypophysectomized or bromocriptine (dopamine agonist)-treated rats do not develop AA, and exogenous prolactin or GH blocks the effect of hypophysectomy;[9] (3) bromocriptine therapy is also effective in EAE and SLE;[43] and (4) hyperprolactemia has been detected in association with several AID in man.[11,50] Moreover, the decreased noradrenaline content of the spleen before the onset of EAE has been interpreted as a reduction of neural release.[68] Because catecholamines inhibit EAE,[21] the early reduced autonomic tone in lymphoid organs may allow the immune processes to develop to antigens.

C. HYPOTHESES CONCERNING THE ORIGIN OF AUTOIMMUNE DISEASES

Random rearrangement of the T cell receptor (TCR) gene segments at the α and β loci, contribution of N region diversity, and combinatorial association of the two chains could lead to a large T cell repertoire (estimated at 10^9

different specificities).[12] Thus predetermined TCR is able to react with a wide array of antigens both foreign and self. Normally, different mechanisms eliminate, paralyze, or suppress autoreactive T cells. Indeed, the origin of autoimmune disease is still controversial and two nonexclusive hypotheses have been put forward.

The first hypothesis is that of the failure of self-tolerance induction (clonal deletion and anergy, immunosuppression). During the expression of alpha/beta TCR genes in the thymus and after cell proliferation, the majority the T cells undergo clonal deletion. Immature T cells with TCR that bind to self-MHC molecules are rescued from cell death (positive selection).[88,98] Thymocytes with TCR that react with both antigen and MHC molecules are eliminated as potentially injurious (negative selection).[88,98] Immature T cells that escape from both selections (<5%) include two types: those that present TCR that link self-MHC molecules but not antigen presented in the thymus, and those that link MHC class I or MHC class II molecules mature into CD4-CD8+ or CD4+CD8- lymphocytes.[24] The major site of the clonal deletion is the thymus. There is some evidence that clonal deletion may be also occur extrathymically. For example, the nature of the antigen presenting cell (APC) interactions may favor deletion (strong interaction) or also anergy (weak interaction).[88] The avidity of cell-to-cell interactions may also vary with the endocrine milieu (GH, prolactin).[10]

The second mechanism of self-tolerance induction is clonal anergy. Occupancy of the TCR is sufficient for the full activation of certain genes (e.g., IL-4). In contrast, other cytokine genes (e.g., IL-2) require additional signaling events (costimulatory signals) provided by soluble ligands or by direct cell-cell interactions, for example via CD28-B7 linkage.[24,84] Without these second signals, the cell is induced into an anergic or unresponsive state, thus making the lymphocyte refractory to antigen challenge and to providing immunological help to other cells. Clonal anergy is thought to be realized peripherally. Cruse and Lewis[24] suggest that peripheral autoreactive cells may be stimulated from the anergy state by adjuvant and self-tissue administration, with adjuvant providing the second signal.

The third mechanism of self-tolerance induction is immunosuppression by cytokines produced by mutually antagonist T cell subsets (Th1 and Th2).[3,101] However, failure of self-tolerance induction is not completely successful since peripheral autoreactive cells have been demonstrated in healthy individuals.[24]

The second hypothesis is that AID result from avoidance of self-tolerance induction. Derived from the understanding of EAE, it has been suggested that autoimmunity is not due to the breakdown of self-tolerance mechanisms but rather circumvention by the display of antigenic determinants to which the host is never tolerant.[58] Antigen presentation in the context of autoimmunity differs from that in the physiological situation. Several mechanisms can lead to new peptide generation and presentation, such as the initiation or upregulation after infection.[58] Presentation of determinants not previously displayed will activate a naive T cell, assuming that self-tolerance is limited to the set of peptides presented at a thymic or extra thymic site of tolerance induction.

III. STRESS/EXERCISE MODULATION OF AUTOIMMUNE DISEASES

In this section, the evidence for a relationship between AID and exercise is reviewed using the models of experimental arthritis, EAE, autoimmune myocarditis, and IDDM. Data for other autoimmune diseases and exercise are more limited. For example, recently it has been demonstrated that endurance training (running, 10 weeks) does not affect brain autoimmunity (brain anti-body production) that appears with aging.[4] Numerous studies provide some evidence that various stressors, and probably exercise, affect the other AID, such as autoimmune thyroidis, Grave's disease, and systemic lupus erythematosus (SLE).[40, 42, 56, 99]

A. RHEUMATOID ARTHRITIS AND ANIMAL MODELS

There are three animal models of rheumatoid arthritis (RA): adjuvant arthritis (AA), collagen-induced arthritis (CIA), and streptococcal cell wall induced arthritis (SCWA). These are induced in rats by a single injection of *Mycobaterium tuberculosis* (or butyricum), collagen, and streptococcal cell wall in an adjuvant. These experimental models of arthritis lead to an inflam-matory reaction with subsequent joint destruction. Their autoimmune nature is based on the fact that the diseases can be transferred by T cells from arthritic rats and that arthritic T cell clones have been described.[96] Further, these experimental arthritic states can be modulated by hormones. It is demonstrated that ACTH injection blocks the inhibition of AA induced by hypophysectomy.[9] Clinical signs of AA and CIA are also lowered by estrogen administration.[42, 51, 73] In contrast, estrogen treatment and castration of male rats increases clinical symptamology of SCWA.[1] This sex steroid regulation in AA and CIA agree with the reports of improvement in clinical signs of RA with contraceptive use, pregnancy, and testosterone injection in male patients,[35,42,55] but not with the higher female:male ratio incidence of RA. It is unlikely that this immunomodulatory effect of sex steroids is direct since evidence of sex steroid receptors is not generally found in lymphocytes (macrophages have these receptors).[34,43] How-ever, it is well known that sex steroids influence the IS since a hypothalamic-pituitary-gonadal-thymic axis can be demonstrated.[25,36] Moreover, prolactin, GH, or melatonin increase the clinical signs of AA or are needed for the development of AA.[9,43]

The association of RA with particular psychological characteristics has been raised.[85,86] Solomon[87] found that patients with RA tend to have a special interest in physical activities before the onset of the disease. Several epidemiological studies have shown that prior to the onset of the first clinical episode RA patients experienced stressful life events.[53,99] In contrast, well-controlled studies have failed to demonstrate this relationship.[41,53,65]

In the earliest animal studies (1970–1982), it is difficult to decide whether experimental stress before the appearance of the clinical signs of experimental arthritis inhibits or enhances the disease. These early studies have been critically reviewed elsewhere.[53] The maximal severity of AA in stressed rats is higher than in control rats.[2] In contrast, stress abrogates the development of CIA since only 3 to 10% of stressed rats develops arthritis compared to 40% of the control rats.[80] Other studies by this group showed the opposite effect: an increased incidence and severity of the disease with stress.[81] These discrepancies may be due to experimental differences (strain, kind of experimental arthritis, nature of the stressor): the same stressor (electric shocks) increased clinical signs of AA in Wistar rats but decreased AA in Long Evans rats.[52] Half of the experiments published by this group[52] did not affect significantly the severity of the disease.[52] Moreover, conditioned aversive stimuli (electric shocks) suppress the development of AA; this indirect effect of stress is blocked by beta-adrenergic antagonist administration.[67]

The effect of muscular exercise as stressor on the development of experimental arthritis is not well known. We have shown that ten bouts of exercise on a treadmill performed between immunization and the onset of the disease increased the incidence of AA in female rats (74% of exercised rats developed AA vs. 45% of unexercised rats), but decreased the incidence of AA in of male rats (27 vs. 59%).[29] The decreased incidence of AA in exercised male rats seems to be blocked by administration of a beta-adrenergic antagonist (Le Page and Ferry, unpublished results). Exercised or sedentary AA rats do not exhibit differences in the development of clinical signs (that are evaluated by the number of inflamed joints and paw thickness), day of onset and of peak severity of the disease, and maximal severity.[29]

It is widely believed that stressful events can aggravate preexisting RA. Some but not all studies support this belief.[99] In the case of muscular exercise, physical training in RA does not exacerbate the activity of the disease.[7,39] Butler et al.[18] found no aggravation of clinical signs in arthritic rats submitted to mild exercise (swimming). In contrast, Lyngberg et al.[66] demonstrated that 13 of 18 trained RA patients (with moderately active disease) exhibited a decrease in number of swollen joints (2 were unchanged and 3 had a small increase in number of affected joints). They suggested that physical exercise (submaximal and strength exercise) over an 8-week period could have beneficial effects on clinical measures without affecting immunological parameters (serum cytokines and in vitro NK activity or lymphoblastic response).[5]

B. MULTIPLE SCLEROSIS AND ANIMAL MODELS

Experimental encephalomyelitis autoimmune (EAE) is an autoimmune disease of the central nervous system mediated by CD4+ T lymphocytes leading to demyelinization.[78] It is induced in susceptible rats by injection of guinea spinal cord (GPSC), basic myelin protein (MBP), or an encephalitogenic peptide in adjuvant. It is also transferred by T cell clones. EAE that follows GPSC injection is the most clinically applicable model of EAE characterized by several bouts of disease and remission (CR-EAE). As with experimental AA, glucocorticoid (GC) administration inhibits the development of the disease.[15,61,62,64] Contraceptive hormone administration in female rats decreases EAE,[34] as do catecholamines (beta-agonists).[21,61] That estrogens reduce EAE[94] agrees with the higher incidence of EAE (or MS) in females compared to males. Further, it is likely that prolactin increases EAE since bromocriptine administration, a dopamine agonist controlling prolactin release, inhibits development of the disease.[79]

To our knowledge, there are no published reports of a relationship between stressful life events and the onset of MS. However, several animal studies provide evidence that stressors applied before the onset of the disease inhibit the clinical signs of experimental paralytic autoimmune disease. The first demonstration of this was by Levine et al.[61] who found that the incidence of EAE was markedly reduced by restraint stress. Restraint stress also had the capacity to suppress the development of passive EAE induced by transfer of lymph node cells of donors with EAE.[62] This effect of restraint stress was recently confirmed by several others authors.[17,33,54] Moreover, Griffin et al.[33] showed that the effect of restraint stress (for 9h/d) on EAE was not observed when rats were challenged with MBP encephalitogenic peptide. They suggested that stress may affect the processing of MBP (processing of the peptide is not required). The effects of stress on EAE can vary with the experimental condition. Sound stress has little inhibitory consequences on the development of EAE compared to electric shocks.[17] Shorter duration to a stressor (1 h/d of restraint stress) increases rather than suppresses EAE, as does longer duration exposure (9 h/d).[33] We have shown that muscular exercise applied between the immunization and onset of disease has negligible effects on EAE.[60] Exercise (10 d) slightly delays the onset of the first bout of CR-EAE induced by GPSC in rats of both sexes and reduces its duration. Moreover, the incidence of CR-EAE is lowered in female rats by exercise (that of monophasic EAE, a milder form of EAE, is increased). We have recently confirmed these results since the onset of passive EAE induced by cellular transfer of encephalitogenic clone is slightly delayed by exercise performed after the cellular transfer and before the disease (Le Page and Ferry, unpublished results).

The effect of exercise or other stressors in patients with MS is not known. Only one animal study reports that restraint stress applied after the first remission, following the incident episode of CR-EAE, prevents relapses as does GC administration.[64]

C. VIRAL-INDUCED MYOCARDITIS

Murine cardiomyopathy induced by Coxsackie virus B (CVB myocarditis) provides an effective model to study acute myocarditis and chronic complement, dilated cardiomyopathy. Both virus- and immune cell-mediated pathogenic mechanisms are implicated in the myocardium destruction.[69] At the start of the disease direct damage is virally mediated. The peak of infiltration of immune cells, particularly CD4+ and CD8+ cells, occurs by day 12; this coincides with the most severe myocardial damage. An autoimmune etiology of this disease is supported by the following facts: (1) cytotoxic T lymphocytes are able *in vitro* to lyse uninfected and virus-infected cardiocytes;[69] and (2) myosin challenge induces similar disease manifestations to those induced by CVB inoculation.[76] That an estrogenic environment is involved is supported by the findings of Huber and Pfaeffle;[46] they demonstrate that susceptibility to CVB myocarditis is increased by estradiol treatment of female mice (they do not normally develop this disease).

The detrimental effect of exercise on the course of CVB myocarditis is well known, associated with an increase mortality of animals with the disease.[19,32] In a study of Cabinian et al.,[19] overall mortality was 52% in exercised mice vs. 4% in unexercised mice. This decreased survival, induced by swim exercise and performed after virus inoculation, was not found by Ilback et al.[48] using treadmill exercise. This suggests that the effects of exercise on physiological systems vary with animal models of muscular exercise.[30] However, all of these studies demonstrate higher inflammatory and necrotic lesions and immune cell infiltration in exercised animals.[19,48] The number of CD4+ and CD8+ in myocardium is increased threefold,[48] and the inflammed area increases by 70%.[19,48] Treadmill exercise was not found to increase histological destruction of myocardium in experimental autoimmune myocarditis induced in the guinea pig by heterologous heart protein.[44] However, these authors did demonstrate that exercise augments left ventricular dilatation (i.e., an increase in *in vitro* left ventricular pressure to volume relation) and presumably the ventricular dysfunction that occurs in this autoimmune disease. It is likely that this detrimental effect of exercise is not due to exercise-induced immunosuppression since the exercise effect is blocked by cyclosporine A and antithymocyte antibody,[19] and exercised animals exhibit increased serum virus neutralizing antibody and circulating antiheart antibody compared to control animals.[19,44]

D. INSULIN-DEPENDENT DIABETES MELLITUS AND ANIMAL MODELS

Insulin-dependent diabetes mellitus (IDDM) of type I is characterized by autoimmune-mediated destruction of beta cells of the pancreatic islets that release insulin. Spontaneous onset of diabetes appears in bio-breeding (BB) rats or nonobese diabetic (NOD) mice; it may be induced by streptozocin (STZ, a pancreatic beta-cell cytotoxin) injection in mice or rats or transferred by T cells.[14] IDDM may be regulated by hormones since exogenous GC attenuates the effect of STZ diabetes[82] and adrenalectomy accelerates the onset of diabetes in NOD mice.[28]

Stress has been suspected to play a role in the onset of IDDM. A number of studies suggest that diabetic patients may be exposed to stressful life events before the onset of symptoms.[57,92] However, these findings are far from conclusive since a control group does not generally exist and there is the problem of recall bias. Animal research shows various effects of stress in terms of disease incidence, day of onset, and insulitis. Stressors applied before the onset of IDDM symptoms have been characterized experimentally. In the case of STZ-induced diabetes in mice, the stress effects are complex. Mazelis et al.[71] found that stress accelerates the onset of disease and Huang et al.[45] demonstrated a decrease in the prevalence of IDDM in stressed mice. Two studies determining the effects of stress on IDDM in BB rats have produced contradictory results. Onset of IDDM symptoms was delayed in stressed female rats,[57] accelerated in stressed rats of both sexes,[20] or unchanged in male rats.[57] The effects of stress on incidence of diabetes are more consistent with reports of increased incidence in stressed female and male rats.[20,57] Recently, Durant et al.[28] confirmed previous studies[17,33,52] showing that the effects of stress on autoimmune responses vary with the stress paradigm used (for example, nature of the stressor, duration, intensity, timing). Long-term chronic stress (26 weeks of either restraint or overcrowding), but not short-term stress (8 d, overcrowding + restraint + anesthesia), inhibits IDDM in NOD mice.[28] Long-term chronic restraint stress diminishes the incidence of IDDM by 29%, delays the onset of symptoms, and tends to reduce the insulitis; overcrowding provides similar and comparable protection with regard to prevalence and onset of disease. Only one study addressed the effect of muscular exercise in BB rats. Physical training over several weeks (5 to 11 weeks) did not affect IDDM in female rats.[77] Running on a treadmill had no influence on the incidence (11/12 trained rats vs. 11/11 control rats), onset of symptoms, and survival duration after the onset of hyperglycemia and insulitis (32 or 35 intact islets were identified in trained or untrained rats).[77] It is not known whether exercise (or other stressors) applied to diabetic animals affects the subclinical signs or ultimate course of IDDM.

IV. POTENTIAL MECHANISMS

The stress system composed of the corticotropin-releasing hormone (CRH) and the locus ceruleus-norepinephrine (LC-NE)/autonomic nervous systems regulates immune responses, as well as other physiological responses through (in part) hypothalamic-pituitary-adrenal (H-P-A) axis activation.[23] H-P-A axis products exert a negative control of inflammatory/AID since GCs mimic all processes involved in self-tolerance induction (i.e., clonal deletion and anergy, suppressor mechanism).[101] Hypoactivity of the H-P-A axis in response to antigen challenge has been recently proposed as the cause of development of AID,[23, 31, 90] together with a genetic prerequisite.[101] There is strong evidence from animal models that a defect or defects occur in several autoimmune diseases: EAE, SCWA, AA, IDDM, autoimmune thyroidis, and SLE.[37,83,95,101] Abnormal immune-H-P-A axis activity is also suggested in humans with these AID.[22,49,50,90,102]

Since experimental stress generally does not accelerate or aggravate experimental arthritis, EAE, or IDDM, it is possible that physical or psychological stressors act to increase the weak negative feedback exerted by GC in AID-susceptible animals. The stimulations of the H-P-A axis by these and immune stressors could be cumulative and partly restore H-P-A axis activation. Moreover, it is possible that a weak H-P-A axis activation would occur only in response to an immune stressor and not in response to other stressors; indeed, the mechanisms of H-P-A axis stimulation may vary with the kind of stressor (immune or nonimmune). Villas et al.[97] demonstrated that AID-susceptible animals (Lewis rat) exhibit a GC response to ether stress that is similar to the GC response of AID-resistant rats. However, this observation was not confirmed by Sternberg et al.[91] It is also possible that physical or psychological stressors alter the prolactin and growth hormone responses to an immune stressor: a decrease in these hormone reponses could lead to a weak generation of autoreactive cells and activation of lymphocytes. This potential mechanism is further supported by finding that prolactin and growth hormone modulate both self-tolerance induction[10] and lymphocyte functions.[43]

V. CONCLUSIONS

To date, there is little evidence to support or explain the effect of stress on autoimmune diseases (AID) that involved dysfunction of cellular immunity. There is a striking contrast between the anecdotal clinical observations or opinions (stressful life events accelerate AID appearance and aggravate prexisting AID) and the results from systematic experimental studies. In humans, the effect of exercise on AID has not been well studied, and the role of other stressors is unclear. In animals, exercise before the onset of disease generally does not exacerbate the clinical signs of AID (except autoimmune myocarditis). The field of AID and exercise requires further investigations. Well-controlled studies to address potentially important clinical questions, such as whether physical activity prevents physical detrerioration in patients with AID without exacerbating clinical manifestations, remain to be conducted.

ACKNOWLEDGMENTS

I wish thank Françoise Homo-Delarche for his critical reading of the manuscript and bibliographical help, and Christine Le Page for assistance.

REFERENCES

1. Allen, J. B., Blatter, D., Calandra, G. B., and Wilder, R. L., Sex hormonal effects on the severity of streptococcal cell wall-induced polyarthritis in the rat, *Arthritis Rheum.*, 26, 560, 1983.

2. Amkraut, A. A., Solomon, G. F., and Kraemer, H. C., Stress, early experience and adjuvant-induced arthritis in the rat, *Psychosom., Med.*, 33, 203, 1971.

3. Arnon, R. and Teitelbaum, D., On the existence of suppressor cells, *Int. Arch. Allergy Appl. Immunol.*, 100, 2, 1993.

4. Barnes, C. A., Forster, M. J., Fleshner, M., Ahanotu, E. N., Laudenslager, M. L., Mazzeo, R. S., Maier, S. F., and Lal, H., Exercise does not modify spatial memory, brain autoimmunity, or antibody response in agged F-344 rats, *Neurobiol. Aging*, 12, 47, 1991.

5. Baslund, B., Lyngberg, K., Andersen, V., Kristensen, J. H., Hansen, M., Klokker, M., and Pedersen, B. K., Effect of 8 wk of bicycle training on the immune system of patients with rheumatoid arthritis, *J. Appl. Physiol.*, 75, 1691, 1993.

6. Bateman, A., Singh, A., Kral, T., and Solomon, S., The immune-hypothalamic-adrenal axis, *Endocr. Rev.*, 10, 92, 1989.

7. Beals, C., Lampman, R. M., Banwell, B. F., Braustein, E. M., Albers, J. W., and Castor, W., Measurement of exercise tolerance in patients with rheumatoid arthritis and osteoarthritis, *J. Rheumatol.*, 12, 3, 1985.

8. Bellinger, D. L., Lorton, D. Felten, S. Y., and Felten, D. L., Innervation of lymphoid organs and implications in development, aging, and autoimmunity, *Int. J. Immunopharmacol.*, 14, 329, 1992.

9. Berczi, I., Nagy, E., Asa, S. L., and Kovacs, K., The influence of pituary hormones on adjuvant arthritis, *Arthritis Rheum.*, 27, 682, 1984.

10. Berczi, I., Baragar, F. D., Chalmers, I. M., Keystone, E. C., Nagy, E., and Warrington, R. J., Hormones in self tolerance and autoimmunity: a role in the pathogenesis of rheumatoid arthritis, *Autoimmunity*, 16, 45, 1993.

11. Besedowsky, H. O. and del Rey, A., Immune-neuroendocrine circuits: integrative role of cytokines, *Frontiers Neuroendocrinol.*, 13, 61, 1992.

12. Blackman, M., Kappler, J., and Marrack, P., The role of the T cell receptor in positive and negative selection of developing T cells, *Science*, 248, 1335, 1990.

13. Blalock, J. E., A molecular basis for bidirectional communication between the immune and neuroendocrine systems, *Phyiol. Rev.*, 69, 1, 1989.

14. Boitard, C. and Bach, J. F., Pathogénie du diabète insulinodependant, maladie polygénique d'origine auto-immune, *Med. Sci.*, 7, 226, 1991.

15. Bolton, C. and Flower, R. L., The effects of the anti-glucorticoid RU 38486 on steroid-mediated suppression of experimental allergic encephalomyelitis (EAE) in the Lewis rat, *Life Sci.*, 45, 97, 1989.

16. Bruot, B. C. and Clemens, J. W., Effect of adjuvant-induced arthritis on serum luteinizing hormone and testosterone concentrations in the male rat, *Life Sci.*, 41, 1559, 1987.

17. Bukilika, M., Djordjevic, S., Maric, I., Dimitrijevic, M., Markovic, B. M., and Jankovic, B. D., Stress-induced suppression of experimental allergic encephalomyelitis in the rat, *Intern. J. Neurosci.*, 59, 167, 1991.

18. Butler, S. H., Godefroy, F., Besson, J. M., and Weil-Fugazza, J., Increase in "pain sensitivity" induced by exercise applied during the onset of arthritis in a model of monoarthritis in the rat, *Int. J. Tissue React.*, 13, 299, 1991.

19. Cabinian, A., Kiel, R. J., Smith, F., Ho, K. L., Khatib, R., and Ryes, M. P., Modification of exercise-aggravated coxsackievirus B3 myocarditis by T lymphocyte suppression in an inbred model., *J. Lab. Clin. Med.*, 115, 454, 1990.

20. Carter, W. R., Hermman, J., Sokes, K., and Cox, D. J., Promotion of diabetes onset by stress in the BB rat, *Diabetologia*, 30, 674, 1987.

21. Chelmicka-Schorr, E., Kwasniewski, M. N., Thomas, B. E., and Arnason, B. G. W., The beta-adrenergic agonist isoproterenol suppresses experimental allergic encephalomyelitis in Lewis rat, *J. Neuroimmunol.*, 25, 203, 1989.

22. Chikanza, C., Chrousos, G., and Panayi, G. S., Abnormal neuroendocrine immune communications in patients with rheumatoid arthritis, *Eur. J. Clin. Invest.*, 22, 635, 1992.

23. Chrousos, G. P. and Gold, P. W., The concept of stress and stress system disorders, *JAMA*, 267, 1244, 1992.

24. Cruse, J. M. and Lewis, R. E., The immune system victorious: selective preservation of self, *Immunol. Res.*, 12, 101, 1993.

25. Deschaux, P. and Rouabhia, M., The thymus. Key organ between endocrinologic and immunologic system, *Ann. N.Y. Acad. Sci.*, 496, 49, 1987.

26. Deschaux, P. A., Immunité et physiologie, *Arch. Int. Physiol. Biochem. Biophy.*, 101, A3, 1993.

27. Derijk, R. and Berkenbosch, F., The immune-hypothalamo-pituary-adrenal axis and autoimmunity, *Int. J. Neurosci.*, 59, 91, 1991.

28. Durant, S., Coulaud, J., Amrani, A., El Hasnaoui, A., Dardenne, M., and Homo-Delarche, F., Effects of various environmental stress paradigms and adrenalectomy on the expression of autoimmune type 1 diabetes in the non-obese diabetic (NOD) mouse, *J. Autoimmunity*, 6, 735, 1993.

29. Ferry, A., Le Page, C., and Rieu, M., Sex as a determining factor in the effect of exercise on an in vivo autoimune response, adjuvant arthritis, *J. Appl. Physiol.*, 76, 1172, 1994.

30. Ferry, A. and Rieu, M., Adaptations des systèmes physiologiques à l'activité physique. *Méd. Sci.*, 10, 863, 1994.

31. Fricchione, G. L. and Stefano, G. B., The stress response and autoimmunoregulation, *Adv. Neuroimmunol.*, 4, 13, 1994.

32. Gatmaitan, B. G., Chason, J. L., and Lerner, A. M., Augmentation of the virulence of murine coxsackievirus B3 myocarditis by exercise, *J. Exp. Med.*, 131, 1121, 1970.

33. Griffin, A. C., Lo, W. D., Wolny, A. C., Whitacre, C. C., Suppression of experimental autoimmune encephalomyelitis by restraint stress: sex differences, *J. Neuroimmunol.*, 44, 103, 1993.

34. Grossman, C. J., Regulation of the immune system by sex steroid, *Endocr. Rev.*, 5, 435, 1984.

35. Grossman, C. J., Roselle, G. A., and Mendenhall, C. L., Sex steroid regulation of autoimmunity, *J. Steroid Biochem. Mol. Biol.*, 40, 649, 1991.

36. Hadden, J. W., Thymic endocrinology, *Int. J. Immunopharmacol.*, 14, 345, 1992.

37. Harbuz, M. S., Rees, R. G., Eckland, D., Jessop, D. S., Brewerton, D., and Lightman, S. L., Paradoxical responses of hypothalamic corticotropin-releasing factor (CRF) messenger ribonucleic acid (mRNA) and CRF-41 peptide and adenohypophysial proopiomelanocortin mRNA during chronic inflammatory stress, *Endocrinology*, 130, 1394, 1992.

38. Harbuz, M. S., Rees, R. G., and Lightman, S. L., HPA axis responses to acute stress and adrenalectomy during adjuvant-induced arthritis in the rat, *Am. J. Physiol.*, 264, R179, 1993.

39. Harkom, T. M., Lampman, R. M., Banwell, B. F., and Castor, C. W., Therapeutic value of graded aerobic exercise training in rheumatoid arthritis, *Arthritis Rheum.*, 28, 32, 1985.

40. Harris, T., Creed, F., and Brugha, T. S., Stressful life events and Grave's disease, *Br. J. Psychiatry*, 161, 535, 1991.

41. Hendrie, H. C., Paraskevas, F., Baragar, F. D., and Adamson, J. D., Stress immunoglobulin levels and early polyarthritis, *J. Psychosom. Res.*, 15, 337, 1971.

42. Homo-Delarche, F., Fitzpatrick, F., Christeff, N., Nunez, E. A., Bach, J. F., and Dardenne, M., Sex steroids, glucocorticoids, stress and autoimmunity, *J. Steroid Biochem. Mol.*, 40, 619, 1991.

43. Homo-Delarche, F. and Durant, S., Hormones, neurotransmitters and neuropeptides as modulators of lymphocyte functions, in *Immunopharmacology of Lymphocytes*, Rola-Pleszczynski, M. R., Eds., Academic Press, London, 1994, 170.

44. Hosenpud, J. D., Campbell, S. M., Niles, N. R., Lee, J., Mendelson, D., and Hart, M. V., Exercise induced augmentation of cellular and humoral associated with increased cardiac dilatation in experimental autoimmune myocarditis, *Cardiovas. Res.*, 21, 217, 1987.

45. Huang, S. W., Plaut, S. M., Taylor, G., and Varenheim, L. E., Effect of stressful stimulation on the incidence of streptozotocin-induced diabetes in mice, *Psychosom. Med.*, 43, 431, 1981.

46. Huber, S. A. and Pfaeffle, B., Differential Th1 and Th2 cell responses in male and female BALBC/c mice infected with coxsackievirus group B type 3, *J. Virol.*, 68, 5126, 1994.

47. Hughes, F. W., Richards, A. B., and Solow, E. A., Similar factors occurring in the "ordinary" and the hyperacute form of experimental allergic encephalomyelitis in the rat and dog, *Life Sci.*, 5, 137, 1966.

48. Ilback, N. L., Fohlman, J., and Friman, G., Exercise in coxsackievirus B3 myocarditis: effects on heart lymphocyte populations and the inflammatory reaction, *Am. Heart J.*, 117, 1298, 1989.

49. Johnson, E. O., Neuroimmunological axis and rheumatic diseases, *Eur. J. Clin. Invest.*, 22, 2, 1992.

50. Jorgensen, C. and Sany, J., Modulation of the immune response by the neuroendocrine axis in rheumatoid arthritis, *Clin. Exp. Rheumatol.*, 12, 435, 1994.

51. Josefsson, E., Tarkowski, A., and Cralsten, H., Anti-inflammatory properties of estrogen. I. In vivo suppression of leucocyte production in bone marrow and redistribution of peripheral blood neutrophils, *Cell. Immunol.*, 142, 67, 1992.

52. Klosterhalfen, W. and Klosterhalfen, S., Evaluation of stress effects in an experimental autoimmune disease, *Ann. N.Y. Acad. Sci.*, 650, 293, 1992.

53. Koehler, T., Stress and rheumatoid arthritis: a survey of empirical evidence in human and animal studies, *J. Psychom. Res.*, 29, 655, 1985.

54. Kuroda, Y., Mori, T., and Hori, T., Restraint stress suppresses experimental allergic encephalomyelitis in Lewis rats, *Brain Res. Bull.*, 34, 15, 1994.

55. Lahita, R. G., Sex steroids and the rheumatic diseases, *Arthritis Rheum.*, 28, 121, 1985.

56. Leclère, J. and Weryha, G., Stress and auto-immune endocrine diseases, *Horm. Res.*, 31, 90, 1989.

57. Lehman, C. D., Rodin, J., McEwen, B. and Brinton, R., Impact of environmental stress on the expression of insulin-dependent diabetes mellitus, *Behav. Neurosci.*, 105, 241, 1991.

58. Lehmann, P. V., Sercarz, E. E., Forsthuber, T., Dayan, C. M., and Gammon, G., Determinant spreading and the dynamics of autoimmune T-cell repertoire, *Immunol. Today*, 14, 203, 1993.

59. Leonard, J. P., MacKensie, F. J., Patel, H. A., and Cuzner, M. L., Splenic noradrenergic and adrenocortical responses during the preclinical and clinical stages of adoptively transferred experimental autoimmune encephalomyelitis, *J. Neuroimmunol.*, 26, 183, 1990.

60. Le Page, C., Ferry, A., and Rieu, M., Effect of muscular exercise on chronic relapsing experimental autoimmune encephalomyelitis, *J. Appl. Physiol.*, 77, 2341, 1994.

61. Levine, S., Strebel, R., Wenk, E. J., and Harman, P. J., Suppression of experimental allergic encephalomyelitis by stress, *Proc. Soc. Exp. Biol. Med.*, 109, 294, 1962.

62. Levine, S. and Strebel, R., Allergic encephalomyelitis: inhibition of cellular passive transfer by exogenous and endogenous steroids, *Experentia*, 25, 189, 1969.

63. Levine, S., Sowinski, R., and Steinetz, B., Effects of experimental allergic encephalomyelitis on thymus and adrenal: relation to remission and relapse, *Proc. Soc. Exp. Biol. Med.*, 165, 218, 1980.

64. Levine, S. and Saltzman, A. Nonspecific stress prevents relapses of experimental allergic encephalomyelitis in rats, *Brain Behav. Immunity*, 1, 336, 1987.

65. Lewis-Faning, E., Report on an enquiry into the etiological factors associated with rheumatoid arthritis, *Ann. Rheum. Dis.*, 9 (Suppl), 94, 1950.

66. Lyngberg, K., Danneskiold-Samsoe, B., and Halskov, O., The effects of physical training on patients with rheumatoid arthritis: changes in disease activity, muscle strength and aerobic capacity. A clinically controlled minimized study, *Clin. Exp. Rheumatol.*, 6, 253, 1988.

67. Lysle, D. T., Luecken, L. J., and Maslonek, K. A., Suppression of the development of adjuvant arthritis by a conditioned aversive stimulus, *Brain Behav. Immunity*, 6, 64, 1992.

68. MacKensie, F. J., Leonard, J. P., and Cuzner, M. L., Changes in lymphocyte beta-adrenergic receptor density and noradrenaline content of the spleen are early indicators of immune reactivity in acute experimental allergic encephalomyelitis in the Lewis rat, *J. Neuroimmunol.*, 23, 93, 1989.

69. Martino, T. A., Liu, P., and Sole, M. J., Viral infection and the pathogenesis of dilated cardiomyopathy, *Circ. Res.*, 74, 182, 1994.

70. Mason, D., MacPhee, I., and Antony, F., The role of the neuroendocrine system in determining genetic susceptibility to experimental allergic encephalomyelitis in the rat, *Immunology*, 70, 1, 1990.

71. Mazelis, A. G. D., Albert, D., Crisa, C., Fiore, H., Parasaram, D., Franklin, B., Ginsberg-fellner, F., and McEvoy, R. C., Relationship of stressful housing conditions to the onset of diabetes mellitus induced by multiple, sub-diabetogenic doses of streptozotocin in mice, *Diabetes Res.*, 6, 195, 1987.

72. Michelson, D., Stone, L., Galliven, E., Magiakou, M. A., Chrousos, G. P., Strenberg, E. M., and Gold, P. W., Multiple sclerosis is associated with alterations in hypothalamic-pituary-adrenal axis function, *J. Clin. Endocrinol. Metab.*, 79, 848, 1994.

73. Mueller, M. N. and Kapas, A., Estrogen pharmacology. II. Supression of experimental polyarthtitis, *Proc. Soc. Exp. Biol. Med.*, 117, 845, 1964.

74. Munck, A., Guyre, P. M., and Holbrook, N. K., Physiological functions of glucocorticoids in stress and their relation to pharmacological actions, *Endocr. Rev.*, 5, 25, 1984.

75. Neidhart, M. and Larson, D. F., Freund's complete adjuvant induces ornithine carboxylase activity in the central nervous system of male rats and triggers the release of pituary hormones, *J. Neuroimmunol.*, 26, 97, 1990.

76. Neuman, D. A., Rose, N. R., Ansari, A. A., and Herskowitz, A., Induction of multiple heart antibodies in mice with coxsackievirus B3- and cardiac myosin-induced autoimmune myocarditis, *J. Immunol.*, 152, 343, 1994.

77. Noble, J. D. and Farelli, P. A., Effect of exercise training on the onset of type 1 diabetes in the BB/wor rat, *Med. Sci. Sports Exerc.*, 26, 1130, 1994.

78. Paterson, P. Y. and Swanborg, R. H., Demyelinating diseases of the central and peripheral nervous system, in *Immunological Disease*, Tlmage, D. W., Franck, M. M., Austen, K. F., and Claman, H. N., Eds., Little Brown, Boston, 1988, 1877.

79. Riskind, P. N., Massacesi, L., Doolittle, T. H., and Hauser, S. L., The role of prolactine in autoimmune demyelination: suppression of experimental allergic encephalomyelitis by bromocriptine, *Ann. Neurol.*, 29, 542, 1991.

80. Rogers, M. P., Trentham, D. E., McCune, W. J., Ginsberg, B. I., Rennke, H. G., Reich, P., and David, J. R., Effect of psychological stress on the induction of arthritis in rats, *Arthritis Rheum.*, 23, 1337, 1980.

81. Rogers, M. P., Trentham, D. E., Dynesius-Trentham, R., Daffner, K., and Reich, P., Exacerbation of collagen arthritis by noise stress, *J. Rheum.*, 10, 651, 1983.

82. Roudier, M., Portha, B., and Picon, L., Glucocorticoid-induced recovery from streptozocin diabetes in the adult rat, *Diabetes*, 29, 201, 1980.

83. Sarlis, N. J., Chowdrey, H. S., Stephanou, A., and Lightman, S. L., Chronic activation of the hypothalamo-pituary-adrenal axis and loss of circadian rhytm during adjuvant-induced arthritis in the rat, *Endocrinology*, 130, 1775, 1992.

84. Schwartz, R. H., A cell culture model for T lymphocyte clonal anergy, *Science*, 248, 1349, 1990.

85. Siedl, O., Psychosomatic considerations in physical activity of rheumatic patients, in *Rheum. Diseases and Sport*, Baenkler, H. W., Eds., Karger, Basel, 1992, 58.

86. Solomon, G. F., Emotional and personality factors in the onset and course of autoimmune disease, particularly rheumatoid arthritis, in *Psychoneuroimmunology*, Ader, R., Ed., Academic Press, New York, 1981, 159.

87. Solomon, G. F., Psychosocial factors, exercise, and immunity: athletes, elderly persons, and AIDS patients, *Int. J. Sports Med.*, 12 (Suppl 1), S50, 1991.

88. Sprent, J., Gao, E. K., and Webb, S. R., T cell reactivity to MHC molecules: immunity versus tolerance, *Science*, 248, 1357, 1990.

89. Sternberg, E. M., Hill, J. M., Crousos, G. P., Kamilaris, T., Listwak, S. J., Gold, P. W., and Wilder, R. L., Inflammatory mediator-induced hypothalamic-pituary-adrenal axis activation is defective in streptococcal cell wall arthtitis-susceptible rats, *Proc. Natl. Acad. Sci. U.S.A.*, 86, 2374, 1989.

90. Sternberg, E. M., Chrousos, G. P., Wilder, R. L., and Gold, P. W., The stress response and the regulation of inflammatory disease, *Ann. Int. Med.*, 117, 854, 1992.

91. Sternberg, E. S., Glowa, J. R., Smith, M. A., Calogero, A. E., Listwak, S. J., Aksentijevich, S., Chrousos, G. P., Wilder, R. L., and Gold, P. W., Corticotropin releasing hormone related behavorial and neuroendocrine responses to stress in Lewis and Fischer rats, *Brain Res.*, 570, 54, 1992.

92. Surwitt, R. S., Schneider, M. S., and Feinglos, M. N., Stress and diabetes mellitus, *Diabetes Care*, 15, 1413, 1992.

93. Takasu, N., Ohara, N., Yauada, T., and Komiya, I. Development of autoimmune thyroid dysfunction after bilateral adrenalectomy in a patient with Carney's complex and after removal of ACTH-producing pituary adenoma in a patient with Cushing's disease, *J. Endocrinol. Invest.*, 16, 691, 1993.

94. Trooster, W. J., Teeklen, A. W., Kampinga, J., Loof, J. G., Nieuwenhuis, P., and Minderhoud, J. M., Suppression of acute experimental allergic encephalomyelitis by the synthetic sex hormone 17-alpha-ethinyestradiol: an immunological study in the lewis rat, *Int. Arch. Allergy Immunol.*, 102, 133, 1993.

95. van de Langerijt, A. G. M., van Lent, P. L.E. M., Hermus, A. R. M. M. M., Sweep, C. G. J., Cools, A. R., and van den Berg, W. B., Susceptibility to adjuvant arthtitis: relative importance of adrenal activity and bacterial flora, *Clin. Exp. Immunol.*, 97, 33, 1994.

96. van Eden, W., Holoshitz, J., Nero, Z., Frenkel, A., Klajman, A., and Cohen, I. R., Arthritis induced by a T-lymphocyte clone that responds to *Mycobacterium tuberculosis* and to a cartilage proteoglycan, *Proc. Natl. Acad. Sci. U.S.A.*, 82, 5117, 1985.

97. Villas, P. A., Dronsfield, M. J., and Blankenhorn, E. P., Experimental allergic encephalomyelitis and corticosterone studies in resistant and susceptible rat strains, *Clin. Immunol. Immupathol.*, 61, 29, 1991.

98. von Boehmer, H., Developmental biology of T cells in T cell-receptor transgenic mice, *Annu. Rev. Immunol.*, 8, 531, 1990.

99. Wallace, D. J., The role of stress and trauma in rheumatoid arthritis and systemic lupus erythematosus, *Semin. Arthritis Rheum.*, 16, 153, 1987.

100. Weiss, J. M., Sundar, S. K., Becker, K. J., and Cierpial, M. A., Behavioral and neural influences on cellular immune responses: effects of stress and interleukin-1, *J. Clin. Psychiatry*, 50, 43, 1989.

101. Wick, G., Hu, Y., Schwarz, S., and Kroemer, G., Immunoendocrine communication via the hypothalamic-pituary-adrenal axis in autoimmune diseases, *Endocr. Rev.*, 14, 539, 1993.

102. Wilder, R. L., Corticotropin releasing hormone and the hypothalamic-pituary-adrenal axis in the regulation of inflammatory arthritis, *Inflammatory Dis. Ther.*, 41, 3, 1993.

Chapter **10**

EXERCISE, IMMUNITY, AND COLON CANCER

Laurie Hoffman-Goetz
Janice Husted

CONTENTS

I. INTRODUCTION

Considerable scientific efforts have focused on cancer prevention with the aim of identifying lifestyle-related risk factors. One factor which has received increasing attention is physical activity. Based on data supporting (1) a link between higher levels of exercise and longevity and (2) a link between moderate energy restriction and slower tumor growth, it has been hypothesized that physical activity may influence the incidence of and mortality from cancer. [39] Although the empirical evidence concerning physical activity and most types of cancer remains limited,[31,85] over 25 epidemiological and at least 4 animal studies have been conducted to investigate the link between exercise and colorectal cancer risk. Thus it seems timely to briefly summarize their findings, to examine the consistency of the human and animal evidence, to discuss the biological plausibility of the findings, and to consider the implementation of intervention strategies.

A. PUBLIC HEALTH SIGNIFICANCE OF COLORECTAL CANCER

Colorectal cancer is one of the most common cancers in developed societies, affecting 3 to 5% of the population.[100] In Canada alone, an estimated 16,300 new cases and 6,300 deaths occurred in 1994,[53] making colorectal cancer the third leading cause of cancer incidence and mortality in both men and women. Because only a minority of colorectal cancers are detected at an early stage, when curative-based treatments are most likely to halt disease progression, scientific efforts have increasingly focused on identification of biobehavioral risk factors to reduce the heavy burden of morbidity and mortality associated with colorectal cancer.

B. COLON CARCINOGENESIS

The sequence of events in the malignant transformation to colon carcinoma of normal gut mucosa has been well characterized genetically and histologically. The defined changes in the progression from normal epithelium include hyperproliferative epithelium and glandular dysplasia, benign, small tubular adenoma (polyp formation), large tubular adenoma, *in situ* carcinoma, and final metastatic carcinoma.[83] This sequence of events has been experimentally replicated in rodents by administration of dimethylhydrazine (DMH); precancerous changes can be observed before the development of overt carcinomas, with the type and extent of epithelial involvement dependent on carcinogen dose and duration of exposure.

There are several types of human colorectal cancer, including hereditary and nonhereditary (sporadic) forms. The genetic changes and their correlation with histological abnormalities have been best documented for two of the inherited forms of colon cancer: familial adenomatous polyposis (FAP) and hereditary nonpolyposis colon cancer (HNPCC).[50,51,83] In addition, a number of genetic alterations have been documented for sporadic forms of colon cancer. The types of genomic lesions found in different types of colon cancer include alterations of genes involved in ensuring the fidelity of DNA during cellular replication (e.g., *p53*) and those involved in replication-signaling pathways (e.g., the deleted in colon cancer or *DCC*). The order of appearance of these genetic alterations appears to be less important to the development of colon cancer than is the cumulative total of genetic lesions.[99]

There are two important implications of these findings for the area of exercise, immunology, and cancer. First, since colonic carcinogenesis in animal models effectively mimics the sequence of events in human colon cancer, progression to the malignant phenotype as a function of varying exercise dosages over time can be evaluated experimentally. Second, it is theoretically possible to identify mechanisms of action for exercise (or the associated hormonal and immunological consequences) on the expression of specific oncogenes and tumor suppressor genes which underlie the basic pathology of disordered cell growth control.

II. EPIDEMIOLOGICAL STUDIES ON EXERCISE AND COLON CANCER

Numerous analytic studies have investigated the link between exercise and cancers of the colon and rectum. Despite their use of different designs, study populations, and measures of exercise, the vast majority have shown that physical inactivity is associated with an increased risk of colon cancer (for a detailed review of the studies, see Sternfeld[85] and Potter et al.[64]). While the magnitude of the observed association appeared to be small, with relative risk estimates ranging from 1.1 to 2.0, it did not materially change once important confounders such as dietary factors, age, and body weight had been controlled. In contrast, the findings of most studies have not indicated a consistent association between physical activity and rectal cancer risk.

A. RETROSPECTIVE STUDIES

One of the first studies was conducted by Vena et al.[96] who used a retrospective or case–control design to examine whether lifetime job activity was associated with incidence of colon cancer in men. Included in this study were 210 and 276 hospital patients diagnosed with colon and rectal cancer, respectively. The 1431 controls consisted of hospital patients diagnosed with a range of nonneoplastic and nongastrointestinal disorders. In the preadmission questionnaire, all study participants were asked to provide detailed information on their lifetime occupation history. This information allowed a comparison of cases and controls on the number and proportion of years worked in a sedentary or light job. While no consistent association was found between physical inactivity and rectal cancer, the findings indicated that the risk of colon cancer increased with increasing amount and proportion of time spent in sedentary or light work. Individuals who were employed for more then 20 years in sedentary or light work jobs, who spent all their work years in sedentary or light work jobs, or who had spent at least 40% of their life in sedentary or light jobs had a twofold risk of colon cancer compared with those were never employed in low activity jobs. At least seven case–control studies using different populations and measures of occupational physical activity have replicated the findings of Vena et al.[3,10,23,24,61,97,98]

In a more recent case-control study, Slattery et al.[81] collected detailed information on both occupational and leisure time physical activity for 229 incident cases of colon cancer and 384 controls. The activity data were obtained for the 2 years prior to the date of diagnosis for the cases and 2 years prior to the interview for the controls. Individual leisure and occupational activities were converted to calories expended per week and then summed to calculate the total physical activity measure. Higher levels of total activity were associated with a reduced risk of colon cancer. Among men, individuals in the highest quartile of activity had approximately three quarters the risk of developing colon cancer compared with men in the lowest quartile (odds ratio [OR] = 0.72, 90% confidence intervals [CI] = 0.41 to 1.36), whereas women in the highest quartile of activity had approximately half the risk compared to those in the lowest quartile (OR = 0.49, 90% CI = 0.29 to 0.91). Adjustments for age, body mass index, fiber, and kilocalorie intake did not materially change the results.

At least two other case–control studies have used a total physical activity measure. Whittemore et al.[103] showed that a sedentary lifestyle among Chinese Americans was associated with a statistically significant elevated risk for colon cancer and with a statistically nonsignificant elevated risk for rectal cancer in both men and women. In contrast, Kune and colleagues[41] did not find a significant association between total physical activity and colorectal cancer. In general, studies which have investigated the link between physical activity and cancers of the colon and rectum combined have not shown a consistent association.[64]

B. PROSPECTIVE STUDIES

The findings of prospective studies, which provide a higher degree of methodological rigor since the measure of physical activity is unlikely to be confounded by the presence of cancer or faulty recall by respondents, are consistent with the results of case–control studies.

In 1960 Gerhardsson et al.[27] initiated a 19-year follow-up study of 1.1 million employed Swedish males between the ages of 20 to 64. Current occupation was used to determine level of physical activity. During the follow-up period, 7115 cases of colon cancer and 5290 cases of rectal cancer developed among the cohort. Men who held sedentary jobs were found to have an increased risk of colon cancer compared with those in physically active jobs (age adjusted relative risk [RR] = 1.4, 90% CI = 1.3 to 1.5). No increased risk was observed for rectal cancer. The findings did not materially change when age, population density, and social class were simultaneously controlled in the analyses.

Severson et al.[78] examined the association between physical activity and colon cancer in 8006 Japanese men residing in Hawaii in 1965. At study intake, participants were asked to rate occupational physical activity as sedentary, moderate, or heavy. During the 21-year follow-up period, there were 192 incident cases of colon cancer and 95 cases of rectal cancer. Compared with sedentary jobs, moderate or heavy activity at work was found to be associated with a reduced risk of colon cancer (RR = 0.72, 95% CI = 0.52 to 1.00), but not with rectal cancer. By contrast, Paffenbarger et al.[57] followed 6351 San Francisco longshoremen over a 22-year period and found no significant relationship between level of occupational physical activity and colorectal mortality risk.

Other prospective studies have focused exclusively on the link between leisure-time or recreational physical activity and colon cancer. Wu et al.[105] followed 11,888 residents of a retirement community located near Los Angeles over a 4-year period. Most of the residents were Caucasian and members of the upper middle socioeconomic class. Among men, decreasing risks of colorectal cancers were found with increasing levels of recreational physical activity. Men who spent more than 2 h a day in recreational physical activities such as swimming, biking, and dancing had 40% risk of developing colorectal cancer than men who spent less than 1 h a day in such activities ($p < 0.05$). A similar trend was observed in women, but it did not achieve statistical significance.

Lee et al.[43,44] used data from the Harvard Alumni Health Study to examine the relationship between leisure-time physical activity and colorectal cancer. Physical activity was assessed in 1962/1966 and again in 1977. All cohort members were followed through 1988 to determine colorectal cancer incidence and mortality. They found that men who reported being highly active or moderately active (i.e., expended >2500 kcal/week or 1000 to 2500 kcal/week, respectively) at both assessments had approximately half the risk of developing colon cancer relative to those who were inactive (expended <1000 kcal/week) at both assessments ($p < 0.05$). However, in subsequent analyses of this population using the same measure of physical activity, no association was found between physical activity and colon cancer risk. In addition, no consistent pattern was observed between physical activity and rectal cancer incidence.

A handful of prospective studies have used a combined measure of occupational and leisure-time physical activity. Using data from the Framingham

Heart Study, Ballard-Barbash et al.[4] followed 4214 individuals (1906 men and 2308 women) between the ages of 30 and 62 over a 28-year period. Total activity was calculated based on the weighted sum of the usual amount of time the participant reported to have spent per 24 h in the following types of activity: sleeping (weight of 1); sedentary, as in sitting and standing (weight of 1.1); slight, as in walking (weight of 1.5); moderate, as in gardening (weight of 2.4); and heavy, as in shoveling (weight of 5). Compared with highly active men, inactive men had a statistically nonsignificant elevated risk of colon cancer (age-adjusted RR = 1.8, 95% CI = 1.0 to 3.2). No relationship was found for women. Other prospective studies which have used a combined measure of occupational and recreational physical activity have also found that inactivity was associated with an increased risk of colon cancer.[26,78]

C. SUMMARY OF FINDINGS

The epidemiological evidence is remarkably consistent. Sedentary jobs, decreased participation in leisure or recreational activities, or minimal total physical activity all seemed to increase the risk of colon cancer. From a public health perspective, these findings merit serious consideration. They suggest that promoting exercise in healthy individuals has the potential to reduce the incidence of colon cancer. This may be particularly the case in westernized countries which tend to have high rates of both colon cancer and sedentary lifestyles.

III. ANIMAL STUDIES OF EXERCISE AND COLON CANCER

A. PHYSICAL STRESS AND TUMORIGENESIS

The observation that stress influences the development of experimental tumors has been repeatedly confirmed in animals. Such studies show that the effect of stress is bimodal: inhibition as well as enhancement of neoplastic process.[37,42,79] A wide range of physical stressors including restraint,[84] surgery and anesthesia,[62,63,75] tail or footshock,[28] cold water immersion,[11] and mechanical shaking[89] have been shown to influence tumorigenesis in animals. Physical exercise can be considered a subset of the wider category of physical stress[34] and should, therefore, elicit effects on tumor development as other physical stressors.

Despite the repeated demonstration of an interaction between stress and experimental tumors, conceptual models for divergent outcomes in terms of tumor burden in response to physical stressors have not been incorporated in most studies. It is should be emphasized that theoretical models are important to the area of exercise, immunology, and cancer because they provide a framework for testing hypothesis about mechanisms of action. Implicit, if not explicit, assumptions about the etiology and pathogenesis of colon cancer based on such models will contribute to the design of exercise intervention strategies to prevent colon cancer. It must also be recognized that even if the physical activity evidence as a whole is persuasive and the underlying mechanisms of action identified, such modifiable risk factors may contribute only a small portion of the variance in colon cancer incidence.

Newberry and colleagues[54,55] proposed that two models might be used to predict whether stress (including exercise) will reduce or enhance experimental tumor growth. These are (1) the opponent process model which emphasizes cross-baseline rebound following cessation of the stressor protocol.[37] This model suggests that for tumors whose growth is stimulated by stress, the termination of stress will result in inhibition of tumor growth, and (2) the chronicity–controllability model which emphasizes that tumor growth in response to stress will mirror the degree of individual control and the duration of stress exposure and adaptation.[79,80] This model recognizes that opposite tumor outcomes can occur at different times on a single continuum of stress exposure. Moreover, issues related to the (exercise) stressor characteristics, the mediating variables, the tumor characteristics, and the tumor–host interactions have not been conceptually linked in most of the animal studies.[30]

B. EXERCISE AND EXPERIMENTAL TUMORS

The idea that exercise, a common physical stressor, modifies experimental tumor growth in animals is not new. Most of the early studies (while demonstrating reduced experimental tumor burden in rats and mice with exercise) used unrealistic exercise protocols, did not allow time for rest and feeding, and introduced a variety of other confounding stressors into the design.[29,74] More recently, studies of experimental tumorigenesis in animals given varying exercise protocols have tended to focus on mammary,[16,17,90,91] pancreatic,[73] and hepatic[87] carcinogenesis. Studies of the late neoplastic processes have been focused on mammary tumor cell[33,104] or H-*ras* transformed fibroblast cell[32,48] metastasis. For the most part, these studies tend to show that regular exercise reduces tumor burden, although issues related to controllability (forced vs. voluntary exercise), chronicity (single exercise exposure vs. training), and where in the continuum the exercise stress is introduced (prior to tumor, concurrent with tumor, after tumor exposure) have not been systematically addressed.

C. EXERCISE AND EXPERIMENTAL COLON CARCINOGENESIS

There have been only a handful of studies which evaluated the impact of exercise on experimental colon carcinogenesis. Andrianopoulos and colleagues[2] injected rats (n = 33) intraperitoneally with dimethylhydrazine (DMH) weekly for 6 weeks; one third of the animals were randomized to an activity condition (access to in-cage activity wheel) and two thirds were maintained in the control condition (standard caging). Following the first confirmed tumor death in the controls, all rats were sacrificed; the number, location, and histology of the tumors were determined. The physically active rats had significantly fewer tumors (6/11) than did control rats (18/20), and there was a mild (but not significant) positive association between physical activity and left colorectal tumor incidence ($r = 0.57$, $p = 0.07$.) While these results are intriguing, absence of measures of actual physical activity attained, of energy expenditure, and of fecal composition and frequency limits the usefulness of this study in pointing to biological mechanisms for the association.

The effects of voluntary[70] and forced treadmill running[92,93] on azoxymethane (AOM)-induced colon carcinogenesis in rats suggests that both regimens are protective. Voluntary wheel exercise (peaking at 2.3 mi/d at week 6 and dropping to 0.2 mi/d by week 32) was associated with a significant reduction in the incidence (percentage of rats with tumors: 52% in sedentary; 19% in physically active) and multiplicity (number of tumors/rat: 0.78 in sedentary; 0.22 in physically active) of adenocarcinomas compared with the sedentary controls; there was no difference in measures of tumor burden for (nonmalignant) adenomas of the colon as a function of exercise. Low intensity treadmill exercise (7 m/min, 5 h/d for 38 weeks) coupled with high fat corn oil diet completely protected rats from colon carcinomas compared with sedentary rats also fed the high fat corn oil diet (0/30 tumors in exercised rats; 10/30 tumors in sedentary rats). There were no significant differences in the number of rats showing dysplastic changes in colonic mucosa or in the distribution of colonic carcinomas within the gut (proximal vs. distal colon) as a function of exercise. These findings suggest that regular, low-intensity exercise protects against the progression toward the invasive/malignant phenotype rather than in the initiation or promotion of transformed epithelium. A protective effect of higher intensity treadmill exercise (24 m/min, 1 h/d, 5 d/week) during the promotion phase of dimethylhydrazine-induced colon cancer was noted by Klurfeld et al.;[38] this protective effect was not related to concentration of fecal bile acids or to stool volume as a function of exercise.

IV. IMMUNE EFFECTORS

It is often suggested that human cancers are nonimmunogenic in nature. Nevertheless, human cancers are to some degree susceptible to immunological control by cellular mechanisms (lymphokine-activated killer cells, tumor-specific cytolytic T cells, tumor-infiltrating macrophages) and by secreted products of these cells (cytokines, eicosanoids).[102,106,107] That immune reactions to cancer cells are an important aspect of host defense is evidenced by the immunological role in maintaining cancer dormancy during remission.[86] Furthermore, many studies have shown that as tumors grow, qualitative and quantitative impairments in host cellular immunity occur (e.g., Reference 21 and reviewed in Reference 107) and such changes are often associated with poor prognosis.

This section considers three broad immunomodulatory mechanisms that may underscore the exercise–cancer association. However, the role of exercise-induced immune changes in tumorigenesis is tentative at best. It is not our intent to provide a catalog of all exercise–immunology studies or to imply that exercise-induced changes in immune functions are a definitive mechanism for the exercise–cancer association. Finally, it is not possible in this brief review to consider competing, nonimmunological mechanisms. However, it is our opinion that multiple and overlapping biological effects of exercise (e.g., changes in secondary bile acid composition + increased peristalsis + altered gut cytokine levels), rather than single immunological effects (e.g., changes in IL-1 levels in the gut mucosa), will likely prove to be important as explanatory variables for the exercise–colon cancer association. In addition, exercise-associated effects on colon cancer risk may be secondary to changes in diet or nutritional patterns, or other health variables. Both short- and long-term caloric restriction, without malnutrition, reduce experimental tumor risk in animals, by altering immune profiles or by slowing the rate of cell division.[76]

A. CYTOKINES

The biological importance of cytokines and the effect of exercise on blood and tissue cytokine levels and synthesis have been reviewed elsewhere in this volume. In this section, the impact of only one cytokine — interleukin-1 (IL-1) — on tumor growth and progression is considered with specific reference to potential mediating roles in exercise–colon cancer associations. The focus on IL-1 is not to imply that other cytokines (IL-6, tumor necrosis factor [TNF], interferon [IFN]) are not potentially important in explaining the exercise–colon cancer association. Rather, by focusing on one cytokine only, the complexity of its role in neoplasia can be illustrated.

The impact of exercise on IL-1 levels varies with concentric and eccentric exercise. Several early studies[12,14] reported increased circulating levels of IL-1 after moderate intensity concentric exercise; other studies failed to detect increases (above basal) in plasma IL-1ß levels after moderate intensity cycle ergometry exercise.[67,82,95] Cycle exercise to exhaustion was associated with increased *in vitro* levels of IL-1 from mononuclear cells.[45] Thus, intensity and/or duration of concentric exercise is likely predictive for increases in circulating IL-1 levels. Eccentric exercise which produces skeletal muscle damage and an inflammatory infiltrate has been consistently associated with increased levels of IL-1.[13,20,22]

Could exercise-mediated changes in IL-1 levels (either acutely or chronically) influence the growth and progression of tumors, in general, and colon cancer, in particular? IL-1 promotes the adhesion of tumor cells to vascular endothelium.[5,8,18,71] This finding is of considerable importance in understanding metastasis, a process which characterizes many solid tumors. Liotta[46] proposed a three-step theory of invasion and metastasis which involves attachment of tumor cells, via cell surface receptors, to a matrix (e.g., basement membrane or stroma); the secretion of hydrolytic enzymes by tumor cells leading to degradation of the matrix; and finally tumor cell locomotion into the region following matrix proteolysis. Locomotion could be in the direction of intravasation or extravasation. Given this model, high local concentrations of IL-1 might result in greater adhesivity of tumor cells (or immunocompetent cells) to the extracelluar matrix underlying vascular endothelium. Considering the complex process of tumor metastasis, there are potentially many biological mechanisms by which IL-1 might mediate an effect on tumorigenesis. For example, high levels of IL-1 (as a result of exercise) could act by encouraging adhesion of tumor cells to extracellular matrix and provide opportunities for innate immune responses such as surface phagocytosis or increased natural killer (NK) cell recycling for tumor target. IL-1 mediated up-regulation of integrin molecules, which promote adhesion and trigger regulatory intracellular signals involved in cell proliferation,[77] could act in an inhibitory fashion for tumor detachment. Given this scenario, an exercise-mediated increase in IL-1 levels might be expected to reduce tumor metastasis. Recent studies also suggest that with increasing tumorigenicity of some cell lines, there is an acquired resistance to cellular regulatory signals medited by cytokines including IL-1.[52] This suggests that if there is a role for exercise, mediated through cytokines, the effect would more likely be apparent prior to than after the acquisition of a highly metastatic phenoytpe. There are, however, no studies of IL-1 levels or the expression of adhesion molecules as a consequence of exercise and in relation to tumor metastasis.

What we do know is that the number of experimental pulmonary metastases that develop in rodents is higher if intensive exercise occurs after tumor cell injection rather than before injection.[33] Uhlenbrück and Order[94] found that the incidence of lung tumors in BALB/c mice that continued run training after tumor inoculation was less than in mice that had rested or were sedentary. Again, cytokine levels were not measured.The metastatic potential of the tumor is likely an important consideration as well. Primary work from our lab shows that exercise-trained mice injected with a weakly metastatic tumor (CIRAS 1) had lower tumor retention in the lungs than their sedentary counterparts; in contrast, in mice injected with a highly aggressive tumor (CIRAS 3), an exercise effect was not demonstrated.[108] This suggests that the timing of exercise and the characteristics of the tumor are significant factors in the metastasis of tumors, perhaps through an IL-1-mediated mechanism.

Ravikumar et al.[69] reported that the ability to generate IL-1 declines during the growth of DMH-induced colon adenocarcinoma isografts in W/Fu rats; further, this decline in IL-1 levels was significantly correlated with greater tumor growth. Hoffmann and Pollack[35] have shown that IL-1 release by peripheral blood mononuclear cells to LPS is decreased in many cancer patients. This points to an extremely complex role for IL-1 in tumor growth and metastasis. Understanding the possible roles and mechanisms of action of IL-1 and exercise-associated changes in other cytokine levels is complicated by the multistage nature of carcinogenesis.

B. EICOSANOIDS

Prostaglandins, mainly of the E series but also F series, have long been implicated in the immune suppression which occurs in both cancer patients and in animal tumor models. The source of the prostaglandins includes tumor cells, including human colorectal cancers[40,72] and tissue macrophages which infiltrate colon tumors.[1] Although there is a strong argument for an immunosuppressive role of prostaglandins, especially of the E series, there are also provocative reports of immune facilitating actions of prostaglandins.[107] While some studies demonstrate inhibition in cancer patients of NK-mediated cytolysis by prostaglandin E_2 (PGE_2),[7] the reverse effects have also been observed with pharmacological antagonism of high-affinity PGE_2 receptors on tumor cells resulting in reduced NK cell–tumor conjugate formation.[25] Administration of a PGE_2 analog to healthy volunteers stimulated T cell function and $TNF\alpha$ production,[101] and nitric oxide production by macrophages can be stimulated by PGE_2.[66]

Prostaglandin biosynthesis has also been associated with the generation of a direct-acting mutagen, malondialdehyde (MDA), from enzymatic and nonenzymatic breakdown of PGH_2.[6] In addition, PGH synthase (prostaglandin endoperoxide synthase) which oxygenates arachidonic acid to PGG_2 and reduces PGG_2 to PGH_2 may play a role in the extrahepatic metabolism of xenobiotics and carcinogens (including aromatic and heterocyclic amines).[49] Thus, arachidonic acid metabolism and prostaglandin generation as a consequence of inflammatory damage arising from eccentric exercise might contribute to tumorigenesis, in the bowel and at other sites.

That exercise alters prostaglandin levels and transiently suppresses natural killer cell function has been suggested by Pedersen and colleagues.[59] Infusion of indomethacin, a cyclooxgenase inhibitor, prevents the exercise-associated reduction in cellular cytotoxicity functions.[60] There is some limited evidence that increases in the concentration of prostaglandins of the F series prostaglandins occur with exercise.[19,68] The effect of 8 weeks of exercise (9 to 15 mi of walking or jogging each week) in middle-aged men on serum PGE levels was not significantly different from preexercise values.[68] Unfortunately, there are no studies that test whether regular, moderate intensity exercise influences prostaglandin concentrations in the villi of the small intestine and/or the mucosa of the colon. Thus, it remains an interesting but untested hypothesis that exercise induces increases in prostaglandin levels in the gut leading to changes in colon cancer risk (in either direction).

C. MUCOSAL IMMUNITY

A potentially important, but overlooked, immunological mechanism for the association between exercise and reduced colon cancer risk is that of the exercise-induced changes in mucosal immunity in the gut. Secretory immunoglobulin A (sIgA) produced by epithelial cells of the mucous membrane of the gastrointestinal tract provides an important barrier function for attachment or entry of pathogens. Intense exercise has been shown to acutely reduce the concentrations of sIgA at other mucosal surfaces[36,47] whereas regular moderate exercise increases serum IgA levels.[56] How does this relate to colon cancer risk? One perspective suggests that increased cell division induced by external or internal stimulation is a common denominator in the pathogenesis of many cancers[65] and infectious agents are one such route leading to a hyperproliferative response. It has been documented that the excess of colorectal cancers in certain areas of China is correlated with endemic *Schistosoma japonicum*.[15] The course of schistosomiasis on the mucosal epithelium of the colon is a thickening of the stroma and excess proliferation of the epithelium where tumors usually develop.[65] Additional evidence for chronic irritation preceding neoplasia also comes from the association of chronic ulcerative colitis as a risk factor for colon cancer.[9]

D. OTHER MECHANISMS

We have recently reviewed the potential mechanisms through which exercise might confer a protective effect against colon cancer.[31] These mechanisms are largely independent of the immune system and include exercise-associated changes in gut peristalsis, fecal transit time, and concentration of fecal bile acids in stool.[88]

V. PROPOSAL FOR DEVELOPMENT OF INTERVENTION STRATEGIES

Epidemiological research in the area of exercise and colon cancer appears to have reached a crossroads. Numerous observational studies have been conducted to investigate this relationship. Their findings are remarkably consistent, suggesting that a sedentary lifestyle leads to a modest increase in colon cancer risk. The evidence from available animal studies supports the epidemiological findings, suggesting that chronic exercise reduces the development of experimental colon tumors. At this stage in the research, it seems reasonable to ask whether an intervention trial is warranted. In our view an intervention study has at least two distinct advantages over another observational study. One relates to its ability to manipulate the exercise regimen, which would allow for a better understanding of the type, intensity, and duration of exercise that confers protection against colon cancer. The other advantage relates to the randomization of the study participants to various levels of exercise, thereby controlling the influences of known and unknown confounders more adequately than past observational studies. Given the prevalence of sedentary lifestyle in western populations, the potential public health impact of such an intervention could be substantial. However, while an intervention trial is viewed as a promising future direction, many issues will need to be addressed or seriously considered in designing such a trial.

One issue relates to the composition of the study population. From both a scientific and public health perspective, it makes sense to target high-risk groups. One potential group may be those individuals with a genetic predisposition, for instance those with a family history of hereditary nonpolyposis colon cancer (HNPCC). An exercise intervention trial in such a population would allow a careful examination of the interplay between genetic and environmental influences on the development of colon cancer. However, one problem with focusing on a genetically predisposed group is the potential lack of generalizability of the findings. Although HNPCC contributes to overall colon cancer burden, the majority of individuals who will develop colon cancer have no prior family history of the disease.

An alternative high-risk strategy would be to include individuals who live a sedentary lifestyle. If this were the approach taken, some age restrictions should be considered and should be consistent with hypotheses concerning where in the carcinogenesis process exercise has its effect. For instance, if it is hypothesized that the effect of exercise operates early in the carcinogenesis process (for example, during promotion or corresponding to the appearance of glandular dysplasia), then a relatively young population should be studied. If, on the other hand, the primary role of exercise is in the prevention of metastatic spread (tertiary prevention), then an older age population would be suitable.

Another issue to consider relates to the size of the study population. Given the uncertainties about whether the effect of exercise is modified by gender, diet, and anatomic site within the colon, it seems important to ascertain an adequate number of study participants to address these issues.

A final issue is the exercise intervention itself. The greatest risk of colon cancer is associated with sedentary lifestyle. In designing an exercise intervention, relatively modest increases in exercise patterns may confer the greatest protection from colon cancer. Likelihood of adherence to a moderate exercise intervention would also be more likely to occur, especially if such an intervention occurs over several years. A moderate exercise intervention, stressing an accumulation of 30 min or more of physical activity/day on most days, would follow the recent recommendations of the Centers for Disease Control and the American College of Sports Medicine.[58] On the other hand, if a genetically predisposed group were selected (for example, those prone to the rare familial adenomatous polyposis disease with the defective *APC* genotype), then the effects of a modest exercise intervention might not be apparent given the overwhelming genetic burden. Here, a more intense exercise protocol might be appropriate. Consideration of these interrelated issues, as well as others detailed in Table 1, would be crucial in designing an exercise intervention trial for colon cancer.

TABLE 1   Representative Issues to Consider in Designing Exercise Intervention for Colon Cancer

Study Population
- If it is a genetic high-risk population with high probability of allelic loss and expression of genetic abnormalities, what type of exercise intervention is needed?
- If it is a general population, is there sufficient evidence about exercise dose to warrant an intervention?

Exercise Program
- How would an intervention be designed to test exercise dose effects?
- What type of exercise intervention would be appropriate (endurance, strength training); and what should be the frequency, duration, and intensity?
- How would low vs. high intensity physical activity be measured in the study sample?
- Would the exercise need to be regular; and, if so, how is regular defined?
- What is the stability of the exercise behavior over time?
- When would the exercise intervention be initiated, and how does it correspond to the carcinogenesis process?

Biological Endpoints
- What is the type of biological endpoint or intermediate biomarker (e.g., histological appearance of dysplasia, identification of *APC* gene)?
- What are the frequency and timing of measurements?
- What are the sensitivity and specificity of the intermediate biomarker or endpoint?

Ethical Considerations
- When should the study be terminated and treatment initiated?
- If the population is high risk (genetic predisposition), what are the ethics of randomizing to the no treatment (no exercise) group? What are the implications for the control group?

Other Issues
- What is the feasbility of monitoring biomarkers/endpoints? What is the cost vs. benefit for public health?
- Is the exercise intervention hypothesis-driven (e.g., tests, biological mechanisms)?

REFERENCES

1. Alleva, D. G., Burger, C. J., and Elgert, K. D., Interferon-γ reduces tumor-induced Ia-macrophage-mediated suppression: role of prostaglandin E_2, Ia, and tumor necrosis factor-α. *Immunopharmacology*, 25, 215, 1993.
2. Andrianopoulos, G., Nelson, R. L., Bombeck, C. T., and Souza, G., The influence of physical activity in 1,2 dimethylhydrazine induced colon carcinogenesis in the rat, *Anticancer Res.*, 7, 849, 1987.
3. Arbman, G., Axelson, O., Fredriksson, M., Nilsson, E., and Sjodahl, R., Do occupational factors influence the risk of colon cancer and rectal cancer in different ways?, *Cancer*, 72, 2543, 1993.

4. Ballard-Barbash, R., Schatzkin, A., Albanes, D., Schiffman, M. H., Kreger, B. E., Kannel, W. B., Anderson, K. M., and Helsel, W. E., Physical activity and risk of large bowel cancer in the Framingham study, *Cancer Res.*, 50, 3610, 1990.
5. Bani, M. R., Garofalo, A., Scanziani, E., and Giavazzi, R., Effect of interleukin-1-β on metastasis formation in different tumor systems, *J. Natl. Cancer Inst.*, 83, 119, 1991.
6. Basu, A. K. and Marnett, L. J., Unequivocal demonstration that malondialdehyde is a mutagen, *Carcinogenesis (London)*, 4, 331, 1983.
7. Baxevanis, C. N., Reclos, G. J., Gritzapis, A. D., Dedousis, G. V., Mitsitzis, I., and Papamichail, M., Elevated prostaglandin E_2 production by monocytes is responsible for the depressed levels of natural killer and lymphokine-activated killer cell function in patients with breast cancer, *Cancer*, 72, 491, 1993.
8. Bertomeu, M. C., Gallo, S., Lauri, D., Haas, T. A., Orr, F. W., Bastida, E., and Buchanan, M. R., Interleukin 1-induced cancer cell/endotheial cell adhesion in vitro and its relationship to metastasis in vivo: role of vessel wall 13-HODE synthesis and integrin expression, *Clin. Exp. Metastasis*, 11, 243, 1993.
9. Biasco, G., Paganelli, G. M., Miglioli, M., Brillanti, S., Di Febo, G., Gizzi, G., Ponz De Leon, M., Campieri, M., and Barbara, L., Rectal cell proliferation and colon cancer risk in ulcerative colitis, *Cancer Res.*, 50, 1156, 1990.
10. Brownson, R. C., Chang, J. C., Davis, J. R., and Smith, C. A., Physical activity on the job and cancer in Missouri, *Am. J. Public Health*, 81, 639, 1991.
11. Burchfield, S. R., Woods, S. C., and Elich, M. S., Effects of cold stress on tumor growth, *Physiol. Behav.*, 21, 537, 1978.
12. Cannon, J. G., Evans, W. J., Hughes, V. A., Meredith, C. N., and Dinarello, C. A., Physiological mechanisms contributing to increased interleukin-1 secretion, *J. Appl. Physiol.*, 61, 1869, 1986.
13. Cannon, J. G., Fielding, R. A., Fiatarone, M. A., Orencole, S. F., Dinarello, C. A., and Evans, W. J., Increased interleukin 1β in human skeletal muscle after exercise, *Am. J. Physiol.*, 257, R451, 1989.
14. Cannon, J. G. and Kluger, M. J., Endogenous pyrogen activity in human plasma after exercise, *Science*, 220, 617, 1983.
15. Chen, M. and Mott, K., Progress in assessment of morbidity due to *Schistosoma japonicum* infection, *Trop. Dis. Bull.*, 85, 2, 1988.
16. Cohen, L. A., Boylan, E., Epstein, M., and Zang, E., Voluntary exercise and experimental mammary cancer, in *Exercise, Calories, Fat and Cancer*, Jacobs, M. M., Ed., Plenum Press, New York, 1992, 41.
17. Cohen, L. A., Choi, K. W., and Wang, C. X., Influence of dietary fat, caloric restriction, and voluntary exercise on N-nitrosomethylurea-induced mammary tumorigenesis in rats, *Cancer Res.*, 48, 4276, 1988.
18. Dejana, E., Bertocchi, F., Bortolami, M. C., Regonesi, A., Tonta, A., Breviario, F., and Giavazzi, R., Interleukin 1 promotes tumor cell adhesion to cultured human endothelial cells, *J. Clin. Invest.*, 82, 1466, 1988.
19. Demers, L. M., Harrison, T. S., and Halbert, D. R., Effect of prolonged exercise on plasma prostaglandin levels, *Prostaglandins Med.*, 6, 413, 1981.
20. Evans, W. J., Meredith, C. N., Cannon, J. G., Dinarello, C. A., Frontera, W. R., Hughes, V. A., Jones, B. H., and Knuttgen, H. G., Metabolic changes following eccentric exercise in trained and untrained men, *J. Appl. Physiol.*, 61, 1864, 1986.
21. Farinas, M. C., Rodriguez-Valverde, V., Zarrabeitia, M. T., Parra-Blanco, J. A., and Sanz-Ortiz, J., Contribution of monocytes to the decreased lymphoproliferative response to phytohemagglutinin in patients with lung cancer, *Cancer*, 68, 1279, 1991.
22. Fielding, R., Manfredi, T. J., Ding, W., Fiatarone, M. A., Evans, W. J., and Cannon, J. G., Acute phase response in exercise. III. Neutrophil and IL-1β accumulation in skeletal muscle, *Am. J. Physiol.*, 265, R166, 1993.

23. Fraser, G. and Pearce, N., Occupational physical activity and risk of cancer of the colon and rectum in New Zealand males, *Cancer Causes Contr.*, 4, 45, 1993.
24. Fredriksson, M., Bengtsoon, N. O., Hardell, L., and Axelson, O., Colon cancer, physcial activity, and occupational exposures. A case study, *Cancer*, 63, 1838, 1989.
25. Fulton, A. M. and Chong, Y. C., Prostaglandin E_2 receptor activity and susceptibility to natural killer cells, *J. Leuk. Biol.*, 51, 176, 1992.
26. Gerhardsson de Verdier, M., Steineck, G., Hagman, U., Rieger, A., and Norell, S. E., Physical activity and colon cancer: a case referent study in Stockholm, *Int. J. Cancer*, 46, 985, 1990.
27. Gerhardsson, M., Norell, S. E., Kiviranta, H., Pedersen, N. L., and Ahlbom, A., Sedentary jobs and colon cancer, *Am. J. Epidemiol.*, 123, 775, 1986.
28. Greenberg, A. H., Dyck, D. G., and Sandler L. S., Opponent processes, neurohormones and natural resistance, in *Impact of Psychoendocrine Systems in Cancer and Immunity*, Fox, B. H. and Newberry, B. H., Eds., C. J. Hogrefe, Toronto, 1984, 225.
29. Hoffman, S. A., Paschkis, K. E., DeBias, D. A., Cantarow, A., and Williams, T. L., The influence of exercise on the growth of transplanted rat tumors, *Cancer Res.*, 22, 597, 1962.
30. Hoffman-Goetz, L., Exercise, natural immunity, and experimental tumor metastasis, *Med. Sci. Sports Exerc.*, 26, 157, 1994.
31. Hoffman-Goetz, L. and Husted, J., Exercise and cancer: do the biology and epidemiology correspond?, *Ex. Immunol. Rev.*, 1, 81, 1995.
32. Hoffman-Goetz, L., MacNeil, B., and Arumugam, Y., Tissue distribution of radiolabelled tumor cells in wheel exercised and sedentary mice, *Int. J. Sports Med.*, 15, 249, 1994.
33. Hoffman-Goetz, L., May, K. M., and Arumugam, Y., Exercise training and mouse mammary tumour metastasis, *Anticancer Res.*, 14, 2627, 1994.
34. Hoffman-Goetz, L. and Pedersen, B. K., Exercise and the immune system: a model of the stress response?, *Immunol. Today*, 15, 382, 1994.
35. Hoffmann, M. and Pollack, S., Interleukin-1 release by cancer patients' monocytes, in *Interleukins, Lymphokines, and Cytokines*, Oppenheim, J. J. and Cohen, S., Eds., Academic Press, New York, 1983, 707.
36. Housh, T. J., Johnson, G. O., Housh, D. J., Evans, S. L., and Tharp, G. D., The effect of exercise at various temperatures on salivary levels of immunoglobulin A, *Int. J. Sports Med.*, 12, 498, 1991.
37. Justice, A., Review of the effects of stress on cancer in laboratory animals: importance of time of stress application and type of tumor, *Psych. Bull.*, 98, 108, 1985.
38. Klurfeld, D. M., Welch, C. B., Einhorn, E., and Kritchevsky, D., Inhibition of colon tumor promotion by caloric restriction or exercise in rats, *FASEB J.*, 2, A433, 1988.
39. Kohl, H. W., LaPorte, R. E., and Blair, S. N., Physical activity and cancer: an epidemiologic perspective, *Sports Med.*, 6, 222, 1988.
40. Kubota, Y., Sunouchi, K., Ono, M., Sawada, T., and Muto, T., Local immunity and metastasis of colorectal carcinoma, *Dis. Colon Rectum*, 35, 645, 1992.
41. Kune, G. A., Kune, S., and Watson, L. F., Body weight and physical activity as predictors of colorectal cancer risk, *Nutr. Cancer*, 13, 9, 1990.
42. LaBarba, R. C., Experiential and environmental factors in cancer: a review of research with animals, *Psychosom. Med.*, 32, 259, 1970.
43. Lee, I.-M. and Paffenbarger, R. S., Jr., Physical activity and risk of developing colorectal cancer among college alumni, *Med. Sci. Sports Exerc.*, 26, 831, 1994.
44. Lee, I.-M., Paffenbarger, R. S., Jr. and Hsieh, C.-C., Physical activity and risk of developing colorectal cancer among college alumni, *J. Natl. Cancer Inst.*, 83, 1324, 1991.
45. Lewicki, R., Tchórzewski, H., Majewska, E., Nowak, Z., and Baj, Z., Effect of maximal physical exercise on T-lymphocyte subpopulations and on interleukin 1 (IL 1) and interleukin 2 (IL 2) production in vitro, *Int. J. Sports Med.*, 9, 114, 1988.
46. Liotta, L. A., Tumor invasion and metastases-role of the extracellular matrix, *Cancer Res.*, 46, 1, 1986.

47. Mackinnon, L. T., Chick, T. W., van As, A., and Tomasi, A., The effect of exercise on secretory and natural immunity, *Adv. Exp. Med. Biol.*, 216A, 869, 1987.
48. MacNeil, B. and Hoffman-Goetz, L., Chronic exercise enhances in vivo and in vitro cytotoxic mechanisms of natural immunity in mice, *J. Appl. Physiol.*, 74, 388, 1993.
49. Marnett, L. J., Aspirin and the potential role of prostaglandins in colon cancer, *Cancer Res.*, 52, 5575, 1992.
50. Marx, J., New colon cancer gene discovered, *Science*, 260, 751, 1993.
51. Marx, J., New tumor suppressor may rival p53, *Science*, 264, 344, 1994.
52. McCann, J., Clues about metastasis may lead to better cancer drugs, *J. Natl. Cancer Inst.*, 87, 636, 1995.
53. National Cancer Institute of Canada, *Canadian Cancer Statistics 1994*, NCIC, Toronto, 1994, 1.
54. Newberry, B. H., Gordon, T. L., and Meehan, S. M., Animal studies of stress and cancer, in *Cancer and Stress. Psychological, Biological and Coping Studies*, Cooper, C. L. and Watson, M., Eds., John Wiley & Sons, Chichester, England, 1991, 27.
55. Newberry, B. H., Liebelt, A. G., and Boyle, D. A., Variables in behavioral oncology: overview and assessment of current issues, in *Impact of Psychoendocrine Systems in Cancer and Immunity*, Fox, B. H. and Newberry, B. H., Eds., C.J. Hogrefe, Lewiston, NY, 1984.
56. Nieman, D. C. and Nehlsen-Cannarella, S. L., The effects of acute and chronic exercise on immunoglobulins, *Sports Med.*, 11, 183, 1991.
57. Paffenbarger, R. S., Jr., Hyde, R. T., and Wing, A. L., Physical activity and incidence of cancer in diverse populations: a preliminary report, *Am. J. Clin. Nutr.*, 45, 312, 1987.
58. Pate, R. R., Pratt, M., Blair, S. N., Haskell, W. L., Macera, C. A., Bouchard, C., Buchner, D., Ettinger, W., Heath, G. W., King, A. C., Kriska, A., Leon, A. S., Marcus, B. H., Morris, J., Paffenbarger, R. S., Patrick, K., Pollock, M. L., Rippe, J. M., Sallis, J., and Wilmore, J. H., Physical activity and public health, *J. Am. Med. Assoc.*, 273, 402, 1995.
59. Pedersen, B. K., Tvede, N., Hansen, F. R., Andersen, V., Bendix, T., Bendixen, G., Galbo, H., Haahr, P. M., Klarlund, K., Sylvest, J., Thomsen, B. S., and Halkjaer-Kristensen, J., Modulation of natural killer cell activity in peripheral blood by physical exercise, *Scand. J. Immunol.*, 27, 673, 1988.
60. Pedersen, B. K., Tvede, N., Klarlund, K., Christensen, L. D., Hansen, F. R., Galbo, H., Kharazmi, A., and Halkjaer-Kristensen, J., Indomethacin in vitro and in vivo abolishes post-exercise suppression of natural killer cell activity in peripheral blood, *Int. J. Sports Med.*, 11, 127, 1990.
61. Peters, R. K., Garabrant, D. H., Yu, M. C., and Mack, T. M., A case control study of occupational and dietry factors in colon rectal cancer in young men by subsite, *Cancer Res.*, 49, 5459, 1989.
62. Pollack, R. E., Babcock, G. F., Romsdahl, M. M., and Nishioka, K., Surgical stress-mediated suppression of murine natural killer cell cytotoxicity, *Cancer Res.*, 44, 3888, 1984.
63. Pollack, R. E. and Lotzová, E., Surgical-stress-related suppression of natural killer cell activity: a possible role in tumor metastasis, *Nat. Immununity Cell Growth Regul.*, 6, 269, 1987.
64. Potter, J. D., Slattery, M. L., Bostick, R. M., and Gapstur, S. M., Colon cancer: a review of the epidemiology, *Epidemiol. Rev.*, 15, 499, 1993.
65. Preston-Martin, S., Pike, M. C., Ross, R. K., Jones, P. A., and Henderson, B. E., Increased cell division as a cause of human cancer, *Cancer Res.*, 50, 7415, 1990.
66. Raddassi, K., Petit, J. F., and Lemaire, G., LPS-induced activation of primed murine peritoneal macrophages is modulated by prostaglandins and cyclic nucleotides, *Cell. Immunol.*, 149, 50, 1993.
67. Randall-Simpson, J. and Hoffman-Goetz, L., Exercise, serum zinc, and interleukin-1 concentrations in man: some methodological considerations, *Nutr. Res.*, 11, 309, 1991.

68. Rauramaa, R., Salonen, J. T., and Kukkonen-Harjula, K., Effects of mild physical exercise on serum lipoproteins and metabolites of arachidonic acid: a controlled trial in middle-aged men, *Br. Med. J.*, 288, 603, 1984.

69. Ravikumar, T., Rodrick, M., Steele, G., Jr., Marrazo, J., O'Dwyer, P., Dodson, T., and King, V., Interleukin generation in experimental colon cancer of rats: effects of tumor growth and tumor therapy, *J. Natl. Cancer Inst.*, 74, 893, 1985.

70. Reddy, B. S., Sugie, S., and Lowenfels, A., Effect of voluntary exercise on azoxymethane-induced colon carcinogenesis in male F344 rats, *Cancer Res.*, 48, 7079, 1988.

71. Rice, G. E. and Bevilacqua, M. P., An inducible endothelial cell surface glycoprotein mediates melanoma adhesion, *Science*, 246, 1303, 1989.

72. Rigas, B., Goldman, I. S., and Levine, L., Altered eicosanoid levels in human colon cancer, *J. Lab. Clin. Med.*, 122, 518, 1993.

73. Roebuck, B. D., McCaffrey, J., and Baumgartner, K. J., Protective effects of voluntary exercise during the postinitiation phase of pancreatic carcinogenesis in the rat, *Cancer Res.*, 50, 6811, 1990.

74. Rusch, H. P. and Kline, B. E., The effect of exercise on the growth of a mouse tumor, *Cancer Res.*, 4, 116, 1944.

75. Saba, T. M. and Antikatzides, T. G., Decreased resistance to intravenous tumor-cell challenge during reticuloendothelial depression following surgery, *Br. J. Cancer*, 34, 381, 1976.

76. Schlenker, E. D., Obesity and the lifespan, in *Nutrition, Physiology, and Obesity*, Schemmel, R., Ed., CRC Press, Boca Raton, FL, 1980, 151.

77. Schwartz, M. A., Signaling by integrins: implications for tumorigenesis, *Cancer Res.*, 53, 1503, 1993.

78. Severson, R. K., Nomura, A. M. Y., Grove, J. S., and Stemmermann, G. N., A prospective analysis of physical activity and cancer, *Am. J. Epidemiol.*, 130, 522, 1989.

79. Sklar, L. S. and Anisman, H., Stress and cancer, *Psych. Bull.*, 89, 369, 1981.

80. Sklar, L. S., Bruto, V., and Anisman, H., Adaptation to the tumor-enhancing effects of stress, *Psychosom. Med.*, 43, 331, 1981.

81. Slattery, M. L., Schumacher, M. C., Smith, K. R., West, D. W., and Abd-Elghany, N., Physical activity, diet, and risk of colon cancer in Utah, *Am. J. Epidemiol.*, 128, 989, 1988.

82. Smith, J. A., Telford, R. D., Baker, M. S., Hapel, A. J., and Weidemann, M. J., Cytokine immunoreactivity in plasma does not change after moderate endurance exercise, *J. Appl. Physiol.*, 73, 1396, 1992.

83. Stanbridge, E. J., Identifying tumor suppressor genes in human colorectal cancer, *Science*, 247, 12, 1989.

84. Steplewski, Z., Vogel, W. H., Ehya, H., Poropatich, C., and McDonald-Smith, J., Effects of restraint stress on innoculated tumor growth and immune response, *Cancer Res.*, 45, 5126, 1985.

85. Sternfeld, B., Cancer and the protective effect of physical activity: the epidemiological evidence, *Med. Sci. Sports Exerc.*, 24, 1195, 1992.

86. Stewart, T. H., Hollinshead, A. C., and Raman, S., Tumor dormancy: initiation, maintenance and termination in animals and humans, *Can. J. Surg.*, 34, 321, 1991.

87. Sugie, S., Reddy, B. S., Lowenfels, A., Tanaka, T., and Mori, H., Effect of voluntary exercise on azoxymethane-induced hepatocarcinogenesis in male F344 rats, *Cancer Lett.*, 63, 67, 1992.

88. Sutherland, W. H. F., Nye, E. R., Macfarlane, D. J., Robertson, M. C., and Williamson, S. A., Fecal bile acid concentration in distance runners, *Int. J. Sports Med.*, 12, 533, 1991.

89. Temoshok, L., Peeke, H. V. S., Mehard, C. W., Axelsson, K., and Sweet, D. M., Stress-behavior interactions in hamster tumor growth, *Ann. N.Y. Acad. Sci.*, 496, 501, 1987.

90. Thompson, H. J., Effect of exercise intensity and duration on the induction of mammary carcinogenesis, *Cancer Res.*, 54, 1960s, 1994.

91. Thompson, H. J., Ronan, A. M., Ritacco, K. A., Tagliaferro, A. R., and Meeker, L. D., Effect of exercise on the induction of mammary carcinogenesis, *Cancer Res.*, 48, 2720, 1988.

92. Thorling, E. B., Jacobsen, N. O., and Overvad, K., Effect of exercise on intestinal tumor development in the male Fischer rat after exposure to azoxymethane, *Eur. J. Cancer Prev.*, 2, 77, 1993.

93. Thorling, E. B., Jacobsen, N. O., and Overvad, K., The effect of treadmill exercise on azoxymethane-induced intestinal neoplasia in the male Fischer rat on two different high-fat diets, *Nutr. Cancer*, 22, 31, 1994.

94. Uhlenbrück, G. and Order, U., Can endurance sports stimulate immune mechanisms against cancer and metastasis?, *Int. J. Sports Med.*, 12, S53, 1991.

95. Ullum, H., Haahr, P. M., Diamant, M., Palmo, J., Halkjaer-Kristensen, J., Kjaer, M., Galbo, H., and Pedersen, B. K., Bicycle exercise enhances plasma IL-6 but does not change IL-1α, IL-1β, or TNFα- pre-mRNA in BMNC, *J. Appl. Physiol.*, 77, 93, 1994.

96. Vena, J. E., Graham, S., Zielezny, M., Swanson, M. K., Barnes, R. E., and Nolan, J., Lifetime occupational exercise and colon cancer, *Am. J. Epidemiol.*, 122, 357, 1985.

97. Vetter, R., Dosemeci, M., Blair, A., Wacholder, S., Unsal, M., Engin, K., and Fraumeni, J. F., Occupational physical activity and colon cancer risk in Turkey, *Eur. J. Epidemiol.*, 8, 845, 1992.

98. Vineis, P., Ciccone, G., and Magnino, A., Asbestos exposure, physical activity and colon cancer: a case-control study, *Tumori*, 19, 301, 1993.

99. Vogelstein, B., Fearon, E. R., Hamilton, S. R., Kern, S. E., Preisinger, A. C., Leppert, M., Nakamura, Y., White, R., Smits, A. M., and Bos, J. L., Genetic alterations during colorectal-tumor development, *New Engl. J. Med.*, 319, 525, 1988.

100. Walker, A. R. P., Walker, B. F., and Segal, I., Can the risk of colon cancer be lessened?, *Dig. Dis.*, 11, 325, 1993.

101. Waymack, J. P., Klimpel, G., Haithcoat, J., Rutan, R. J., and Herndon, D. N., Effect of prostaglandin E on immune function in normal healthy volunteers, *Surg. Gynecol. Obstet.*, 175, 329, 1992.

102. Whiteside, T. L., Letessier, E., Hirabayashi, H., Vitolo, D., Bryant, J., Barnmes, L., Snyderman, C., Johnson, J. T., Myers, E., Herbermann, R. B., Rubin, J., Kirkwood, J. M., and Vlock, D. R., Evidence for local and systemic activation of immune cells by peritoneum-oral injections of interleukin 2 in patients with advanced squamous cell carcinoma of the head and neck, *Cancer Res.*, 53, 5654, 1993.

103. Whittemore, A. S., Wu-Williams, A. H., Lee, M., Shu, Z., Gallagher, R. P., Deng-ao, J., Lun, Z., Xianghui, W., Kun, C., Jung, D., Teh, C.-Z., Chengde, L., Yao, X. J., Paffenberger, R. S., and Henderson, B. E., Diet, physical activity, and colorectal cancer among Chinese in North America and China, *J. Natl. Cancer Inst.*, 82, 915, 1990.

104. Woods, J. A., Davis, M. J., Mayer, E. P., Ghaffar, A., and Pate, R. R., Exercise increases inflammatory macrophage antitumor cytotoxicity, *J. Appl. Physiol.*, 75, 879, 1993.

105. Wu, A. H., Paganini-Hill, A., Ross, R. K., and Henderson, B. E., Alcohol, physical activity and other risk factors for colorectal cancer: a prospective study, *Br. J. Cancer*, 55, 687, 1987.

106. Yoshino, I., Yano, T., Murata, M., Ishida, T., Sugimachi, K., and Kimura, G., Tumor-reactive T-cells accumulate in lung cancer tissues but fail to respond due to tumor cell-derived factor, *Cancer Res.*, 52, 775, 1992.

107. Young, M. R. I., Eicosanoids and the immunology of cancer, *Cancer Metast. Rev.*, 13, 337, 1994.

108. Jadeski, L. and Hoffman-Goetz, L., Exercise and in vivo natural cytotoxicity against tumor cells of varying metastic capacity, *Clin. Exp. Metastasis*, 14 (2), in press.

Chapter 11

EXERCISE, IMMUNITY, AND AGING

Robert S. Mazzeo

CONTENTS

I. INTRODUCTION

Aging is associated with a functional decline in several components of the immune system.[17,29,34] As a result, the elderly are more vulnerable and are at greater risk for a variety of infectious diseases, tumorigenesis, and autoimmune disorders. Cell-mediated immune function is most adversely affected which is directly related to the well-documented involution of the thymus.[18,21,50] Consequently, total T cell numbers, subset distributions, and T cell responsiveness are compromised with aging. Additional age-related defects in immune function have been reported in cytokine production, receptor number and expression, signal transduction, antigen recognition, and cell differentiation and blastogenesis.[38,42,47,48,52]

Attempts to prevent and/or reverse this immunosenescence have yielded interesting results. Caloric restriction has been shown to prevent or delay dysfunctions of the immune system as determined by increased mitogen-induced proliferation, interleukin-2 (IL-2) induction and synthesis, cytotoxic

0-8493-8190-8/96/$0.00+$.50

T cell function, and greater percentage of T cells in spleen.[43,49,53,54] Dietary restriction has also been documented to lower tumor incidence associated with advancing age, improve immune responsiveness after inoculation with an infectious agent, and to reduce autoimmune disorders.[7,15,24] It has also been suggested that the improvement in immune function accounts, in part, for the increased longevity associated with caloric restriction.

Additionally, partial restoration of immune function has been observed from other techniques including thymic and bone marrow cell grafts,[19,20] administration of thymic hormones as well as IL-2, and the addition of calcium ionophores.[8,14,32,33,47,48]

Participation in a regular aerobic exercise program is well documented to reduce the onset and risk factors associated with a number of serious diseases associated with aging including coronary heart disease, diabetes, and cancer. The extent to which such an endurance training program may have a similar effect in altering the age-related decline in immune function is less understood. The major reason for this uncertainty is related to the scarcity of data in the literature addressing the issue of exercise and immune function in the elderly. A similar lack of knowledge also exists regarding the influence that a single bout of acute exercise has on immune function in this population. This has both physiological as well as clinical implications when one considers that an acute bout of exercise is known to be immunosuppressive and the elderly are at greater risk from infectious diseases. Thus, this chapter will review what is known regarding the interaction between exercise, training, and aging with special attention directed toward possible underlying neuroendocrine regulation.

II. ACUTE EXERCISE AND IMMUNE FUNCTION IN THE ELDERLY

It is generally agreed that an acute bout of exercise is immunosuppressive (for review see References 23, 26, and 37). Depending on the intensity and duration, this exercise-induced modulation of immune function can persist long into the recovery period. To date, however, the majority of these studies have been performed in young populations only, with very little information available regarding the response in the elderly (Table 1). How the elderly can respond and adapt to the stress imposed by an acute bout of exercise not only is important from a mechanistic standpoint, but also there are significant clinical implications because infectious diseases can be more debilitating in this age group and because acute exercise is immunosuppressive.

Fiatarone et al.[12] examined the effect of an acute bout of maximal cycling in young (30 ± 1 years) and old (71 ± 1 years) women. No differences between age groups were observed in baseline natural killer (NK) cell numbers and function in peripheral blood lymphocytes. In response to exercise NK cell activity increased significantly in both groups; however, no difference was

Table 1   Studies Examining the Influence of Age and Exercise on Immune Function

Species	Variables Measured	Condition	Change with Age	Ref.
		Acute Exercise		
Human	NK cell cytotoxic activity	Rest and acute exercise (treadmill walking)	↑ In activity after exercise	5
BALB/c mice	Proliferation (PHA) spleen and thymus	Rest and acute exercise (swim to exhaustion)	↓ With age and exercise	6
Human	NK cell cytotoxic activity	Rest and acute exercise (maximal bicycling)	No change with age or exercise	12
		Chronic Exercise		
Fischer 344 rat	Antibody production to specific antigen	Rest	↓ With age, no training effect	1
Human	NK cell cytotoxic activity	Rest and acute exercise	↑ With training at rest and after exercise compared to age-matched control	5
BALB/c mice	Proliferation (PHA) spleen and thymus	Rest and acute exercise	↓ With age, ↑ with training response to acute exercise	6

Table 1 (continued) Studies Examining the Influence of Age and Exercise on Immune Function

Species	Variables Measured	Condition	Change with Age	Ref.
Fischer 344 rat	Proliferation (Con A), IL-2 production, cytotoxicity (spleen)	Rest	↓ with age, ↓ with training in young and middle-aged but not old	35
Human	NK and T cell function function (blood lymphocytes)	Rest	No change after 12-week training but ↑ in highly trained age matched	36
Fischer 344 rat	Proliferation (Con A), IL-2 production (spleen)	Rest	↓ with age, ↓ with training in young and middle-aged but not old	40

Note: NK = natural killer cell, PHA = phytohemagglutinin, Con A = concanavalin A, IL-2 = interleukin-2.

observed between age groups. Thus, NK cell activity was enhanced immediately postexercise, as is generally reported in young populations; and the effect was similar in both age groups.

The response of NK cell activity in elderly women to acute exercise was also examined by Crist et al.[5] In addition, this study compared individuals who had participated in 16 weeks of aerobic training with age-matched sedentary controls (72 ± 1 years). Women participating in the training program demonstrated a 33% increase in baseline NK cell tumor cytotoxicity in peripheral blood lymphocytes when compared with age-matched sedentary controls. An acute bout of progressive treadmill exercise produced an increase in NK cell activity in both groups; however, the trained women achieved significantly greater values of NK cell activity compared to controls (50.3 vs. 31.1%, respectively). No comparisons were made with younger women of either training status.

When young and old BALB/c mice were required to swim until exhaustion (194 ± 28 min), spleen, thymus, and axillary node lymphocyte responsiveness to phytohemagglutinin (PHA) was suppressed in both groups.[6] However, it is of interest that while baseline responsiveness to mitogen was significantly lower in old vs. young mice (↓ 68% for splenocytes), the bout of exhaustive exercise had a greater immunosuppressive effect in the young (↓ 62% for splenocytes) when compared to the old (↓ 26% for splenocytes) mice.

Along this line, we have recently performed similar pilot experiments in human subjects to examine the influence of an acute bout of exercise on immune function. Peripheral blood lymphocyte numbers and percentages as well as responsiveness to PHA were studied in young (n = 6, 23 ± 2 years) and old (n = 7, 68 ± 3 years) male subjects both immediately prior to and after 20 min of supine bicycle ergometry at approximately 60% of maximal work capacity. As indicated in Figure 1, prior to exercise, responsiveness to PHA was significantly lower in old subjects when compared to the young. Immediately after the acute exercise stimulus, the PHA response was suppressed 22% in young subjects when compared to their preexercise values; however, similar to the findings for mice mentioned above,[6] the suppressive effect of exercise was attenuated in the old subjects (↓ 10%). Mechanisms responsible for this observation remain unknown, but may be related to the fact that baseline PHA responsiveness was already significantly reduced in the elderly subjects prior to exercise and thus a smaller margin existed for suppression. A more likely explanation pertains to the contribution as well as sensitivity to a number of neuroendocrine regulators released in response to the exercise stress which are known to be immunosuppressive (see discussion below). With advancing age, the responsiveness to these neuroendocrine regulators is significantly altered; and this may contribute to the attenuated immune responses observed during acute exercise in the elderly.

In these same subjects, we did not observe any age-related difference in the percentage of CD3+, CD4+, and CD19+ peripheral blood lymphocytes;

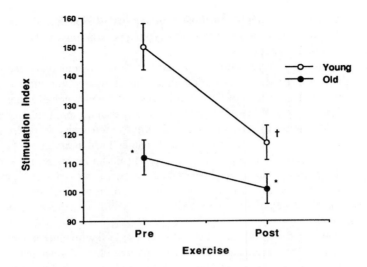

FIGURE 1   Stimulation index in young (23 ± 2 years) and old (68 ± 3 years) male subjects in response to PHA-induced stimulation of peripheral blood lymphocytes at rest and immediately after 20 min of supine cycling. * Significant difference between young and old. † Significant difference between pre- and postexercise ($p < 0.05$).

however, the percentage of CD8+ cells was significantly reduced in the old subjects. As total number of lymphocytes declined with age, this resulted in a lower number of cells expressing CD3+, CD4+, and CD8+ with age (Figure 2). These findings are consistent with the majority of literature examining T cell subsets as a function of age.[18,21,50] Total lymphocyte numbers as well as individual T cell subsets measured increased in response to the 20-min bout of submaximal exercise. This lymphocytosis, which is associated with an acute bout of exercise,[10,11,13,23,26] occurred to the same extent in both age groups, suggesting that the mechanisms responsible are unaffected by age.

III. CHRONIC EXERCISE AND IMMUNE FUNCTION IN THE ELDERLY

There have been very few studies examining the effect of endurance training in the elderly, and these primarily have examined the influence of training on baseline immune function only (Table 1). Two training studies involving human subjects are available. As cited above, Crist et al.[5] examined the influence of 16 weeks of aerobic training (3 d/week at 50% heart rate reserve) in elderly women. It was reported that, compared to age-matched sedentary controls, trained women demonstrated 33% increase in basal NK cell cytotoxic activity. Further, an incremental treadmill exercise test elicited a 32%

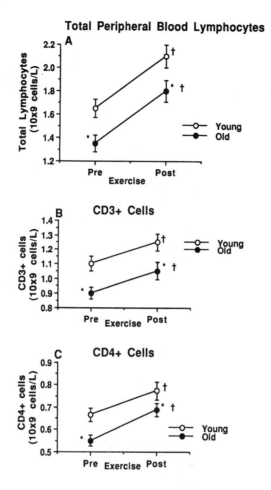

FIGURE 2 Total peripheral blood lymphocyte (A), CD3+ (B), and CD4+ (C) subpopulations at rest and immediately after 20 min of supine cycling in young and old subjects. * Significant difference between young and old. † Significant difference between pre- and postexercise ($p < 0.05$).

increase in NK cell activity in the control group, but a significantly greater increase in the trained women (↑ 50%). Thus, it was concluded that long-term aerobic training enhances NK cell-mediated cytotoxicity in elderly women.

However, Nieman et al.[36] have found that 12 weeks of moderate aerobic training (5 d/week at 60% heart rate reserve) had no effect on basal NK cell activity and T cell function (PHA responsiveness) in previously sedentary women (73 ± 1 years). These investigators did find that T cell function was significantly greater in a group of highly conditioned female endurance competitors (n = 12, 73 ± 2 years) when compared to age-matched sedentary controls, but remained below the level for young, sedentary women (n = 13, 22 ± 1 year). The mechanisms responsible for the differences in immune function between the moderately trained and highly conditioned women remain uncertain, but may be related to differences in the training intensity, duration, and frequency. Alternatively, the age at which exercise training is initiated may be a factor because the highly conditioned women had begun an exercise program earlier in life.

Results from animal studies allow for a more invasive approach (analysis of spleen, thymus, and axillary nodes). Unfortunately, as is the case with human experiments, very few studies exist which address the relationship between aging and endurance training on immune function.

Pahlavani et al.[40] investigated the role of exercise training on immunosenescence in male Fischer 344 rats. Rats of four different age groups (1, 6, 12, and 18 months of age, initially) were examined after a 6-month training program (swimming for 60 min, twice daily, 5 d/week). Interleukin-2 production and lymphocyte proliferation (both with concanavalin A [Con A] and lipopolysaccharide stimulation) were measured in isolated splenocytes. Unstimulated as well as mitogen-induced proliferation of lymphocytes in both trained (↓ 41%) and untrained (↓ 52%) rats declined significantly with increasing age. Con A-stimulated lymphocyte proliferation was significantly reduced with training in the 7- and 12-month-old rats (32 and 23%, respectively) when compared to age-matched control groups. However, in the 18- and 24-month-old rats, no differences were observed between groups. An age-related decline in IL-2 synthesis was observed in both the trained and the untrained rats. The 24-month-old rats from both groups exhibited significantly less IL-2 production than their younger counterparts. Training was associated with significantly lower IL-2 production when compared to controls, but only for the 7-month-old rats. It was concluded that exercise training did not prevent the age-related decline in lymphocyte proliferation as well as IL-2 production. Further, training had an adverse effect on mitogen-induced proliferation and for IL-2 production in the younger animals.

We have also measured immune function in endurance trained (15 weeks at 75% maximal running capacity) male Fischer 344 rats across age groups.[35] Con A-mediated lymphocyte proliferation, IL-2 production, and NK cell cytotoxicity were determined in splenocytes from 8-, 17-, and 27-month-old rats under resting conditions. Mitogen-induced proliferation and IL-2 production were found to decrease significantly with age in both trained and untrained animals. Training significantly reduced proliferation and IL-2 production in 8- and 17-month-old animals; however, these variables were found to increase in the 27-month group compared to age-matched controls. NK cell activity declined significantly with age, and training did not alter this response.

In an attempt to measure immune function *in vivo*, we have previously administered keyhole limpet hemocyanin ([KLH] a T cell-dependent antigen) in young and old Fischer 344 rats and determined antibody production 10 and

17 d thereafter.[1] KLH antibody production was found to be significantly reduced in old compared to young animals ($\downarrow$ 77%). Endurance training by treadmill running for 10 weeks did not improve this response in old animals.

Recent pilot studies from our laboratory have examined the influence of both age and training on lymphocyte subsets in young (7 months), middle-aged (15 months), and old (25 months) Fischer 344 rats. Training consisted of 12 weeks of treadmill running at 75% maximal capacity. Splenocyte subpopulations were determined by dual label flow cytometry (FACScan). When adjusted for spleen weights, total T cell numbers were lower for old animals regardless of training status (Figure 3). Training reduced T cell numbers for the young and middle-aged, but increased numbers in the old animals. As indicated in Figure 4, CD4+ and CD8+ T cells followed a similar pattern to that of total T cells such that percentages and numbers declined with age. Similarly, a reduction in CD4+ and CD8+ T cell numbers was observed with training for young ($\downarrow$ 25%) and middle-aged ($\downarrow$ 47%) animals, but increased in the old rats ($\uparrow$ 53%). These results indicate that splenocyte subpopulations are altered with age and training; however, a significant interaction was observed such that these immunological markers decreased with training in the younger groups, but increased in the old trained animals. This is similar to the findings reported previously from our laboratory on Con A-induced splenocyte proliferation and IL-2 production.[35] Further, the training-induced reduction in spleen weight observed may contribute to the diminished T cell numbers reported.

In the only study to examine the influence of endurance training on acute exercise in aged animals, De la Fuente et al.[6] measured mitogen-induced proliferative response in spleen, thymus, and axillary nodes from young (15 ± 2 weeks) and old (60 ± 5 weeks) BALB/c mice. In response to a swim until exhaustion, both young and old untrained mice demonstrated a suppressed proliferative response to PHA when compared to control mice that did not exercise. However, mice from both age groups that had been swim trained (90 min/d for 20 d) not only achieved greater proliferative responses than did the untrained mice after exhaustive swimmimg, but also had significantly greater values compared to the resting control mice. Thus, the acute bout of exercise was not immunosuppressive in the swim-trained group. This response was found to be greater in the young compared to the old animals.

IV. NEUROENDOCRINE REGULATION, IMMUNE FUNCTION, AND AGING

Evidence is emerging implicating a number of neuroendocrine factors to be associated with exercise-induced immunosuppression in young populations. When this observation is coupled with the growing body of literature suggesting neuroendocrine alterations/insensitivity affiliated with aging, an extremely intriguing relationship between exercise, aging, and immune function becomes apparent.

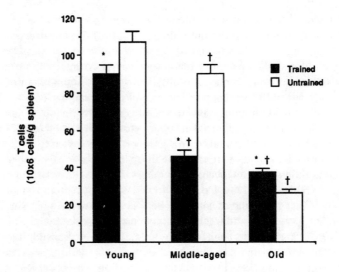

FIGURE 3   The influence of 12 weeks of endurance training on total T cell numbers from spleen in young (7 months), middle-aged (15 months) and old (25 months) male Fischer 344 rats. * Significant aging effect . † Significant training effect ($p < 0.05$).

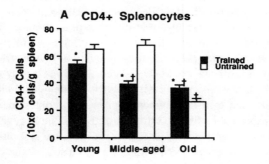

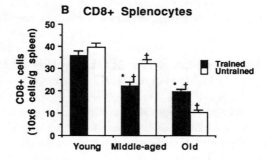

FIGURE 4   Number of CD4+ (A) and CD8+ (B) cells from spleen in Fischer 344 rats across age and training status. * Significant aging effect . † Significant training effect ($p < 0.05$)

An acute bout of exercise is a stressor that elicits a number of neuroendocrine responses which help the individual to adjust, both physiologically and metabolically, to the exercise-induced disruptions in homeostasis. These same neuroendocrine responses are now believed to play a central role in modulating immune function during exercise. Sympathetic nerve and adrenal medullary activity increases progressively as a function of exercise intensity leading to an exponential rise in circulating catecholamines. Additionally, direct stimulation of sympathetic nerves innervating the spleen also contributes to the immunomodulation associated with acute exercise. In general, the sympathoadrenal responses to exercise have been shown to play a role in modulating exercise-induced changes in immune function including leukocytosis and lymphocytosis from lung and splenic reservoirs; alterations in lymphocyte subsets (numbers and percentages), as well as redistribution of lymphocytes that differ in their beta-adrenergic receptor number; and changes in NK cell cytotoxic activity, number, and function.[13,22,23,28] These responses can also be elicited by the infusion of epinephrine, norepinephrine, and isoproterenol in the resting state but using concentrations similar to those found during exercise.[51] The observation that beta-blockade prevents a number of these exercise-related responses suggests beta-receptor regulation.[22,23] Additionally, beta-receptor function (and associated signal transduction) on circulating lymphocytes can be directly stimulated by the catecholamines resulting in an inhibition of both T and B cell proliferative capacity.[3,4,28,46] During recovery from a strenuous bout of acute exercise, beta-receptor density and responsiveness of lymphocytes are significantly increased in human subjects which contribute to the immunosuppression observed during this period.[3,4] Endurance training can result in down-regulation of the beta-receptors located on lymphocytes thereby making them less responsive to catecholamine stimulation.[4] This may, in part, account for the reduction in immunosuppression associated with acute exercise reported to occur with endurance training.

Corticosteroids are also known to suppress immune function as demonstrated by a reduction in T lymphocyte proliferation, production of IL-2 and mRNA synthesis for IL-2, and diminished IL-2 receptor expression.[11,16,23,44] Plasma corticosteroid concentrations increase as a function of the intensity and duration of exercise. Elevation of plasma corticosteroid levels has been shown to be directly involved in the exercised-induced suppression of T cell proliferation associated with acute physical activity. This is further supported by the observation that administration of a corticosteroid inhibitor, aminoglutethimide, was able to block the suppression of T cell proliferation induced by exercise in the rat.[11]

Recent evidence has suggested a regulatory role for prostaglandins, in particular prostaglandin E_2 (PGE$_2$), produced and released by monocytes and neutrophils, on immune function during exercise.[22,27,41] Mitogen-induced T cell responsiveness as well as B lymphocyte proliferation is inhibited by the addition of physiological concentrations of PGE$_2$. Prostaglandins also suppress lymphokine production and induce nonspecific suppressor–T cell activity. In response to stress, PGE_2 has been shown to contribute to the down-regulation observed for NK cell cytotoxic activity. The suppression of NK cell function documented to occur during the postexercise recovery period also appears to be related to PGE_2 mechanisms.[22,27,41] The addition of indomethacin, a prostaglandin inhibitor, can prevent the postexercise suppression of NK cell activity. Interestingly, Mahan and Young[27] have provided evidence to suggest that the training-induced improvement in immune function in response to acute exercise is mediated, in part, via PGE_2 mechanisms. In response to an exhaustive bout of swimming, splenocytes from untrained rats were more sensitive to the suppressive effect of PGE_2 than from nonexercised controls; however, trained animals demonstrated an insensitivity to the suppressive effects of PGE_2 resulting in a lesser degree of lymphocyte suppressive activity postexercise.

It is clear that the neuroendocrine system plays a critical role in modulating immune function in response to both an acute bout as well as a chronic endurance exercise in young populations. However, the aging process is associated with functional declines in many facets of the neuroendocrine system including alterations in receptor number, density, and affinity; diminished receptor responsiveness; and various components of signal transduction as well as a reduction in the ability to synthesize and release hormones and neurotransmitters. Consequently, elderly individuals are likely to respond differently to both acute and chronic exercise stimulation. Specifically, age-related changes exist in overall catecholamine metabolism and receptor responsiveness, tissue-specific sympathetic nerve activity, stress-induced corticosteroid production and effectiveness, and sensitivity to PGE_2, including T lymphocytes.[25,30,31,39,45]

While the sympathoadrenal responses to acute exercise are similar, for the most part, between young and old individuals, the elderly are less responsive for a given amount of stimulation as measured by cardiovascular and biochemical reactions.[25,30,31] With regard to immune function, an age-related decline in functional sympathetic nerve terminals in the spleen has been directly associated with the immunosenescence of T lymphocytes (T-dependent antigen challenge), suggesting a causal relationship between these variables.[2,9] It is unknown, however, to what extent that this observation influences exercise-induced immune function in the elderly. We have previously reported a decline in norepinephrine content in the spleen with age in Fischer 344 rats which correlated with the age-related immunosenescence.

Growth hormone production, as determined by pulse frequency and amplitude, declines significantly with advancing age. The physiological implications associated with this age-related decline in growth hormone response include reductions in the ability for protein synthesis and maintenance of cell homeostasis, as well as in liver and immune function.[31,45] This is further supported by the observation that administration of growth hormone to aged rats restores thymic structure and size, increases thymic hormone production, and spleen weight. This results in direct improvement in immune function as measured by increases in T cell proliferation and IL-2 production in old rats.

V. CONCLUSIONS

In summary, the evidence to date suggests that (1) an acute bout of exercise is a stressor that modulates many aspects of immune function; (2) endurance training can alter both basal and exercise-induced immune responsiveness; and (3) immune function, primarily T cell-mediated events, decline significantly with advancing age. Unfortunately, very little is known regarding the interaction between acute exercise, training, and aging. Additionally, the mechanisms responsible for the exercise-induced alterations in immune function, the extent to which neuroendocrine regulation contributes to these responses, and the determination of whether young and elderly individuals respond equally to these regulatory factors remain to be discovered.

ACKNOWLEDGMENTS

Data pertaining to immune function in young and old human subjects were collected at the Baker Medical Research Institute, Melbourne, Australia, in collaboration with Drs. Murray Esler and C. Rajkumar. T cell subsets in Fischer 344 rats were determined with the assistance of Dr. Monica Fleshner, University of Colorado, Boulder, CO.

REFERENCES

1. Barnes, C. A., Forster, M. J., Fleshner, M., Ahanotu, E. N., Laudenslager, M. L., Mazzeo, R. S., Maier, S. F., and Lal, H., Exercise does not modify spatial memory, brain autoimmunity, or antibody response in aged F-344 rats, *Neurobiol. Aging*, 12, 47, 1991.
2. Bellinger, D. L., Ackerman, K. D., Felten, S. Y., and Felten, D. L., A longitudinal study of age-related loss of noradrenergic nerves and lymphoid cells in the rat spleen, *Exp. Neurol.*, 116, 295, 1992.
3. Butler, J., Kelly, J. G., O'Malley, K., and Pidgeon, F., β-Adrenoceptor adaptation to acute exercise, *J. Physiol. (London)*, 344, 113, 1983.
4. Butler, J., O'Brien, J., and Pidgeon, F., Relationship of β-adrenoreceptor density to fitness in athletes, *Nature (London)*, 298, 60, 1982.
5. Crist, D. M., MacKinnon, L. T., Thompson, R. F., Atterborn, H. A., and Egan, P. A., Physical exercise increases natural cellular-mediated tumor cytoxicity in elderly women, *Gerontolology*, 35, 66, 1989.
6. De la Fuente, M., Ferrandez, M. D., Miquel, J., and Hernanz, A., Changes with aging and physical activity in ascorbic acid content and prolieative response of murine lymphocytes, *Mech. Aging Dev.*, 65, 177, 1992.

7. Effros, R. B., Walford, R. L., Weindruch, R., and Mitcheltree, C., Influence of dietary restriction on immunity to influenza in aged mice, *L. Gerontol.*, 46, B142, 1991.

8. Fagiolo, U., Amadori, A., Borghesan, F., Zamarchi, R., Veronese, M. L., De Silvestro, G., Passarella, E., and Crepaldi, G., Immune dysfunction in the elderly: effect of thymic hormone administration on several in vivo and in vitro immune function parameters, *Aging*, 2, 347, 1990.

9. Felten, S. Y., Bellinger, D. L., Collier, T. J., Coleman, P. D., and Felten, D. L., Decreased sympathetic innervation of spleen in aged Fischer 344 rats, *Neurobiol. Aging*, 8, 159, 1987.

10. Ferry, A., Picard, F., Duvallet, A., Weill, B., and Rieu, M., Changes in blood leukocyte populations induced by acute maximal and chronic submaximal exercise, *Eur. J. Appl. Physiol.*, 59, 435, 1990.

11. Ferry, A., Weill, B. L., and Rieu, M., Immunomodulations induced in rats by exercise on a treadmill, *J. Appl. Physiol.*, 69, 1912, 1990.

12. Fiatarone, M. A., Morley, J. E., Bloom, E. T., Benton, D., Solomon, G. F., and Makinodan, T., The effect of exercise on natural killer cell activity in young and old subjects, *J. Gerontol.*, 44, m37, 1989.

13. Foster, N. K., Martyn, J. B., Rangno, R. E., Hogg, J. C., and Pardy, R. L., Leukocytosis of exercise: role of cardiac output and catecholamines, *J. Appl. Physiol.*, 61, 2218, 1986.

14. Frasca, D., Adorini, L., Mancini, C., et al., Reconstruction of T-cell functions in aging mice by thymosin alpha one, *Immunopharmacology*, 11, 155, 1986.

15. Gilman-Sachs, A., Kim, Y. B., Pollard, M., and Snyder, D. L., Influence of aging, environmental antigens, and dietary restriction on expression of lymphocyte subsets in germ-free and conventional Lobound-Wistar rats, *J. Gerontol.*, 46, B101, 1991.

16. Goodwin, J. S., Atluru, D., Sierakowski, S., and Lianos, E. A., Mechanism of action of glucocorticoids. Inhibition of T cell proliferation and interleukin 2 production by hydrocortisone is reversed by leukotriene B4, *J. Clin. Invest.*, 77, 1244, 1986.

17. Hausman, P. B. and Weksler, M. E., Changes in the immune response with age, in *Handbook Biology of Aging*, Finch, C. E. and Schneider, E. L., Eds., Van Nostrand Reinhold, New York, 1985, 414.

18. Hirokawa, K. and Makinodan, T., Thymic involution: effect on T cell differentiation, *J. Immunol.*, 114, 1659, 1975.

19. Hirokawa, K., Sato, K., and Makinodan, T., Influence of age of thymic grafts on the differentiation of T cells in nude mice, *Clin. Immunol. Immunopathol.*, 24, 251, 1982.

20. Hirokawa, K. and Utsuyama, M., Combined grafting of bone marrow and thymus, and sequential multiple thymus graftings in various strains of mice. The effect on immune functions and life span, *Mech. Aging Dev.*, 49, 49, 1989.

21. Hirokawa, K., Utsuyama, M., and Kasai, M., Role of the thymus in aging of the immune system, in *Biomedical Advances in Aging*, Goldstein, A. L., Ed., Plenum Press, 1990, 375.

22. Kappel, M., Tvede, N., Galbo, H., Haahr, P. M., Kjaer, M., Linstow, M., Klarlund, K., and Pedersen, B. K., Evidence that the effect of physical exercise on NK cell activity is mediated by epinephrine, *J. Appl. Physiol.*, 70, 2530, 1991.

23. Keast, D., Cameron, K., and Morton, A. R., Exercise and the immune response, *Sports Med.*, 5, 248, 1988.

24. Kubo, C., Day, N. K., and Good, R. A., Influence of early or late dietary restriction on life span and immunological parameters in MRL/Mp-Ipr/Ipr mice, *Proc. Natl. Acad. Sci.*, 81, 5831, 1984.

25. Lakatta, E. G., Age-related alterations in the cardiovascular responses to adrenergic mediated stress, *Fed. Proc.*, 39, 3173, 1980.

26. MacKinnon, L. T. and Tomasi, T. B., Immunology of exercise, in *Sports Med. Fitness, Training, Injuries*, Urban & Schwarzenberg, Baltimore, MD, 1988, 30, 273.

27. Mahan, M. P. and Young, M. R., Immune parameters of untrained or exercise-trained rats after exhaustive exercise, *J. Appl. Physiol.*, 66, 282, 1989.

28. Maki, T., Density and functioning of human lymphocytic β-adrenergic receptors during prolonged physical exercise, *Acta Physiol. Scand.*, 136, 569, 1989.

29. Makinodan, T. and Kay, M. M. B., Age influence on the immune system, *Adv. Immunol.*, 29, 87, 1980.

30. Mazzeo, R. S. and Horvath, S. M., A decline in myocardial and hepatic norepinephrine turnover with age in Fischer 344 rats, *Am. J. Phyiol.*, 252, E762, 1987.

31. Meites, J., Neuroendocrine biomarkers of aging in the rat, *Exp. Gerontol.*, 23, 349, 1988.

32. Miller, R. A., Immunodeficiency of aging: restorative effects of phorbol ester combined with calcium ionophore, *J. Immunol.*, 137, 805, 1986.

33. Miller, R. A., Jacobson, B., Weil, G., and Simons, E. R., Diminished calcium influx in lectin-stimulated T cells from old mice, *J. Cell Physiol.*, 132, 337, 1987.

34. Miller, R. A., The cell biology of aging: immunological models, *J. Gerontol.*, 44, B4, 1989.

35. Nasrullah, I. and Mazzeo, R. S., Age-related immunosenescence in Fischer 344 rats: influence of exercise training, *J. Appl. Physiol.*, 73, 1932, 1992.

36. Nieman, D. C., Henson, D. A., Gusewitch, G., Warren, B. J., Dotson, R. C., Butterworth, D. E., and Nehlsen-Cannarella, S. L., Physical activity and immune function in elderly women, *Med. Sci. Sports Exerc.*, 25, 823, 1993.

37. Nieman, D. C. and Nehlsen-Cannarella, S. L., The immune response to exercise, *Semin. Hematol.*, 31, 166, 1994.

38. Nordin, A. A. and Proust, J. J., Signal transduction mechanisms in the immune system: potential implication in immunosenescence, *Endocrinol. Metab. Clinics*, 16, 919, 1987.

39. Odio, M. and Brodish, A., Decreased plasticity of glucoregulatory responses in aged rats: effects of chronic stress, *J. Gerontol.*, 46, B188, 1991.

40. Pahlavani, M. A., Cheung, T. H., Cheskey, J. A., and Richardson, A., Influence of exercise on the immune function of rats at various ages, *J. Appl. Physiol.*, 64, 1997, 1988.

41. Pedersen, B. K., Influence of physical activity on the cellular immune system: mechanisms of action, *Int. J. Sports Med.*, 12, S23, 1991.

42. Proust, J. J., Filburn, C. R., Harrison, S. A., Buchholz, M. A., and Nordin, A. A., Age-related defect in signal transduction during lectin activation of murine T lymphocytes, *J. Immunol.*, 139, 1472, 1987.

43. Richardson, A. and Cheung, H. T., The relationship between age-related changes in gene expression, protein turnover, and the responsiveness of an organism to stimuli, *Life Sci.*, 31, 605, 1984.

44. Smith, K. A., Crabtree, G. R., Kenned, S. J., and Munick, A. V., Glucocorticoid receptors and glucocorticoid sensitivity of mitogen stimulated and unstimulated human lymphocytes, *Nature* (*London*), 267, 523, 1977.

45. Sonntag, W. E., Hormone secretion and action in aging animals and man, *Rev. Biol. Res. Aging*, 3, 299, 1987.

46. Strom, T. B., Lundin, A. P., and Carpenter, C. B., The role of cyclic nucleotides in lymphocyte activation and function, *Prog. Clin. Immunol.*, 3, 115, 1977.

47. Thoman, M. L. and Weigle, W. O., Reconstitution of in vivo cell-mediated lympholysis responses in aged mice with interleukin 2, *J. Immunol.*, 134, 949, 1985.

48. Thoman, M. L. and Weigle, W. O., Partial restoration of Con A-induced proliferation, IL-2 receptor expression, and IL-2 synthesis in aged murine lymphocytes by phorbol myristate acetate and ionomycin, *Cell Immunol.*, 114, 1, 1988.

49. Umezawa, M., Hanada, K., Naiki, H., Chen, W., Hosokawa, M., Hosono, M., Hosokawa, T., and Takeda, T., Effects of dietary restriction on age-related immune dysfunction in the senescence accelerated mouse (SAM), *J. Nutri.*, 120, 1393, 1990.

50. Utsuyama, M., Kasai, M., Kurashima, C., and Hirokawa, K., Age influence on the thymic capacity to promote differentiation of T cells: induction of different composition of T cell subsets by aging thymus, *Mech. Aging Dev.*, 58, 267, 1991.

51. Van Tits, L. J. H., Michel, M. C., Grosse-Wilde, H., Happel, M., Eigler, F. W., Soliman, A., and Brodde, O. E., Catecholamines increase lymphocyte β_2-adrenergic receptors via a β_2-adrenergic, spleen-dependent process, *Am. J. Physiol.*, 258, E191, 1990.
52. Vie, H. and Miller, R. A., Decline, with age, in the proportion of mouse T cells that express IL-2 receptors after mitogen stimulation, *Mech. Aging Dev.*, 33, 313, 1986.
53. Weindruch, R., Kristie, J. A., Naeim, F., Mullen, B., and Walford, R. L., Influence of weaning-initiated dietary restriction on response to T cell mitogens and on splenic T cell levels in a long-lived mouse hybrid, *Exp. Gerontol.*, 17, 49, 1982.
54. Weindruch, R., Gottesman, S. R. S., and Walford, R. L., Modification of age-related immune decline in mice dietarily restricted from or after midadulthood, *Proc. Natl. Acad. Sci.*, 79, 898, 1982.

Chapter **12**

SUBSTANCE ABUSE, EXERCISE, AND IMMUNITY

Sally E. Blank
Gary G. Meadows

CONTENTS

I. INTRODUCTION

Substance abuse is a national problem that affects health care, social systems, and the economy. Alcohol abuse alone is attributed to 100,000 deaths per year and $86 billion in health care and related costs in the U.S.[3] Substance abuse has no economic, social, racial, ethnic, or gender barriers. Modulation of the immune response by alcohol, tobacco, marijuana, cocaine, anabolic steroids, and other drugs of abuse has been actively studied for decades. Each of these drugs has been researched in clinical settings and in laboratories using animal models. Often clinical studies are complicated by multiple drug use, malnourishment, and disease in human subjects.[36,53] Animal models may control for some complications presented in clinical studies, but animal models of substance abuse may not be directly applicable to human subjects if drug metabolism or species-specific responses to drugs differ from that of human subjects. With the exception of research on alcohol consumption, few studies incorporate exercise stress into research designs on immunomodulation by drugs of abuse. Popular opinion and limited epidemiological evidence may lead one to conclude that an inverse relationship exists between frequency of substance abuse and exercise volume (i.e., intensity, duration, and frequency). However, those who regularly engage in physical activity are not exempt from drug addiction or substance abuse. Cocaine has been considered by some as a possible ergogenic aid to enhance physical performance. Too frequently athletic celebrities acknowledge drug addiction. Drug-related deaths of athletes are often portrayed with ironic surprise in the media. The cardiotoxic effects of cocaine and alcohol abuse are well known. Physically active individuals who combine cocaine and other drug use may be at increased risk of fatigue and cardiotoxicity during exercise stress.[21,22] At least 12 million people in the U.S. are estimated to concurrently use cocaine and ethanol.[36]

A significant percentage of the physically active population engages in substance abuse and by doing so may be more inclined for increased risk-taking behavior.[84] These individuals often have a higher incidence of injury, illness, exposure to infectious diseases, and death.[84] In light of the fact that up to 55% of the physically active population engages in substance abuse,[12,74,84] further study of the immunomodulatory implications of exercise stress and substance abuse is warranted.

There is a paucity of research on the impact of substance abuse and exercise stress on the immune response. This review will highlight modulation of natural killer (NK) cells by alcohol abuse and chronic exercise stress. The incidence of substance abuse and the immunomodulatory effects of alcohol, tobacco, marijuana, cocaine, and anabolic steroids are included. Concluding remarks will address the likelihood that exercise stress can attenuate the immunomodulatory effects of substance abuse.

II. SUBSTANCE ABUSE AND RELATED HEALTH PROBLEMS

A. ALCOHOL ABUSE

Alcohol consumption in the U.S. is estimated by the apparent per capita consumption. Alcohol intake is determined relative to the total population aged

14 years and older. There has been a slow progressive decrease in alcohol consumption from 1979 to 1987. The per capita consumption fell from 2.8 to 2.4 gallons of pure ethanol over the 8-year period along with an increasing trend for alcohol abstainers.[3]

Chronic abuse of alcohol is directly related to an increased mortality rate from numerous cardiovascular and hepatic anomalies including alcoholic cardiomyopathy, alcoholic cirrhosis of the liver, and acute alcoholic hepatitis. At least 5 to 75% of malignant cancers of the stomach, head and neck, and liver are indirectly linked to alcohol abuse.[3] Approximately 42 to 46% of alcohol-related deaths are attributed to motor vehicle and nontraffic accidents and to homicide with intent to injure.[3] Alcohol was the drug most used by high-school seniors in 1990, with 90% response rate compared with 64% who tried cigarettes. Heavy binge drinking is more common among college students (41%) than their nonstudent peers (33%), the latter who tend to have higher daily alcohol usage (4.9 vs 3.8%, respectively).[3]

1. Alcohol Abuse and Immunity

Alcohol is a widely investigated immunomodulator (Table 1). Both acute and chronic exposure to excessive alcohol may be immunomodulatory. Assessing the impact of alcohol intake and other drugs of abuse on immune function in human subjects is complicated by factors such as nutritional status, stress, depression, and other drug use.[29,44,47,53] Animal models of alcohol intake do not always reflect realistic patterns of human subjects. Additionally, metabolism of alcohol varies among species.[24,25,52] Commonalties of research findings across alcohol studies indicate that cellular number and function within the immune system can be directly altered by excessive acute and chronic alcohol intake.[53] Moreover, alcohol-mediated changes in psychological and neuroendocrine regulation can indirectly modulate cells of the immune system.[45]

Often immunological abnormalities are not observed in healthy, well-nourished, abstinent alcoholics.[53] However, alcoholics without clinical liver disease are reported to have increased percentages of activated CD8+ cells, and decreased percentages of CD4+, CD45RA+, and CD8hi/ CD45RA+ cells. Normal phenotype may be restored after alcohol withdrawal.[23] The clinical impact would be selective T cell expansion toward cytotoxic T cells vs. regulatory T cells.[23] The percentage of natural killer (NK) cells and *in vitro* NK cell cytolytic activity may be reduced or unchanged in chronic alcohol abusers.[57,70,71]

Alcohol impairs lymphocyte mitogenesis to concanavalin A (Con A),[67] antibody production by antigen-stimulated B lymphocytes,[4] and macrophage-induced antigen-specific proliferation of T cells.[80] Alcoholics with liver disease have increased serum concentrations of interleukin-1 (IL-1), IL-6, and IL-8. The incidence of elevated cytokine concentration in the blood is associated with the progression of alcoholic liver disease.[56] *In vitro* exposure to alcohol decreases stimulated macrophage production of IL-1β and IL-6, but increases transforming

TABLE 1   Drug-Related Immunomodulation

Chronic Substance Abuse	Cell-Mediated Immunity	Humoral Immunity	Cytokine Produccution and Proliferative Responses
Alcohol	↑ %CD8+ ↓ %CD4+[23] ↑↓ % NK cells[57] ↑↓ NK cell activity[57,70,71]	↓ B cell response to antigen[4]	↓ IL-1β,IL-6[80] ↑ TGFβ[80] ↑ TNF[10] ↑ IL-8[10] ↓ T cell proliferative response[67,80]
Tobacco	↑ Alveolar macrophage number[38] ↓ NK cell cytolytic activity[30,42] ↑ Circulating T cells[42]	↓ B cell responses[77] ↓ Salivary and serum IgA[8,30] ↑ Salivary IgM[8] ↑ Bronchoalveolar IgG and ↓ serum IgG[8,30] ↑ Serum IgE and IgD[8,42]	↑ Or ↓ Proliferation of Tcells[42]
Marijuana (see text for interpretation)	↓ NK and T cell cytolytic activities[16,78] ↓ Alveolar macrophage activation and number[17,54]	↓ Serum IgG and ↑ IgD concentrations[60,87]	↓ IL-1 secretion and ↓ IFNγ secretion[87] ↓ Proliferation of T cells to PHA and Con A[60,61,64]
Cocaine	↑ Or ↓ NK cell cytolytic activity[63,83,88]	↓ PFC response[88]	↓ IL-4, IL-2, IL-10, IL-5, IFN production[85] ↓ B cell proliferative response[88] ↑ Or ↓ T cell proliferative response[48]
Anabolic–androgenic steroids and resistive exercise[18]	↑ NK cell cytolytic activity	↓ Serum IgA and IgM concentrations	↑ B cell proliferative response compared to controls

Note: ↑ Increased or stimulated compared to controls; ↓ decreased or inhibited compared to controls.

growth factor beta (TGFβ), and prostaglandin E_2 production by macrophages which is associated with decreased antigen-specific T cell proliferation.[80] Alcoholic hepatitis is linked to increased serum concentrations of tumor necrosis factor (TNF). Increased circulating concentrations of TNF may induce production of IL-8 which is related to peripheral neutrophilia and hepatic accumulation of neutrophils.[10] The pervasive suppression of immune function of alcohol is a primary cause of morbidity and mortality in alcohol abusers.[58] Suppressed immune function and high-risk sexual activity also place alcohol abusers at increased risk of exposure to human immunodeficiency virus (HIV).[91] Acute alcohol intake has been linked to increased *in vitro* HIV replication in peripheral blood mononuclear cells from human subjects.[7]

Alcohol Abuse, Exercise Stress, and Natural Killer Cells

There is no evidence that regular physical activity can restore impaired immune function in substance abusers. In fact, studies on substance abuse, exercise, and immunity are rare. Over the last 6 years, Blank and Meadows[57] have investigated the influence of chronic alcohol intake and moderate intensity endurance exercise on natural immunity. In the absence of exercise, continuous daily intake of at least 20 g of ethanol per kilogram of body weight significantly reduces NK cell cytolytic activity in female C57BL/6 mice given 20% w/v ethanol as the sole fluid source.[57] Cytolytic activity is reduced within 24 h of ethanol exposure and remains suppressed concurrent with ethanol intake.[57] In this model, lymphocyte subsets in peripheral blood and the spleen are selectively modulated over time by ethanol. The loss of the predominate cytolytically active subset of NK cells, the NK1.1+/LGL-1+ cells,[55] is present in the spleen but not in peripheral blood within 4 weeks of the onset of ethanol intake. Loss of the percentage of NK1.1+/LGL-1+ cells from the blood occurs by 8 to 10 weeks of ethanol exposure.[14] The CD8+ population is also reduced in both the blood and the spleen with long-term (8 to 10 weeks) ethanol consumption.[14] Chronic exercise protects against the loss of CD8+ cells in both body compartments.[14] Ethanol can act on NK cells by several mechanisms. Ethanol intake reduces the cytolytic activity of individual NK1.1+ cells as demonstrated by *in vitro* assays of highly enriched (approximately 90% NK1.1+) NK cells from mice given ethanol for 2 weeks.[33] The percentages of splenic and circulating NK1.1+ cells are not altered in mice at this time. With longer term exposure to ethanol, NK cell cytolytic activity is also influenced by the loss of NK1.1+ cells in several body compartments.

Despite evidence that forced treadmill endurance training enhances the clearance of ethanol from the blood in rested rats,[5] mice do not demonstrate a protective effect of chronic exercise against the deleterious effects of chronic ethanol intake on NK cells. Ethanol-consuming mice are capable of sustaining training regimes consisting of forced treadmill running at 12 m/min, 60 min/day, 5 d/week for 10 weeks. A 25% increase in maximal citrate synthase activity of the quadriceps femoris muscle is indicative of metabolic adaptation to endurance training.[13] Following training, splenic NK cell activity is reduced in ethanol-consuming mice by approximately 40% compared with water-drinking sedentary controls.[13] Moderate intensity endurance training does not attenuate the loss of NK1.1+/LGL-1+ cells associated with ethanol intake.[14] The results of these experiments indicate that training-induced adaptations in skeletal muscle oxidative capacity occur in mice having ethanol-related impairment of splenic NK cell activity. Therefore, individuals who abuse alcohol may be capable of engaging in aerobic exercise programs and demonstrate certain expected cardiovascular and skeletal muscle metabolic adaptations to chronic exercise. However, these beneficial adaptations may occur independently of positive modulation of natural immunity by regular endurance-type exercise.

The biological implications of these findings suggest that in the alcohol abuser, chronic endurance-type exercise cannot restore the functional capacity of NK cells or enhance NK cell surveillance. In such cases, the stress of exercise cannot be considered a "eustress" which attenuates the "distressful" consequences of chronic alcohol intake on NK cell function.

B. TOBACCO ABUSE

Initial exposure to tobacco occurs before most Americans reach the age of 18 years.[28] Of the 3 million plus adolescents who smoke, most are addicted to nicotine.[28] Smokeless tobacco consumption is increasing in popularity, particularly among adolescents and young adult males.[34,74] In 1986, over 10 million individuals in the U.S. used smokeless tobacco, one third of which were under 21 years old.[1] A recent report indicated that smokeless tobacco use may be as high as 55% in physically active populations including professional baseball players.[74] In nonalcoholics, cigarette smoking is positively associated with drinking alcohol and approximately 90% of alcohol abusers also use tobacco.[15] A recent survey of college students in Virginia indicated that almost one quarter of the students smoked tobacco for at least 1 year. Smoking was positively linked to recent alcohol binge drinking and use of illegal drugs such as marijuana and cocaine in the previous year.[1] Cigarette smoking is directly linked to increased risk of lung cancer, coronary heart disease, hypertension, and respiratory illnesses.[68,86] Risk of cancer is increased with combined alcohol and tobacco use.[59,72,82,90] Smokeless tobacco use is related to increased risk of gingival recession, oral leukoplakia, oral cancer, and cardiovascular dysfunction, among others.[34,74] Denial of the susceptibility for increased risk for fatal diseases is common among tobacco users. Adolescents and young adult smokers surveyed about their estimates of general susceptibility to fatal and nonfatal diseases generally denied susceptibility to increased risk. Older smokers (>14 years) thought that life-long smoking would increase their risk of nonfatal respiratory dysfunction, such as breathlessness; however, none of the smokers acknowledged increased risk for cancer and heart disease.[37]

1. Tobacco Use and Immunity

Cigarette smoking is often linked to immunosuppression. Due to the interaction of tobacco use with alcohol use, stress, and other complicating factors, assessment of the independent effects of tobacco on *in vivo* immunomodulation is difficult to determine.[2] In particular, cigarette smoking affects mucosal immune function (Table 1). Alveolar macrophage number may increase in lungs exposed to cigarette smoke. [38] Smokers are reported to have reduced salivary immunoglobulin A (IgA) and increased IgM concentrations whereas in bronchoalveolar lavage fluid, a compensatory increase in IgG concentration may be present in smokers compared to nonsmokers.[8] Heavy drinking increases sIgA concentrations and may mask the modulatory effects of cigarette smoking on salivary immunoglobulin concentrations.[8] Circulating immune parameters are also affected by cigarette smoking and may include increased polymorphonuclear neutrophil number, decreased peripheral blood NK cell cytolytic activity, increased absolute number of T cells, decreased CD4+:CD8+ ratio, increased concentrations of serum IgE and IgD, decreased serum IgG and IgA concentrations, and increased or decreased T cell proliferative responses.[8,30,42] *In vitro*, antibody-forming cell (AFC) response to T-dependent and T-independent antigens and plaque forming cell (PFC) responses to sheep red blood cells (SRBC) are inhibited in subjects exposed to cigarette smoke and in cell cultures exposed to nicotine.[69,77] Sopori et al.[77] observed that nicotine plays a major role in the immunosuppressant effects of cigarette smoke on antigen-stimulated B cell responses.

Alcohol, Cigarette Smoking, and Exercise Behaviors

Physical activity is often weakly correlated with smoking in those individuals employed in heavy manual labor and lower socioeconomic occupations.[73] Increased exercise participation and physical fitness are associated with decreases in smoking but not alcohol use.[11,73] Alternatively, alcohol and drug use have been cited by physically active high-school boys but not girls, as barriers to participation in regular exercise programs.[81] Initiation and regular use of alcohol and drugs are often linked to habit and depression.[35,73] Gottlieb and Green[35] observed that smoking, drinking, and exercising are often used as stress-coping mechanisms. In both men and women, initiation of smoking may be associated with life events such as death of a partner. For men, life events also tend to be associated with alcohol consumption and physical activity.[35] Concurrent exercise and drug use behaviors are not limited to the U.S. In Australia, concurrent use of alcohol, cigarette smoking, and regular physical exercise may be common lifestyle behaviors. Arkwright and co-workers[6] reported that cigarette smoking and regular physical exercise were both significantly associated with drinking alcohol among 491 Caucasian male government employees, aged 20 to 45 years. Among these men 18% abstained from alcohol but smoked cigarettes, whereas 50% of the men drank more than 350 ml/week of alcohol (3 to 5 drinks per day, heavy drinkers). Approximately

46% of abstainers indicated that they exercised regularly compared to 65% of the heavy drinkers who also exercised regularly.[6]

In Finland, 1537 monozygotic and 3507 dizygotic twins pairs were surveyed for alcohol use, cigarette smoking, and physical activity. Cigarette smokers consumed at least 5 to 10 packs of cigarettes in a lifetime and smoked daily or nearly daily. Alcohol use and activity levels and volumes were also self-reported. A positive correlation ($r = 0.32$) was observed between cigarette smoking and alcohol intake. However, low negative correlations were reported for alcohol use and physical activity ($r = -0.02$) and for cigarette smoking and physical activity ($r = -0.14$). Approximately 25% of total sample did not smoke and reported low physical activity and low monthly alcohol consumption (80 g alcohol). Of the smokers 20% reported low activity levels and above average alcohol consumption, and 72% of this group binged on alcohol at least once per month. Of the smokers 80% reported low physical activity and high alcohol intake. Approximately 6% of the total sample reported high activity levels (roughly 6 h/week). Of this group, one half were current smokers and reported very high alcohol intake and regular alcohol binges .[46]

C. MARIJUANA ABUSE

In 1976, an estimated 36 million individuals in the U.S. reported at least one episode of marijuana use and 15 million persons smoked marijuana on a regular basis.[62] Marijuana is frequently used by adolescents and young adults (18 to 25 years old). In 1982, 59% of high-school seniors reported using the drug with 35% of these students acknowledging use prior to high school.[26] Biological effects of marijuana are influenced by the route of administration of the drug, predominately, smoking or ingestion.[62] Marijuana users are exposed to numerous chemical substances; the primary psychoactive ingredient is δ-9-tetrahydrocannabinol (THC). Research findings from the last 10 years indicate that chronic marijuana use is linked to cardiac anomalies, impaired lung function and cancer, brain damage, altered cellular metabolism and chromosomal number, and impaired immune function.[41,62] Increased marijuana use by young adults is associated with squamous cell carcinoma of the head and neck, malignant tumors which are predominately associated with chronic tobacco smokers in the sixth decade of life.[26] Coabuse of marijuana and tobacco smoking is prevalent and complicates interpretation of health risks directly associated with marijuana use. Combined smoking of marijuana and tobacco is associated with abnormal cellular morphology, mitosis, and DNA replication in the lung.[49,50]

1. Marijuana and Immunity

Marijuana use is generally associated with suppressed immune responses (Table 1). Among the findings indicating marijuana-related suppression of immunity are decreased lymphocyte blastogenesis to phytohemagglutinin

(PHA),[61] impaired circulating NK cell cytotoxicity,[78] decreased macrophage activation,[17] reduced IL-1 secretion in response to pokeweed mitogen (PWM), decreased interferon-gamma (IFN-γ) secretion in response to PHA,[87] inhibition of Con A- and PHA-induced lymphocyte proliferation,[60,64] decreased number of alveolar macrophages compared to nonsmokers,[54] impaired cytotoxic T cell activity against herpes virus-infected cells without changes in the percentages of CD4+ or CD8+ cells,[16] and decreased antibody production and PFC response to SRBC.[51] Altered serum IgG concentration and IgD concentration may be also present in marijuana smokers.[60,87]

In a recent review of marijuana and immunity, Hollister[41] indicated that research in the past decades was poorly controlled. Marijuana-related immunosuppression in *in vitro* experiments and with *in vivo* animal models occurred predominately when investigators used excessive concentrations of THC and related cannabinoids which were not clinically relevant. Most results from clinical studies produce equivocal findings and do not support laboratory research models of marijuana or cannabinoid exposure. Hollister[41] has challenged popular opinion among marijuana researchers and maintains that direct evidence of immunosuppression by marijuana is unfounded.

D. COCAINE ABUSE

Coabuse of alcohol and cocaine is not uncommon. In 1990, an estimated 11.6 million persons used cocaine and ethanol concurrently.[36] Cocaine use, independent of alcohol intake, is directly linked to cardiovascular abnormalities and cardiac emergencies such as tachycardia, hypertension, acute myocardial infarction, ventricular arrhythmia, and sudden death.[89] HIV infection is not directly linked to cocaine use. However, cocaine users are at high risk of HIV infection due to the nature of sexual activity and intravenous drug use in this group.[19]

1. Cocaine and Immunity

Cocaine is a potent mediator of altered neuroendocrine and immune responses[88] (Table 1). Cytokine production from mitogen-stimulated lymphocytes can be completely inhibited by *in vitro* exposure to 0.1–100 µg/ml of cocaine.[85] Cocaine use can be suppressive or stimulatory for NK cell function. Acute simulation of NK cell cytolytic activity can occur within 5 min of cocaine exposure.[83] The mechanism associated with the rapid change in NK cell function may be altered metabolism of central neurotransmitters which causes increased release of beta endorphins and catecholamines, known activators of NK cell activity.[83]

Inhibition of *in vitro* NK and T cell cytolytic activity by cocaine is dose dependent.[88] Decreased NK cell cytolytic activity may be inversely related to cocaine use.[63] However, the circulating total number and percentages of NK cells may not be altered in cocaine users.[63] Cultured lymphocytes demonstrate biphasic dose-dependent changes in T cell mitogenesis.[48] Catecholamines mediate changes in lymphocyte regulation and trafficking by binding to adrenergic surface receptors on the cells.[9,20] Thus, cocaine may indirectly affect circulating lymphocyte number and function by inducing sympathetic hyperactivity.

E. ANABOLIC–ANDROGENIC STEROID ABUSE

Nonmedical anabolic steroid use is most prevalent among athletic populations. It is estimated that self-administration of anabolic steroids by athletes may exceed 1000 times medically prescribed dosage.[84] Anabolic steroids are typically used as ergogenic aids by athletes and for developing mesomorphic appearance in nonathletes. The extent of use ranges from middle school children to professional athletes and represents at least a $400,000 market.[31] Of those using anabolic steroids for nonmedical purposes, roughly 500,000 are high-school students.[89] Studies indicate that approximately 10% of high-school boys and 6% of high-school girls use anabolic steroids.[92] Estimates of anabolic steroid use among athletes indicate widespread usage, particularly among male and female athletes involved in body building and strength and power sports.[27,84]

The cardiotoxic effects of high-dose and multiple steroid use place the anabolic steroid user at increased risk of myocardial failure and impaired cardiovascular response during exercise stress.[89] Other potential health risks from anabolic steroid use include liver function abnormalities, testicular atrophy, piliosis hepatitis, cancer of the liver and kidneys, HIV infection, and numerous other nonfatal and fatal disorders.[40,43,84]

1. Anabolic–Androgenic Steroids, Resistive Exercise, and Immunity

Research on prevalence of anabolic steroid use is substantial; however, studies on immunomodulation by anabolic steroids in athletes are lacking. Calabrese et al.[18] (Table 1) compared the effects of anabolic steroid use on selective immune variables in 24 male body builders. Thirteen body builders acknowledged self-administration of 2 to 20 times physiological replacement of testosterone by anabolic–androgenic steroids. Anabolic steroid use did not alter the total number of circulating lymphocytes or subpopulations of T cells compared to nonsteroid users who were body builders or controls. Mitogen-stimulated lymphocyte proliferation exhibited variable results among the groups. Only the B cell mitogen, *Staphylococcus aureus*, Cowan strain (SAC) induced higher proliferative values for steroid users compared to controls. However, these values did not differ from body builders who did not take steroids. Compared to controls, proliferative responses for T cell mitogens PHA and PWM, and Con A were unaffected by steroid use. Differences in NK cell cytolytic activity, determined at one effector to target ratio, were present between steroid users and controls. There was a significant trend toward higher

NK cell cytolytic activity in steroid users. Serum immunoglobulins, IgA and IgM, were reduced in steroid users but not nonsteroid users. The authors cautiously hypothesized that changes in NK cell cytolytic activity may indicate either that positive natural immunosurveillance is associated with steroid use or that increased NK cell activity may reflect autoimmune damage. Reductions in serum immunoglobulins and some mitogen-stimulated proliferative responses are consistent with the immunosuppressive effects of anabolic–androgenic steroids. Calabrese et al.[18] concluded that there is potential for immuno-modulation and increased susceptibility to host immunosuppression in individuals self-administering excessive dosages of anabolic–androgenic steroids.

III. CONCLUSIONS

It is unlikely that regular physical exercise can attenuate the adverse effects of substance abuse on immune function. Parallels can be drawn to the combined effects of substance abuse and exercise on the cardiovascular system. Participation in regular exercise programs often does not protect against the deleterious effects of tobacco or alcohol on the myocardium, skeletal muscle, or cardiovascular system.[65,66,76,79] In fact, substance abuse can interfere with beneficial adaptations of the cardiovascular system to chronic endurance exercise. It is therefore relevant to consider whether exercise should be used as an intervention in the substance abuser. If so, are there limits to exercise intensity and duration beyond which susceptibility to infection and disease are increased in the substance abuser? The immunological evidence available to address these questions is scarce. Physical activity has been used as an intervention in alcohol and drug rehabilitation. Often indices of physical fitness, self-concept, and depression improve in abstinent alcoholics enrolled in exercise programs.[32,75] A concern recognized in the encouragement of physical activity as a positive intervention in rehabilitation is that individuals who seek rewards from compulsive behaviors will pursue other addictive, but socially acceptable behaviors in attempt to avoid alcohol or drugs.[39] Examples of possible addictive physical activities are compulsive exercising and bodybuilding. Therefore, understanding the underlying motivation for addictive patterns is imperative when considering adaptation of physical activity in a rehabilitative setting.[39]

ACKNOWLEDGMENTS

The authors acknowledge support, in part, from grants R01AA07293 and K02440138 from the National Institute of Alcohol Abuse and Alcoholism and the State of Washington Fund #171 for research on drug and alcohol abuse.

REFERENCES

1. Consensus conference. Health applications of smokeless tobacco use, *J. Am. Med. Assoc.*, 255, 1045, 1986.
2. Smoking and immunity, *Lancet*, 335, 1561, 1990.
3. Eighth Special Report to the U.S. Congress on Alcohol and Health, Department of Health and Human Services, Alexandria, VA, 1994, 1.
4. Aldo-Benson, M., Mechanisms of alcohol-induced suppression of B-cell response, *Alcoholism: Clin. Exp. Res.*, 13, 469, 1989.
5. Ardies, C. M., Morris, G. S., Erickson, C. K., and Farrara, R. P., Both acute and chronic exercise enhance *in vivo* ethanol clearance in rats, *J. Appl. Physiol.*, 66, 555, 1989.
6. Arkwright, P. D., Beilin, L. J., Rouse, I., Armstrong, B. K., and Vandongen, R., Effects of alcohol use and other aspects of lifestyle on blood pressure levels and prevalence of hypertension in a working population, *Circulation*, 66, 60, 1982.
7. Bagasra, O., Balla, A. K., and Lischner, H. W., Effects of alcohol ingestion in vitro susceptibility of blood mononuclear cells to infection with HIV and of selected T cell functions, *Alcoholism: Clin. Exp. Res.*, 13, 1305, 1989.
8. Barton, J. R., Riad, M. A., Gaze, M. N., Maran, A. G. D., and Ferguson, A., Mucosal immunodeficiency in smokers, and in patients with epithelial head and neck tumors, *Gut*, 31, 378, 1990.
9. Benschop, R. J., Oostveen, F. G., Heijnen, C. J., and Ballieux, R. E., Beta 2-adrenergic stimulation causes detachment of natural killer cells from cultured endothelium, *Eur. J. Immunol.*, 23, 3242, 1993.
10. Bird, G. A., Cytokines — mediators of acute alcoholic hepatitis, in *Alcohol, Drugs of Abuse and Immunomodulation*, Watson, R. R., Ed., Plenum Press, Oxford, 1993, 163.
11. Blair, S. N., Jacobs, D. R., and Powell, K. E., Relationships between exercise or physical activity and other health behaviors, *Public Health Rep.*, 100, 172, 1985.
12. Blank, S. E., DePauw, K. P., Peavy, R. D., and Meadows, G. G., Physical activity and alcohol consumption trends among physically active college students, *Am. J. Health Prom.*, 7, 327, 1993.
13. Blank, S. E., Johansson, J.-O., Origines, M. M., and Meadows, G. G., Modulation of NK cell activity by moderate intensity endurance training and chronic ethanol consumption, *J. Appl. Physiol.*, 72, 8, 1992.
14. Blank, S. E., Johansson, J.-O., Pfister, L., J., Gallucci, R., Lee, E. G., and Meadows, G. G., Mechanistic differences in NK cell cytolytic activity in treadmill-trained and chronic ethanol-consuming mice, *J. Appl. Physiol.*, 76, 2031, 1994.
15. Bobo, J. K., Nicotine dependence and alcoholism epidemiology and treatment, *J. Psychoactive Drugs*, 24, 123, 1992.
16. Cabral, G. A., Dove-Pettit, D. A., and Fischer-Stenger, K., Marijuana inhibition of cytotoxic T-lymphocyte activity, in *Alcohol, Drugs of Abuse and Immunomodulation*, Watson, R. R., Ed., Plenum Press, Oxford, 1993, 653.
17. Cabral, G. A. and Vasquez, R., Effects of marijuana on macrophage function, in *Drugs of Abuse, Immunity, and Immunodeficiency*, Friedman, H., Specter, S., and Klein, T. W., Eds., Plenum Press, New York, 1991, 93.
18. Calabrese, L. H., Kleiner, S. M., Barna, B. P., Skibinski, C. I., Kirkendall, D. T., Lahita, R. G., and Lombardo, J. A., The effects of anabolic steroids and strength training on the human immune response, *Med. Sci. Sports Exerc.*, 21, 386, 1989.
19. Chaisson, R. E., Bacchetti, P., Osmond, D., Brodie, B., Sande, M. A., and Moss, A. R., Cocaine use and HIV infection in intravenous drug users in San Francisco, *J. Am. Med. Assoc.*, 261, 561, 1989.
20. Coffey, R. G. and Hadden, J. W., Neurotransmitters, hormones, and cyclic nucleotides in lymphocyte regulation, *Fed. Proc.*, 44, 112, 1985.

21. Conlee, R. K., Barnett, D. W., Kelly, K. P., and Han, D. H., Effects of cocaine on plasma catecholamine and muscle glycogen concentrations during exercise in the rat, *J. Appl. Physiol.*, 70, 1323, 1991.
22. Conlee, R. K., Barnett, D. W., Kelly, K. P., and Han, D. H., Effects of cocaine, exercise, and resting conditions in plasma corticosterone and catecholamine concentrations in the rat, *Metabolism*, 40, 1043, 1991.
23. Cook, R. T., Ballas, Z. K., Waldschmidt, T. J., Cook, B. L., Labrecque, D. R., and Byers, C., Phenotypic alterations of lymphocyte fine subsets in the alcoholic: implications for function, in *Alcohol, Drugs of Abuse and Immunomodulation*, Watson, R. R., Ed., Pergamon Press, Oxford, 1993, 91.
24. Crabb, D. W., Bosron, W. F., and Li, T.-K., Ethanol metabolism, *Pharmacol. Ther.*, 34, 59, 1987.
25. Dole, V. P., Ho, A., and Gentry, R. T., Toward an analogue of alcoholism in mice: criteria for recognition of pharmacologically motivated drinking, *Proc. Natl. Acad. Sci. U.S.A.*, 82, 3469, 1985.
26. Donald, P. J., Advanced malignancy in the young marijuana smoker, in *Drugs of Abuse, Immunity, and Immunodeficiency*, Friedman, H., Specter, S., and Klein, T. W., Eds., Plenum Press, New York, 1991, 33.
27. Duda, M., Female athletes: targets for drug abuse, *Physician Sports Med.*, 14, 142, 1986.
28. Elders, M. J., Perry, C. L., Eriksen, M. P., and Giovino, G. A., The report of the Surgeon General: preventing tobacco use among young people, *Am. J. Pub. Health*, 84, 543, 1994.
29. Evans, D. L., Leserman, J., Pedersen, C. A., Golden, R. N., Lewis, M. H., Folds, J. A., and Ozer, H., Immune correlates of stress and depression, *Psychopharmcol. Bull.*, 25, 319, 1989.
30. Ferson, M., Edwards, A., Lind, A., Milton, G. W., and Hersey, P., Low natural killer-cell activity and immunoglobulin levels associated with smoking in human subjects, *Int. J. Cancer*, 23, 603, 1979.
31. Fields, R., *Drugs and Alcohol in Perspective*, W. C. Brown, Dubuque, IA, 1992, 127.
32. Frankel, A. and Murphy, J., Physical fitness and personality in alcoholism, *Q. J. Stud. Alcohol*, 35, 1272, 1974.
33. Gallucci, R. M., Pfister, L. J., and Meadows, G. G., The effects of ethanol consumption on enriched natural killer cells from C57BL/6 mice, *Alcoholism: Clin. Exp. Res.*, 18, 625, 1994.
34. Goolsby, M. J., Smokeless tobacco: the health consequences of snuff and chewing tobacco, *Nurse Pract.*, 17, 24, 1992.
35. Gottlieb, N. H. and Green, L. W., Life events, social network, life-style, and health: an analysis of the 1979 survey of personal health practices and consequences, *Health Educ. Q.*, 11, 91, 1984.
36. Grant, B. F. and Hartford, T. C., Concurrent or simultaneous use of alcohol with cocaine: results of national survey, *Drug Alcohol Depend.*, 25, 97, 1990.
37. Hansen, W. B. and Malotte, C. K., Perceived personal immunity: the development of beliefs about susceptibility to the consequences of smoking, *Prev. Med.*, 15, 363, 1986.
38. Harris, J. O., Swenson, E. W., and Johnson, J. E., III, Human alveolar macrophages: comparison of phagocytic ability, glucose utilization, and ultrastructure in smokers and nonsmokers, *J. Clin. Invest.*, 49, 2086, 1970.
39. Hatcher, A. S., From one addiction to another: life after alcohol and drug abuse, *Nurse Pract.*, 14, 13, 1989.
40. Haupt, H. A. and Rovere, G. D., Anabolic steroids: a review of the literature, *Am. J. Sports Med.*, 12, 469, 1984.
41. Hollister, L. E., Marijuana and immunity, *J. Psychoactive Drugs*, 24, 159, 1992.
42. Holt, P. G., Immune and inflammatory function in cigarette smokers, *Thorax*, 42, 241, 1987.

43. Hough, D. O., Anabolic steroids and ergogenic aids, *Am. Fam. Physician*, 41, 1157, 1990.
44. Irwin, M., Caldwell, C., Smith, T. L., Brown, S., Schukit, M. A., and Gillin, J. C., Major depressive disorder, alcoholism, and reduced natural killer cell cytotoxicity, *Arch. Gen. Psychiatry*, 47, 713, 1990.
45. Irwin, M., Hauger, R. L., Brown, M., and Britton, K. T., CRF activates autonomic nervous system and reduces natural killer cytotoxicity, *Am. J. Physiol.*, 255, R744, 1988.
46. Kaprio, J., Koskenvuo, M., and Sarna, S., Cigarette smoking, use of alcohol, and leisure-time physical activity among same-sexed adult male twins, in *Twin Research 3: Epidemiological and Clinical Studies*, Alan R. Liss, New York, 1981, 37.
47. Khansari, D. N., Murgo, A. J., and Faith, R. E., Effects of stress on the immune system, *Immunol. Today*, 11, 170, 1990.
48. Klein, T. W., Newton, C., and Friedman, H., Cocaine effects on cultured lymphocytes, in *Drugs of Abuse, Immunity, and Immunodeficiency*, Friedman, H., Specter, S., and Klein, T. W., Eds., Plenum Press, New York, 1991, 151.
49. Leuchtenberger, C., Leuchtenberger, R., and Ritter, U., Effects of marijuana and tobacco smoke on DNA and chromosomal complement in human lung explants, *Nature (London)*, 242, 403, 1973.
50. Leuchtenberger, C., Leuchtenberger, R., and Schneider, A., Effects of marijuana and tobacco smoke on human lung physiology, *Nature (London)*, 241, 137, 1973.
51. Levy, J. A., Munson, A. E., Harris, L. S., and Dewey, W. L., Effects of Δ^9-THC on the immune response of mice, *Fed. Proc. Exp. Biol.*, 34 (Abstr.), 782, 1975.
52. Lieber, C. S., Seitz, H. K., Garro, A. J., and Worner, T. M., Alcohol-related diseases and carcinogenesis, *Cancer Res.*, 39, 2863, 1979.
53. MacGregor, R. R., Alcohol and immune defense, *J. Am. Med. Assoc.*, 256, 1474, 1986.
54. Mann, P. E. G., Cohen, A. B., Finley, T. N., Ladman, A. J., Alveolar macrophages. Structural and functional differences between nonsmokers and smokers of marijuana and tobacco, *Lab. Invest.*, 25, 111, 1971.
55. Mason, L., Giardina, S. L., Hecht, T., Ortaldo, J., and Mathieson, B. J., LGL-1: a non-polymorphic antigen expressed on a major population of mouse natural killer cells, *J. Immunol.*, 140, 4403, 1988.
56. McClain, C. J., Hill, D. B., Marsano, L., Cohen, D., and Shedlofsky, S., A role for cytokines in alcoholic hepatitis, in *Alcohol, Drugs of Abuse and Immunomodulation*, Watson, R. R., Ed., Plenum Press, Oxford, 1993, 133.
57. Meadows, G. G. and Blank, S. E., Modulation of natural killer cell activity by alcohol, in *Alcohol, Immunity, and Cancer*, Yirmiya, R. and Taylor, A. N., Eds., CRC Press, Boca Raton, FL, 1993, 55.
58. Mitchell, M. C., Overview of effects of liver disease, alcohol consumption and substance abuse on immune response and infection, in *Alcohol, Drugs of Abuse and Immunomodulation*, Watson, R. R., Ed., Plenum Press, Oxford, 1993, 3.
59. Mufti, S. I., Alcohol and cancers of the esophagus, in *Alcohol, Immunity, and Cancer*, Yirmiya, R. and Taylor, A. N., Eds., CRC Press, Boca Raton, FL,, 1993, 159.
60. Nahas, G. G. and Osserman, E. F., Altered serum immunoglobulin concentration in chronic marijuana smokers, in *Drugs of Abuse, Immunity, and Immunodeficiency*, Friedman, H., Specter, S., and Klein, T. W., Eds., Plenum Press, New York, 1991, 25.
61. Nahas, G. G., Suciu-Foca, N., Armand, J.-P., and Morishima, A., Inhibition of cellular mediated immunity in marihuana smokers, *Science*, 183, 419, 1973.
62. Petersen, R. C., Marihuana research findings: 1976, *NIDA Res. Monogr.*, 14, 1, 1977.
63. Pillai, R. and Watson, R. R., Immunotoxicology of drug and alcohol use: relevance to AIDS and cancer, in *Alcohol, Drugs of Abuse and Immunomodulation*, Watson, R. R., Ed., Plenum Press, Oxford, 1993, 427.
64. Pross, S., Newton, C., Klein, T., Widen, R., Smith, J., and Friedman, H., Suppression of T lymphocyte subpopulations by THC, in *Drugs of Abuse, Immunity, and Immunodeficiency*, Friedman, H., Spector, S., and Klein, T. W., Eds., Plenum Press, New York, 1991, 113.

65. Rothstein, J. M. and Rose, S. J., Muscle mutability. II. Adaptation to drugs, metabolic factors, and aging, *Phys. Ther.*, 12, 1788, 1982.
66. Rubin, E., Katz, A. M., Lieber, C. S., Stein, E. P., and Puskin, S., Muscle damage produced by chronic alcohol consumption, *Am. J. Pathol.*, 83, 499, 1976.
67. Saad, A. J. and Jerrells, T. R., Flow cytometric and immunohistochemical evaluation of ethanol-induced changes in splenic and thymic lymphoid cell populations, *Alcoholism: Clin. Exp. Res.*, 15, 796, 1992.
68. Samet, J. M., The epidemiology of lung cancer, *Chest*, 103, 20S, 1993.
69. Savage, S. M., Donaldson, L. A., Cherian, S., Chilukuri, R., White, V. A., and Sopori, M., Effects of cigarette smoke on the immune response, *Toxicol. Appl. Pharmacol.*, 111, 523, 1991.
70. Saxena, Q. B., Mezey, E., and Adler, W. H., Regulation of natural killer activity in vivo. II. The effect of alcohol consumption on human peripheral blood natural killer activity, *Int. J. Cancer*, 26, 413, 1980.
71. Saxena, Q. B., Saxena, R. K., and Adler, W. H., Ethanol and natural killer activity, in *NK Cells and Other Natural Effector Cells*, Herberman, R. B., Eds., Academic Press, New York, 1982, 651.
72. Schmidt, W. and Popham, R. E., The role of drinking and smoking in mortality from cancer and other causes in male alcoholics, *Cancer*, 47, 1037, 1981.
73. Shepard, R. J., Exercise and lifestyle change, *Br. J. Sports Med.*, 23, 11, 1989.
74. Siegel, D., Benowitz, N., Ernster, V. L., Grady, D. G., and Hauck, W. W., Smokeless tobacco, cardiovascular risk factors, and nicotine and cotinine levels in professional baseball players, *Am. J. Public Health*, 82, 417, 1992.
75. Sinyor, D., Brown, T., Rostant, L., and Seraganian, P., The role of physical fitness program in the treatment of alcoholism, *J. Stud. Alcohol*, 43, 380, 1982.
76. Song, S. K. and Rubin, E., Ethanol produces muscle damage in human volunteers, *Science*, 175, 327, 1972.
77. Sopori, M. L., Savage, S. M., Christner, R. F., Geng, Y.-M., and Donaldson, L. A., Cigarette smoke and the immune response: mechanism of nicotine induced immunosuppression, in *Alcohol, Drugs of Abuse and Immunomodulation*, Watson, R. R., Ed., Pergamon Press, Oxford, 1993, 663.
78. Specter, S. and Lancz, G., Effects of marijuana on human natural killer cell activity, in *Drugs of Abuse, Immunity, and Immunodeficiency*, Friedman, H., Specter, S., and Klein, T. W., Eds., Plenum Press, New York, 1991, 47.
79. Stamford, B. A., Matter, S., Fell, R. D., Sady, S., Cresanta, M. K., and Papanek, P., Cigarette smoking, physical activity, and alcohol consumption: relationship to blood lipids, and lipoproteins in premenopausal females, *Metabolism*, 33, 585, 1984.
80. Szabo, G., Monocyte-mediated immunodepression after acute ethanol exposure, in *Alcohol, Drugs of Abuse and Immunomodulation*, Watson, R. R., Ed., Plenum Press, Oxford, 1993, 121.
81. Tappe, M. K., Duda, J. L., and Ehrnwald, P. M., Perceived barriers to exercise among adolescents, *J. School Health*, 59, 153, 1989.
82. Tuyns, A. J., Epidemiology of alcohol and cancer, *Cancer Res.*, 39, 2840, 1979.
83. Van Dyke, C., Stesin, A., Jones, R., Chuntharapai, A., and Seaman, W., Cocaine increases natural killer cell activity, *J. Clin. Invest.*, 77, 1387, 1986.
84. Wadler, G. I. and Hainline, B., *Drugs and the Athlete*, Davis, F. A., Philadelphia, 1989, 55.
85. Wang, Y., Huang, D. S., Giger, P. T., and Watson, R. R., The influence of cocaine *in vivo* and *in vitro* on production of cytokines by Th1 and Th2 cells, in *Alcohol, Drugs of Abuse and Immunomodulation*, Watson, R. R., Ed., Plenum Press, Oxford, 1993, 673.
86. Warner, K. E., Health and economic implications of a tobacco-free society, *J. Am. Med. Assoc.*, 258, 2080, 1987.
87. Watzl, B., Scuder, P., and Watson, R. R., Influence of marijuana components (THC and CBD) on human mononuclear cells cytokine secretion *in vitro*, in *Drugs of Abuse, Immunity, and Immunodeficiency*, Friedman, H., Specter, S., and Klein, T. W., Eds., Plenum Press, New York, 1991, 63.

88. Watzl, B. and Watson, R. R., Immunomodulation by cocaine — a neuroendocrine mediated response, *Life Sci.*, 46, 1319, 1990.
89. Welder, A. A. and Melchert, R. B., Cardiotoxic effects of cocaine and anabolic-androgenic steroids in the athlete, *J. Pharm. Toxicol. Methods*, 29, 61, 1993.
90. Williams, R. R. and Horm, J. W., Association of cancer sites with tobacco and alcohol consumption and socioeconomic status of patients: interview study from the Third National Cancer Survey, *J. Natl. Cancer Inst.*, 58, 525, 1977.
91. Windle, M., High-risk behaviors for AIDS among heterosexual alcoholics: a pilot study, *J. Stud. Alcohol*, 50, 503, 1989.
92. Windsor, R. and Dumitru, D., Prevalence of anabolic steroid use by male and female adolescents, *Med. Sci. Sports Exerc.*, 21, 494, 1989.

Chapter 13

EXERCISE, IMMUNITY, AND DIETING

———————————————————————— Carole A. Conn

CONTENTS

I. INTRODUCTION

Dietary practices and exercise habits are an inevitable part of daily life. We either choose them actively or by default. Epidemiological studies suggest that both have significant influences on our health and longevity.[22,81,113] Evidence linking different choices concerning exercise and diet with well-being or disease has stimulated interest in the study of the interactions of different exercise training regimens and diet alterations on host defense against disease. The issue of how exercise and diet might interact to impact resistance to infectious disease, incidence and modulation of neoplasm, and autoimmune states is complex because of the myriad combinations of factors involved. Table 1 lists individual characteristics that are known to influence immune function. For example, mice are far more tolerant to endotoxin, which can be

0-8493-8190-8/96/$0.00+$.50
© 1996 by CRC Press Inc.

Table 1   Individual Considerations Known to
Impact Resistance to Disease and
Indices of Immune Function

Characteristic	Ref.
Species/strain/genetics	34, 57, 79, 136
Age	15, 42, 59, 91,157
Gender	53, 132
Body size/body composition	43, 134
Fitness level	88, 108, 130
Nutritional status	13, 20
Stress level/other lifestyle factors	67, 94, 77
Circadian rhythms/seasonal cycles	8, 55

a cause of septicemia, than rats or larger species;[79] both childhood and aging are frequently associated with decreased resistance to disease and changes in indices of immune function;[17,42] and women produce more immunoglobin and are more susceptible than men to some autoimmune diseases, e.g. rheumatoid arthritis and lupus erythematosus.[53] Table 2 lists aspects of exercise training or of experimental designs for training studies that might be expected to influence disease outcomes and/or measurements of indices of immune function. Since the two main types of exercise training, i.e., strength and endurance, involve different physiological adaptations, it is likely that they impact immune function in different ways. This has not yet been widely studied, particularly with respect to strength training. However, some of the variables listed in Table 2 are already known to influence resistance to disease. For example, in studies of experimental infections in animals conducted from 1922 to 1989, exercise occurring at the time of the exposure to the pathogen reduced resistance and increased the severity of illness. [88]

In addition to the many variables of exercise regimens that may affect immune function, common alterations in diet used by athletes and by weight watchers are diverse and may include fasting, very low calorie diets, moderate caloric restriction, high protein diets, high carbohydrate diets, very low fat diets or specific changes in the fat content of the diet (i.e., increased consumption of polyunsaturated fats or decreased consumption of saturated fats), and megadoses of selected vitamins and minerals (Table 3). It is quite clear that either excesses or deficiencies in any of several vitamins, particularly vitamin A (the "anti-infection vitamin"),[131] can decrease resistance to disease and can alter many indices of immune function.[14,41,100] Similarly, content and source of protein and fat in the diet have been shown to alter incidence of disease and various measures of immune response.[41,100] How these dietary factors interact with either strength or endurance training to affect resistance to infectious, neoplastic, and autoimmune diseases or to alter immune status has been the focus of a number of studies.

The rationale for measuring indices of immune function to assess the status of the immune system is that the body must be able to synthesize

Table 2   Aspects of Exercise that May Impact Immune Function

Characteristic	Ref.
Type	31, 105, 130, 144
Resistance	
Endurance	
Concentric[a]	
Eccentric[b]	
Intensity	38, 105, 106
Moderate	
Severe	
Duration	26, 64, 95
Short	
Long	
Chronicity	89, 130
Acute	
Chronic	
Frequency	
Other	8, 88, 89
Timing of exercise in relation to infectious exposure	
Timing of exercise in relation to circadian and seasonal cycles	
Forced or voluntary exercise	
Natural exercise for the species	

[a] Concentric contractions occur when muscles shorten as they develop force, e.g., lifting a heavy object from the floor to a table or climbing stairs.

[b] Eccentric contractions occur when muscles lengthen as they develop force, e.g., using muscles to slow the force of gravity when moving a very heavy object from a table to the floor or running downhill. Eccentric exercises are associated with more muscle soreness and inflammatory symptoms.

antibodies and mobilize phagocytes and otherwise alter the internal environment (e.g., increase temperature to produce a fever) to destroy invading organisms. Thus, the capacity to make these responses may indicate the capacity to resist disease. Any condition that alters resistance to disease might be expected to change one or more of these indices. Recently the data documenting the association of the delayed-type hypersensitivity (DTH) test with risk of sepsis or with alterations in other immunological parameters have been reviewed.[140] However, it should be noted that the clinical significance of small alterations in one or more indices of immune function is not altogether clear. Additional research is necessary to relate specific changes in each of these indices to clinically significant immunosuppression or immunoenhancement.[13,75,134] Measurements of these indices have been used to assess the status of individual portions of an immune response and to determine whether that status is altered by the treatment or condition under study. Some indices of immune function that are commonly measured are listed in Table 4 along with the direction of changes that have been documented to occur under conditions of aging and protein/calorie malnutrition, both of which are associated with increased incidence of infection,[13,42,157] as well as the direction of changes that have been reported in studies that examined either the effects of food restriction or exercise. The association of the latter two conditions with incidence of infection will be discussed briefly below. Table 4 is not comprehensive, but is meant to illustrate that the direction of change in many of these indices due to the variable under study is not the same in every report, while clear trends can also appear such as the impairment of T lymphocyte function with aging.

In order to decrease the complexity of the issue somewhat, this review has been limited to examination of current knowledge concerning the interaction of restriction of food intake (i.e., dieting) and regular endurance exercise on

TABLE 3   Diet Alterations Known to Influence Various Aspects of Immune Function

Dietary Condition	Ref.
Undernutrition	
Starvation, fasting	76, 150, 154
Underfeeding[a]	81
Protein/calorie deficiency	16
Low protein content	46, 62
Low carbohydrate content	80, 123
Reduced or altered fat content	51, 81
Single vitamin or mineral deficiencies	14, 41, 100
Adequate nutrition	
Adequate diet[b]	126
Normal diet/self-selected diet[c]	32, 76
Overnutrition	
Excess calories	27, 81, 151
Excess protein/fat	100
Megadoses of vitamins and minerals	100, 131
Experimental conditions	
Timing of feeding with respect to circadian rhythms	54, 101
Undernutrition without malnutrition[d]	151

[a] Underfeeding, or reduced consumption of a normal diet, may result in deficiencies of some vitamins and minerals.
[b] Adequate diet is often considered to be a varied diet adequate in all nutrients at the level of the Recommended Dietary Allowances.
[c] Normal, usual, or self-selected diet is not necessarily adequate or optimal, but is often used as the reference diet in studies of food restriction.
[d] Undernutrition without malnutrition is an experimental, enriched diet which provides the food-restricted animals adequate quantities of all nutrients except calories.

resistance to infectious disease and on indices of immune function in athletes and other adults. There is widespread use for such knowledge. Infectious disease episodes are estimated by the Centers for Disease Control to be more than 700 millon cases annually, resulting in medical costs and production costs due to lost work equivalent to $17.2 billion.[141] Because approximately one third of Americans are overweight,[82] millions of people each year begin to restrict food intake and to exercise in an effort to reduce weight; and athletes modify their diets and train to enhance performance, with little knowledge of the consequences of such behaviors on immune function.

Section II will briefly summarize the independent effects of exercise and food restriction on resistance to infectious disease with a view to predicting how these effects might be expected to interact. Section III.A will describe studies examining the incidence of disease and changes in markers of the immune response in athletes who maintain low body weight in order to

TABLE 4 Common Indices of Immune Function and How Levels of These Indices Have Been Found to Change

	Aging[a]	PCM[b]	Restr[c]	Exercise[d]
Specific (acquired) immunity				
In vivo measures				
Serum immunoglobulins	=/–	=/+	–	=
Serum antibody response	=/–	=/–/+	+	+
Delayed type hypersensitivity	–	–	–	=
T helper:T suppressor ratio	+/–	–	=	=
In vitro measures				
Lymphocyte proliferation	–	–	+/–	=/+
Cytolytic T cell activity	–	–	+	o
Nonspecific (innate) immunity				
In vivo measures				
Resting leukocyte number	=	–	–	=/–
Febrile response	=/–	–	=/+	=/–/+
Acute phase protein response	–	–	=/–	=
Cytokine response	=/–	=/–/+	=/+	=
In vitro measures				
Natural killer cell activity	=/–/+	=/–	+	+
Phagocytic activity	=/–	=	–	=/+
Bactericidal activity	=	=/–	+	=/–/+

Note: No change =, increased +, decreased -, no data o; compared with values in control subjects, under conditions of aging, protein/calorie malnutrition (PCM), food restriction (Restr), and in exercise-trained individuals at rest (Exercise).

[a] Aging — Ref. 15, 18, 29, 33, 36, 39, 59, 97, 107, 109, 119, 120, 129.
[b] PCM — Ref. 18, 23, 24, 25, 41, 43, 69, 71, 75, 85, 122, 124, 128.
[c] Restr — Ref. 19, 30, 35, 45, 69, 78, 118, 128, 134, 151.
[d] Exercise — Ref. 19, 72, 84, 86, 88, 103, 107, 111, 112, 116, 148.

enhance performance. Section III.B considers what is known about resistance to disease and changes in immune function in other populations with predictable combinations of diet and exercise. Section III.C presents several experimental studies of animals that can add to current understanding; and Section IV gives suggestions for further research.

II. INDEPENDENT EFFECTS OF EXERCISE OR FOOD RESTRICTION

A considerable body of information has been generated concerning the independent effects of several paradigms of undernutrition, e.g., fasting, protein–calorie malnutrition, and longevity-enhancing calorie restriction, on resistance to various diseases and on immune function. Similarly, the effect of both moderate and fatiguing endurance exercise has been studied. From what is known about the independent effects of exercise or low levels of food intake on resistance to disease, how might we expect exercise and dieting to influence susceptibility to infections ?

A. EFFECTS OF EXERCISE
Various aspects of exercise and immunity are topics of other chapters in this volume to which the reader is referred. Moderate exercise has been associated with increased resistance to infectious disease while excessive exercise, exercise combined with the stress of competition, or exercise during the course of an infection has been associated with decreased resistance to infections.[8,38,88,127] It has been suggested that regular moderate exercise training, perhaps by causing regular release of small quantities of immunoregulatory cytokines, may prime the immune system to respond more favorably to infectious challenge.[110,133] A recent review discusses the evidence that exogenous administration of low doses of cytokines does modify the course of severe infections in a beneficial manner in the immunocompromised host by stimulating host defense mechanisms.[146] Thus, the independent effect of moderate exercise training during dieting on resistance to infection might be expected to be beneficial.

B. EFFECTS OF FOOD RESTRICTION
The effect of decreased food consumption and/or malnutrition or leanness on resistance to infectious diseases is a controversial topic. Malnourishment (both caloric deficit and multiple nutrient deficiencies) and rampant infectious disease coexist in war-torn nations.[76,87] Soldiers undergoing the rigorous Ranger training course, which includes severe food restriction as well as other stressors, suffer increased incidence of infection.[9] Malnourished children are more likely to suffer infections and to die from them than well-fed children.[17,41] The

immediate causes of death of malnourished children are usually infections.[143] Several indices of immune function are found to be depressed in malnourished children and to increase after weight is regained.[15,16,23,24] However, infections contribute to malnutrition by decreasing appetite and food intake, by interfering with nutrient absorption, and by increasing nutrient utilization in the mounting of host defense responses, e.g., fever and protein synthesis.[2] This decreased food intake during infection is thought to be an important host defense response that is less detrimental to the host than to the invading microorganisms.[56] Murray and Murray[98,99] have reviewed the data supporting their hypotheses that infection may be more related to the period of refeeding than to the period of food deprivation in children; and that starvation or severe caloric limitation in animal studies and in clinical observations in developing countries both are associated with suppression of infections, especially viral infections, while weight gain during refeeding brings recrudescence of malaria, brucellosis, and tuberculosis. In contrast, others have found that the best humoral and cell-mediated responses to antigenic challenge, which might be expected to be protective, can be measured in the first 4 d of refeeding.[140] By reviewing results of many studies in animals, several investigators have concluded that maintenance of low body weight by restriction of calories while supplementing the low calorie diets with an amount of protein, vitamins, and minerals equivalent to the amount that would have been consumed by animals eating *ad libitum*, i.e., undernutrition without malnutrition, is a means of improving resistance to infections, delaying or preventing development of cancer, and increasing longevity.[44,151] Some investigators have found that the most restrictive diet producing the smallest animals resulted in the longest life spans.[153] However, others are unconvinced that leaner is better and note that among animals maintained on a restricted diet those with highest body weights lived the longest.[47,66,138] One of the early longevity studies noted that rats with a maximum lifetime weight of 330 to 450 g lived the longest, whereas those below or above that range died sooner.[95] Similarly, results of a long-term prospective study of 750,000 men and women found little difference in mortality from all causes for those between 80 and 120% of average weight with higher mortality rates for those above and below this range.[83] Thus the relationship between restriction of food intake, body size or leanness, and resistance to disease is at present unclear. Since moderate exercise may improve resistance to infectious illness and food restriction leading to lower body weight may either help or hinder resistance, it might be expected that moderate exercise during dieting may act synergistically with food restriction to enhance resistance to disease or that exercise may alleviate some of the immunosuppressive effects of food restriction.

One study conducted at the University of Minnesota in 1945 is often cited as evidence that severe food restriction, when it is uncomplicated by any of the other deprivations of wartime and famine, such as poor housing and sanitation or the stress of battle, does not increase susceptibility to infectious disease.[76]

In this excellent and comprehensive work, 32 normal-weight healthy young men, volunteers from the conscientious objectors to the Selective Service System were selected to undergo a 25% weight loss over a period of 6 months by severe restriction of caloric intake. The restricted portions of food given were thought to be adequate in all micronutrients. Over the period of food restriction, an average of 1.1 colds per man was recorded among the experimental group, not different from the 1.2 colds observed among a control group of laboratory workers. Severity of these upper respiratory infections was not remarkably different between groups. However, among the experimental group there were 7 cases of persistant cough lasting more than a week after all other symptoms of the cold had disappeared. This did not occur in the control subjects and was thought to be related to decreased mucous secretion in the food-restricted individuals. It should be noted that one subject in this study was hospitalized for tuberculosis near the end of the first 12 weeks of refeeding. These young men led relatively normal social lives, at least during the first months of the experiment, and had assigned tasks in the Laboratory of Physiological Hygiene where they were residing and therefore were considered to have had similar exposure to pathogens as the control subjects. One interesting fact about their daily regimen that usually goes unmentioned is that they were required to walk 22 mi/week out-of-doors for exercise and to participate in a weekly one half hour treadmill walk at 3.5 mi/h, 10% grade. In addition, they walked 2 to 3 mi/d (or 14 to 21 mi/week) to and from the dining hall where their special meals were prepared. Thus they walked on average 5 to 6 mi/d throughout their 6 months of food restriction. These walking exercises were completed even during the last weeks of semistarvation when apathy and lethargy prevented them from completing their laboratory assignments. Although the intensity of the 22-mi walking exercise was not reported, the weekly distance walked was greater than the 3 mi/d, 5 d/week that was found to accelerate recovery from upper respiratory illness in women.[105] Would the young men have suffered increased incidence or duration of infection compared with controls if no exercise had been included in their daily routines? Did the moderate walking exercise alleviate some of the immunosuppressive effects of food restriction or would the incidence and severity of their respiratory infections have been the same had they not exercised?

III. INTERACTIVE EFFECTS OF EXERCISE AND FOOD RESTRICTION

A. STUDIES OF ATHLETES

The most common infectious illness among athletes is viral upper respiratory tract infection, followed by gastrointestinal disorders and skin infections.[125] Is there an increased incidence of these infections, and are there alterations in indices of immune function among athletes most likely to combine caloric restriction with regular exercise training? Low body weight is considered desirable for participants of gymnastics, figure skating, performance dancing, and distance running. Training for the sport of wrestling often involves substantial weight changes during the course of one season.[135]

Wrestlers' diets are likely to be low in calories and under the recommended dietary allowance (RDA[139]) for several micronutrients, particularly vitamins A and C, thiamine, pyridoxine, iron, zinc, and magnesium.[126] Although illness has been identified as a health factor concern among wrestlers,[40] there have been surprisingly few studies of frequency of illness or status of immune function in wrestlers, who regularly lose 4 to 13% of their body weight up to 30 times per season largely through dieting and dehydration but also through exercise to burn calories and to induce sweating.[65] One study of 37 college wrestlers found that 100% of these athletes had an illness during a 2-month period of competition.[137] However, this frequency was not different from that of the competitive swimmers and gymnasts in the study; and there was no comparison group not participating in competitive sport. In another study, parents or guardians of 104 high-school varsity wrestlers and 73 junior and senior boys randomly selected as controls were asked to recall illnesses of the subjects for the preceding 60 d before (November) and after (February) one competitive season.[40] Results were compared between wrestlers and controls and among wrestlers competing in different weight classes, the hypothesis being that those athletes competing in the lower weight classes might report more illnesses because more of these athletes "make weight," the practice of losing weight to compete in a lower weight class. No differences in frequency of illness were found in this study and no measurements of indices of immune function were made. Sevier[125] describes several infectious illnesses that are frequent among wrestlers: impetigo (bacterial infection), molluscum contagiosum and herpes simplex (viral infections), and tinea corporis (fungal infection). Given the high level of exposure to these contagious diseases resulting from their contact sport, it is not clear whether food restriction may increase their susceptibility.

Surveys of dietary intakes of figure skaters, gymnasts, and dancers consistently show low caloric intake and consumption of several nutrents at levels below the RDA.[126] Figure skaters and gymnasts have not yet been studied with respect to infectious illness. Similarly, there are no studies reporting the frequency of incidence of infectious disease among dancers. However, one study reported a decreased relative number of T lymphocytes in blood taken at rest from 32 ballet dancers, compared with the number in blood from 32 age-matched nondancer controls, whereas *in vitro* measurements of immune function were not different between the dancers and nondancers.[156]

Long-distance runners, who are notably lean,[93] have been the population of athletes most studied with regard to the effects of exercise on resistance to infectious illness and the effects of both acute and chronic exercise on indices of immune function. Data from these endurance athletes, and from prospective studies of sedentary individuals who have undergone variable periods of endurance training, have led to the development of the "J" curve model of the relationship between exercise and upper respiratory tract infections.[104] This model summarizes data that support the hypotheses that individuals engaging in moderate endurance exercise have a lower risk of respiratory infection compared with sedentary individuals and that excessive endurance exercise increases the risk of infection. However, there is disagreement as to whether runners consume less or more than sedentary individuals in the maintenance of their lean state. Brownell et al.[7] reviewed studies with data showing that daily energy consumption of runners is greater than that of matched controls, which is intuitively expected based on the substantial energy output of the runners and which might make it easier to consume recommended levels of micronutrients in support of immune function. However, other studies reviewed reported daily caloric intakes of runners, particularly female runners, that are unexpectedly lower than intakes of sedentary women. Subsequent reports have not yet clarified whether an increase in metabolic efficiency develops in female runners, permitting them to maintain body weight on a limited caloric intake, or self-reported food diaries are inappropriate instruments for the quantification of energy intake in female runners who may be sufficiently weight conscious to severely underreport dietary intake.[28,68,92] A recent review of survey studies of food intake of runners also fails to clarify the extent to which male and female runners may restrict their caloric intake.[126] Therefore, it is not known how increased or decreased energy intake by endurance-trained individuals may have influenced the "J" curve relationship between endurance exercise and resistance to upper respiratory infections[104] or the enhanced natural killer (NK) cell activity found in endurance-trained individuals.[61]

One intervention study of athletes documents differences in *in vitro* measurements of selected indices of immune function between a mixed group of nine competitive female athletes (four gymnasts, two swimmers, two volleyball players, and one tennis player) and ten age-matched sedentary women before 2 weeks of caloric restriction leading to weight loss.[78] Phagocytic function was found to be higher in leukocytes from the athletes compared with those from controls before initiation of caloric restriction. Stimulation of mononuclear cells with phytohemagglutinin resulted in significantly higher proliferation of cells from the athletes than from the controls. After a weight reduction of 4% in 2 weeks at 65% of the usual caloric consumption during training, there was no significant decrease in proliferation of cells taken from the athletes. No changes in serum concentrations of immunoglobulins or complement were noted following weight loss. However, weight loss significantly depressed phagocytic function and decreased plasma levels of fibronectin, an opsonizing glycoprotein. Therefore food restriction, or the weight loss resulting from the energy deficit, antagonized the exercise-induced enhancement of phagocytic function in this mixed group of athletes. Unfortunately the control group in this study did not undergo weight loss, nor were they measured twice to assess any change over time in these variables.

B. STUDIES OF OTHER HUMAN SUBJECTS

In addition to athletes desirous of low body weight to enhance performance in their sport, two other populations might be expected to provide insight into the interaction of restriction of caloric intake and regular exercise on resistance to infectious disease and on indices of immune function. Both obese patients and patients with anorexia nervosa have altered body sizes and exercise patterns. For many years clinical observations of individuals with anorexia nervosa have noted that these patients engage in high levels of physical activity while maintaining very low body weights and severely reducing food intake.[76] Recent data confirm these observations: energy expended as physical activity was measured to be 48% of total daily energy expenditure in anorexic patients, significantly greater than the 30% of total expenditure in control subjects.[11] This excess activity returns to normal during weight gain: activity of weight-recovered anorexia nervosa patients was not different from that of normal control subjects.[73] The high level of voluntary activity of the anorexia patients is in contrast to the lethargy and inactivity observed in starving individuals in other situations, such as prisoners of war and the subjects of the semistarvation study of young men previously described.[76] Since the excess activity of the anorexic patients increases the number of calories that must be consumed in order to gain weight, it has been recommended that treatment for anorexia include restriction of exercise in order to maximize the rate of weight gain in individuals averse to eating.[74] On the other hand, obesity is associated with inactivity, and treatment of obesity frequently emphasizes the combination of decreases in food intake with increases in physical activity.[49] Exercise is thought to be particularly important for long-term maintenance of weight loss in previously obese individuals.[155] Therefore, it is of interest to identify what is known concerning the incidence of disease and immune status of anorexic and obese individuals before and after treatment.

1. Anorexia Nervosa Patients

Reviewers of the early literature concerning anorexia nervosa found that less tuberculosis than might be expected from the emaciated state of the patients was reported and that little mention of increased susceptibility to pneumonia or upper respiratory infection was made in accounts of case studies, and therefore concluded that the information available at that time would not support the hypothesis that undernourishment of anorexia nervosa patients leads to a reduction in their resistance to infection.[76] Subsequently, several investigators have noted a low incidence of infectious diseases, particularly colds and influenza, among their anorexia nervosa patients (e.g., References 1, 4, 43, and 115). Severe infection (septicemia, pneumonia) that was unrecognized before death because fever, leukocytosis, and other clinical symptoms were absent was discovered at postmortem examination of anorexia nervosa patients;[147] and raises the caveat that the true incidence of infection among anorexia patients may not be known. Symptoms that are part of the acute phase response to infection, i.e., fever, acute phase protein synthesis, and serum cytokine response, are known to be diminished in children who are malnourished and to return to normal with recovery of weight.[23-25] It has been reported anecdotally that previously anorectic patients who have regained their weight complain that they have become more susceptible to colds and influenza.[21] Did they merely regain the capability to produce symptoms or were they truly more susceptible to infectious illness? If weight-recovered anorexia patients are more susceptible to disease, and if their activity decreases with weight recovery as has already been noted, does the decrease in activity contribute to their newfound susceptibility?

Some studies have tested the hypothesis that enhancements in immune function may mediate the apparently reduced susceptibility to infectious disease in anorexia nervosa patients. The evidence in support of this hypothesis is not strong. In several studies, measurements of indices of immune function in anorexics show that T and B cell functions are normal or enhanced at body weights greater than 60% of normal weight for height,[1,43,117] while subjects weighing less than 60% desirable weight were anergic to a DTH test.[117] However, in another study, DTH was reduced in subjects who were 62 to 84% of desireable weight, and patients' cells required greater doses of mitogens to elicit responses of comparable magnitude to cells from controls in *in vitro* tests of lymphocyte function.[9] Total leukocyte counts have been found to be reduced in anorexic patients,[4,5,50,115,121] and bactericidal activity of polymorphonucleocytes from anorectic patients is diminished.[50,115,121,145] Two studies have documented a return to normal bactericidal activity when weight has been regained.[50,145]

Two other hypotheses have been put forward to explain the lower incidence of infections in anorexia nervosa patients. One hypothesis is that their high level of exercise counteracts the depressive effects of undernutrition on immune function and resistance to disease.[37] The other hypothesis is that the nutrient quality, in particular the high protein content, of the low quantity of food intake of the anorexia nervosa patients contributes to their enhanced resistance.[53,115] In comparison with the usual American diet that is 10 to 12% protein, 50 to 53% carbohydrate, and 35 to 40% fat, the nutrient intake of anorexia patients has been found to be 18 to 35% protein, 20 to 33% carbohydrate, and 49 to 54% fat albeit at the low energy level of 948 to 1031 kcal/d.[70,123] Large quantities of green vegetables, salads, and fruit are consumed while carbohydrates in sweets, bread, and potatoes are avoided;[4,10] however, significant underconsumption of several micronutrients has been documented.[142] Neither of these two hypotheses concerning the low incidence of infectious disease in anorexia patients has been extensively explored.

2. Obese Patients

Obesity is associated with greater incidence and severity of infectious illness.[13,52,134] In a retrospective study of 502 consecutive surgical patients during 1 year, the obese patients, whether or not they had lost weight just prior to surgery, had two to seven times more respiratory and surgical site infections during recovery than the nonobese patients.[32] Results of this study did not support the investigators' hypothesis that prior weight loss would be beneficial in protecting against infection. Two things should be noted in this study: that even with a mean weight loss of 15 kg in approximately 5 weeks, mean body weight at surgery of those who had undergone prior loss was still 8 kg higher than the normal weight individuals and only 2 kg lower than the nonreduced obese; and further that the weight of the obese individuals in this study was only 112% the weight of the normal-weight controls and thus they might not have been classified as obese in many studies. Edelman[27] reviewed older clinical literature and concluded that there is substantial evidence that incidence of postoperative wound infection is increased from 60% to as much as 700% by obesity. However, results from experimental studies with animals that were reviewed were mixed: sometimes obesity was associated with decreased resistance to experimental challenges and sometimes not. In one experiment, normal-weight dogs were overfed and their physical activity was restricted to produce obesity or were underfed to decrease body weight. Obesity increased susceptibility and underfeeding decreased susceptibility to intracerebral inoculation of distemper virus. The protective effect of underfeeding was stronger than the deleterious effect of overfeeding. Strain differences in mice (genetically obese vs. genetically lean) are more important than dietary differences in the resistance to experimental infections.[27,134] Obese individuals are not more susceptible to all infectious diseases. Epidemiological evidence indicated that incidence of death from tuberculosis was only 21% of the expected rate (as compared with 149% of the expected rate for cardiovascular or renal disease) in obese men.[6]

Very few studies of obesity have focused on functions of the immune system; however, among the indices of immune function that have been measured, the following have been found to be depressed in obese compared with nonobese subjects: bactericidal capacity of neutrophils, release of macrophage migration inhibition factor (a cytokine that keeps macrophages at the site of infection), and monocyte maturation into macrophages.[134] Antibody response to hepatitis B vaccine was decreased in healthy obese compared with normal-weight individuals.[149] These investigators suggested that vaccine deposition into fat may be a factor in a poor immunogenic response, but some poor responders among very thin subjects in this study suggests that other factors also may play a role.[149] One study of obese and normal children (6 to 18 years) observed that decreases in indices of immune function in the obese were associated with deficiencies in iron and zinc, and these decreases were reversed by 4 weeks of diet supplementation without any loss in weight.[12] However, it is not known to what extent obesity in adults and perhaps the alterations in their immune function are associated with micronutrient deficiencies.[134]

A few studies have assessed indices of immune function following treatment for obesity with restricted food intake. Fasting (80 kcal/d as carbohydrate, one multivitamin supplement, and water *ad libitum*) by 13 obese women and 2 men for 14 d, resulting in an average weight loss of 9.4 kg, was found to enhance several indices of immune function compared with values obtained prior to initiation of fasting: bactericidal activity of monocytes, natural killer cell cytolytic activity, and serum immunoglobulin concentrations were all increased.[154] The only decrease in an index of immune function in this study was that lymphocyte proliferation to mitogen stimulation was decreased after fasting. In discussing their results, these investigators drew a parallel to results from their animal experiments that showed immunopotentiating effects of fasting in mice, i.e., survival to an experimental infection of *Listeria monocytogenes* was 5% in *ad libitum* fed mice and 95% in fasted mice, likely resulting from enhanced activity of the monocyte–macrophage cells. Both these human and mice studies employed short-term fasting as a method of food restriction, and fasting has often been found to produce results different from long-term decreases in food intake.[76] Long-term food restriction in genetically obese mice showed that they do not respond in the same way as lean mice, and genetic obesity largely eliminated the immunopotentiating effects of food restriction.[3] Chronic treatment of obese humans with very low calorie diets ([VLCD], <800 kcal/d supplemented with 100% RDA for of all micronutrients and relatively rich in protein) lasting 6 weeks[35] and 12 weeks,[96] resulting in losses of 13 and 14 kg, respectively, altered several indices of immune function at the completion of the treatment period. Lymphocyte proliferation decreased in the 6-week study and was not changed or increased (depending on the stimulating agent) in the 12-week study. The ratio of T helper:T suppressor cells fell, but not to a level considered to indicate depressed immunocompetence.[35] Despite these changes in markers of immune function, the investigators noted that no clinical symptoms of infections were apparent during the treatment lasting 6 weeks.[35] There was no mention of any incidence of infection in the 12-week study.[96] Stallone[134] reviews evidence from another study in which DTH was depressed and antibody response to tetanus toxoid booster was depressed in middle-aged obese women after a 21-kg loss resulting from 6 months of sequential treatment (12 weeks of VLCD, 6 weeks of refeeding, and 8 weeks of 1200 to 1500 kcal/d balanced diet). DTH responses remained low in subjects who were studied at follow-up who did not regain their weight.

Thus, the available literature shows some evidence that obesity may be associated with increased susceptibility and altered immune function and that weight loss, or severe caloric restriction leading to weight loss, can further alter immune function. All of these weight reduction studies used diets that were supplemented with 100% RDA of micronutrients, but were low in macronutrient energy. None of these weight reduction studies included nondieting obese controls, nor exercise in combination with food restriction.

Noticeably lacking from the literature are prospective weight reduction studies of either obese or normal-weight individuals in which comparisons of incidence of infectious illness and of changes in indices of immune function over time are made among sedentary individuals who have been randomly assigned to one of four diet and activity intervention groups: a group of sedentary control subjects permitted *ad libitum* food consumption, a sedentary group with restricted food consumption, an exercising group permitted *ad libitum* consumption, and an exercising group with restricted consumption. The exercise training could be either resistance training or endurance training in separate experiments. Nutrient composition of the diets should be controlled with respect to quantities of immunomodulatory fats and micronutrients. Such studies would help to clarify the independent and interactive effects of caloric restriction and exercise on incidence of infectious disease, and changes in immune system status.

Prospective studies in freely living humans do suffer certain limitations, such as unequal exposure to pathogens, inadequate control of adherence to dietary and exercise regimens, and large intersubject variability. Many of these limitations can be avoided by using prospective studies of the influence of caloric restriction and exercise on resistance to disease and on immune function in animal models where subject differences are smaller, more control can be achieved over housing and feeding conditions and exercise regimens, and all animals can be subjected to exact exposure to one pathogen. However, resistance training is difficult to model in animals, and extrapolation from animal models to humans is necessarily done with caution. Understanding of the impact of caloric restriction and exercise on immunity can best be advanced when both human studies and experiments using animal models add to the available data.

C. EXPERIMENTAL STUDIES OF ANIMALS

A few experiments have examined the effects of endurance exercise and food restriction on all causes of death over a lifetime in rats and mice. Although the main focus of these studies was longevity of the animals, they also provide some information on resistance to infectious disease. It should first be noted that the beneficial effect of caloric restriction, whether initiated from birth or in adulthood, on both mean and maximum life span has been clearly established for food-restricted sedentary rodents (reviewed in References 66, 91, and 151). That caloric restriction did not impair resistance to infectious disease was inferred by noting that restricted animals lived longer than *ad libitum* fed animals whether they were housed in conventional animal quarters or specific pathogen free rooms.[151] To my knowledge, no direct challenges with infectious agents have been made to adult rodents on a longevity-enhancing diet (restricted calories with adequate protein and micronutrients) to evaluate incidence or duration of sickness behavior or mortality in comparison with normally fed controls. However, one study has immunized sedentary mice on such a restricted diet with an intraperitoneal injection of influenza virus and has measured serological and cellular immune responses.[30] These investigators found that old animals fed restricted diets were more like young animals than old animals fed control diets in several measures of immune response to influenza: proliferative response of splenocytes, serum antibody response, and antigen presentation. Presumably these old calorie-restricted animals with the greater immune responses would be better able than the old animals receiving additional food to survive an infectious challenge with influenza.

Exercise also has been found to increase life span in both male and female *ad libitum* fed rats, but in many studies exercise also decreased body weight (e.g., References 47 and 64). One study[64] showed that mean life span of freely fed rats given access to running was increased compared with (heavier) sedentary rats pair-fed with the runners, and compared with (much heavier) freely fed sedentary rats; that is, more of the runners attained old-age, and thus better resistance to disease may have occurred in the runners. However, sedentary rats food-restricted to the same weight as the rats permitted to run (i.e., eating 28% less than the runners) lived significantly longer than any of the other groups. Another interesting study, which was actually done to test the hypothesis that exercise mediates the longevity-enhancing effects of mating, nevertheless provides some information on the independent effects of exercise and food restriction on susceptibility to infectious disease in male rats.[26] The most common cause of death in this colony was pneumonia. Underfed rats were allowed access to the same food as the *ad libitum* fed controls for 6 h each day which resulted in a 20% lower mean body weight for the restricted group. Exercised rats were forced to run daily for only 2 min at 19 m/min, which did not result in a lower body weight than that of the sedentary controls fed *ad libitum*. Both exercise and food restriction independently increased life span by approximately 15%. At necropsy 65% of the 48 *ad libitum* fed sedentary controls, 64% of the 44 food-restricted sedentary rats, and (significantly fewer) 38% of the 45 *ad libitum* fed runners had pneumonia. Thus one might speculate that exercise enhanced resistance to the infection that produced pneumonia in these rats while food restriction did not alter susceptibility.

The few studies of longevity which have examined the effects of food restriction combined with voluntary wheel running or forced treadmill exercise can provide some speculative information about resistance to infection. Goodrick et al.[48] fed the same diet to adult male rats either *ad libitum* or every other day and provided half of each dietary group with voluntary running wheels. Both mean and maximum life span of the rats fed every other day, whether they had running wheels or not, were significantly longer than those of the *ad libitum* fed rats. Exercise had no independent effect on survival. Thus, voluntary exercise neither prevented nor facilitated the beneficial effect of food restriction on life span. Although causes of death were not reported in this particular study, the housing of the animals in conventional rather than specific pathogen-free quarters permits speculation that both the exercising and sedentary animals which were food restricted may have been better able than their freely fed counterparts to resist infectious disease during their lifetime. In another investigation, male rats that were both food restricted (fed daily a smaller portion of the same food given the *ad libitum* fed rats) and permitted wheel-running exercise had increased mortality during the early part of the experimental period compared with sedentary food-restricted rats and with both freely fed sedentary and freely fed exercising rats.[63] Causes of these early deaths were not reported, but it seems unlikely that infectious disease contributed to their early mortality because this study was conducted in specific pathogen-free animal quarters and the pathogen-free status of the animals was documented. The maximum life span of the surviving rats in the food-restricted, exercising group was no different from that of the food-restricted, sedentary group. Therefore, in this study, voluntary exercise antagonized the beneficial effect of food restriction on mean life span without preventing the extension of maximum life span by food restriction in the longest-lived animals. In a study conducted 50 years earlier, male rats forced to run for 2 h daily and fed a low protein diet from a liver source showed improved longevity compared with sedentary food-restricted rats fed the same ration, whereas exercise had no effect on survival in any other of several dietary groups either *ad libitum* fed or restricted during the latter half of adult life.[95] Because this colony of animals had a high incidence of respiratory diseases, and therefore one might speculate that those that lived the longest were least susceptible or best able to recover from a mild infection, this is the only study that lends any support to the hypothesis that there may be beneficial synergistic effects of exercise and food restriction on resistance to infectious disease.

There have been very few animal experiments investigating the combined effects of exercise and food restriction on indices of immune function. One study tested the hypothesis that exercise can prevent undernutrition-induced immunodepression in female mice.[37] Mice were fed *ad libitum* or given restricted quantities of the same diet to induce a weight loss of 25% in 3 weeks. Half of each dietary group were exercised on a treadmill 5 d/week at 18 m/min for 30 min, and the other half were brought to the exercise room but kept sedentary. There were no differences among groups in serum antibody response 5 d following immunization with sheep red blood cells, in nonstimulated lymphocyte blastogenesis, or in proliferation induced by phytohemagglutinin or concanavalin A. Immunodepression induced by undernutrition was seen only in decreased spleen and thymus weight and elevated corticosterone levels. One third of the undernourished, sedentary animals displayed intestinal bleeding suggestive of stress-induced ulcers. Exercise did not enhance any of these indices of immune function in the *ad libitum* fed mice. However, exercise in the underfed mice significantly attenuated the decrease in spleen (but not thymus) weight, significantly attenuated the elevation in corticosterone, and significantly enhanced the proliferative response to lipopolysaccharide stimulation. In addition, evidence of intestinal bleeding was found in none of the undernourished mice which were exercised. The investigators concluded that indeed, under the conditions of this experiment, exercise could prevent some aspects of undernutrition-induced immunodepression.

Another study of female hamsters fed *ad libitum* or underfed the same diet to a 20% weight loss, with half of each dietary group provided with a running wheel, assessed the effects of voluntary running on the ability to mount an acute phase response, which is an important component of the nonspecific host defense response to diverse challenges to the immune system.[19] Five markers of the acute phase response were measured: fever, circulating interleukin-6, serum cortisol, serum amyloid A, and serum iron. In response to injection of a low dose of lipopolysaccharide, an experimental model of infection with Gram-negative bacteria, the underfed hamsters, whether permitted exercise or not, had a blunted serum amyloid A response. The underfed hamsters permitted to exercise failed to develop the expected hypoferremic response. Thus the results of this study showed that underfeeding inhibited the ability to mount some portions of an acute phase response and that voluntary exercise exacerbated, rather than prevented, the blunted response due to food restriction.

Most of the the animal experiments discussed here, which have employed the combination of exercise and food restriction, have used underfeeding of the same diet fed to the control animals rather than restricting the energy intake while ensuring adequacy of essential nutrients. Although this approach appears to mirror the usual human experience when weight loss is attempted by dieting,[102,126] additional studies are needed to examine the effects of undernutrition without malnutrition combined with exercise on immune function. No study to date has used pathogens to challenge the immune system of animals both energy restricted and permitted or forced to exercise. Responses are likely to be different for viral, bacterial, and parasitic challenges.[75]

IV. SUMMARY AND IMPLICATIONS FOR RESEARCH

It is clear that there is much to be learned about the impact of dieting and exercise on the incidence of infectious illness and immune response to infection. Because evidence exists that moderate endurance exercise may improve resistance to infectious illness and because food restriction leading to lower body weight may either help or hinder resistance, it is appealing to suggest that moderate exercise during dieting to lose weight may act synergistically with food restriction to enhance resistance to disease or that exercise may alleviate some of the immunosuppressive effects of food restriction. Based on the evidence reviewed here, it is not possible to conclude that dieting and engaging in regular endurance exercise work together to help improve resistance to disease or to cause physiologically important alterations in indices of immune function. Very little direct information is available on this issue. Needed are (1) prospective weight reduction studies combining exercise and food restriction that address the incidence of infectious illness and of changes in indices of immune function over time in human subjects, and (2) experimental studies of exercise and food restriction in animals using controlled exposure to pathogens. The design of those studies can benefit from careful control of the variables listed in Tables 1 to 3.

In closing it should be noted that increased understanding of the interaction of dieting and exercise on immune system function also has importance for diseases other than infectious illness. It is well established in animals that caloric restriction without deficiencies of essential nutrients is associated with decreased incidence of cancer, although the mechanism by which caloric restriction retards cancer onset is unknown.[152] Moderate levels of physical activity are also linked with decreased incidence of cancer, but traditionally exercise has been considered a means of increasing energy use as another way of decreasing energy available to the tumor.[81] Recent data showing that exercise alters indices of immune function that may play a role in suppression of neoplasm[60] suggest other possible mechanisms by which exercise and food restriction might interact. Patients with autoimmune diseases such as rheumatoid arthritis are treated with fasting to suppress inflammation[114] as well as exercise to increase joint motion, muscle strength, and endurance;[58] and represent another population that would benefit greatly from increased understanding of the interaction of exercise and dieting on immune function.

REFERENCES

1. Armstrong-Esther, C. A., Lacey, J. H., Crisp, A. H., and Bryant, T. N., An investigation of the immune response of patients suffering from anorexia nervosa, *Postgrad. Med. J.*, 54, 395, 1978.
2. Beisel, W. R., Impact of infectious disease on the interaction between nutrition and immunity, in *Nutrient Modulation of the Immune Response*, Cunningham-Rundles, S., Ed., Marcel Dekker, New York 1993, 475.
3. Boissonneault, G. A. and Harrison, D. E., Obesity minimizes the immunopotentiation of food restriction in Ob/Ob mice, *J. Nutr.*, 124, 1639, 1994.
4. Bowers, T. K. and Eckert, E., Leukopenia in anorexia nervosa, *Arch. Intern. Med.*, 138, 1520, 1978.
5. Brambilla, F., Ferrari, E., Panerai, A., Manfredi, B., Petraglia, F., Catalano, M., and Sacerdote, P., Psychoimmunoendocrine investigation in anorexia nervosa, *Neuropsychobiology*, 27, 9, 1993.
6. Bray, G., *The Obese Patient*, W. B. Saunders, Philadelphia, 1976, 218.
7. Brownell, K. D., Steen, S. N., and Wilmore, J. H., Weight regulation practices in athletes: analysis of metabolic and health effects, *Med. Sci. Sports Exerc.*, 19, 546, 1987.
8. Cannon, J. G., Exercise and resistance to infection, *J. Appl. Physiol.*, 74, 973, 1993.
9. Cason, J., Ainley, C. C., Wolstencroft, R. A., Norton, K. R. W., and Thompson, R. P. H., Cell-mediated immunity in anorexia nervosa, *Clin. Exp. Immunol.*, 64, 370, 1986.

10. Casper, R. C., Kirschner, B., Sandstead, H. H., Jacob, R. A., and Davis, J. M., An evaluation of trace metals, vitamins, and taste function in anorexia nervosa, *Am. J. Clin. Nutr.*, 33, 1801, 1980.

11. Casper, R. C., Schoeller, D. A., Kushner, R. , Hnilicka, J., and Gold, S. T., Total daily energy expenditure and activity level in anorexia nervosa, *Am. J. Clin. Nutr.*, 53, 1143, 1991.

12. Chandra, R. K. and Kutty, K. M., Immunocompetence in obesity, *Acta Pediatr. Scand.*, 69, 25, 1980.

13. Chandra, R. K., Immunodeficiency in undernutrition and overnutrition, *Nutr. Rev.*, 39, 225, 1981.

14. Chandra, R. K., Micronutrients and immune functions: an overview, *Ann. N.Y. Acad. Sci.*, 587, 9, 1990.

15. Chandra, R. K., Nutrition and immunity in the elderly, *Nutr. Rev.*, 50, 367, 1992.

16. Chandra, R. K., Protein-energy malnutrition and immunological responses, *J. Nutr.*, 122, 597, 1992.

17. Chandra, R. K., The nutrition-immunity-infection nexis: the enumeration and functional assessment of lymphocyte subsets in nutritional deficiency, *Nutr. Res.*, 3, 605, 1983.

18. Chandra, R. K., Influence of nutrition on immunocompetence in the elderly, in *Nutrient Modulation of the Immune Response*, Cunningham-Rundles., S., Ed., Marcel Dekker, New York, 1993, 455.

19. Conn, C. A., Kozak, W., Tooten, P., Gruys, E., Borer, K. T., and Kluger, M. J., Effect of voluntary exercise and food restriction on response to lipopolysaccharide in hamsters, *J. Appl. Physiol.*, 78(2), 466, 1995.

20. Cruickshank, A. M., Hansell, D. T., Burns, H. J. G., and Shenkin, A., Effect of nutritional status on acute phase response to elective surgery, *Br. J. Surg.*, 76, 165, 1989.

21. Dally, P., *Anorexia Nervosa*. Grune & Stratton, New York, 1969, 45.

22. Davis, M. A., Neuhaus, J. M., Moritz, D. J., Lein, D., Barclay, J. D., and Murphy, S. P., Health behaviors and survival among middle-aged and older men and women in the NHANES I epidemiologic follow-up study, *Prevent. Med.*, 23, 369, 1994.

23. Doherty, J. F., Golden, M. H. N., Remick, D. G., and Griffin, G. E., Production of interleukin-6 and tumour necrosis factor-a in vitro is reduced in whole blood of severely malnourished children, *Clin. Sci.*, 86, 347, 1994.

24. Doherty, J. F., Golden, M. H. N., Griffin, G. E., and McAdam, K. P. W. J., Febrile response in malnutrition, *W. I. Med. J.*, 38, 209, 1989.

25. Doherty, J. F., Golden, M. H. N., Raynes, J. G., Griffin, G. E., and McAdam, K. P. W. J., Acute-phase protein response is impaired in severely malnourished children, *Clin. Sci.*, 84, 169, 1993.

26. Drori, D. and Folman, Y. Environmental effects on longevity in the male rat: exercise, mating, castration, and restricted feeding, *Exp. Gerontol.*, 11, 25, 1976.

27. Edelman, R., Obesity: does it modulate infectious disease and immunity?, *Prog. Clin. Biol. Res.*, 67, 327, 1981.

28. Edwards, J. E., Lindeman, A. K., Mikesky, A. E., and Stager, J. M., Energy balance in highly trained female endurance runners, *Med. Sci. Sports Exerc.*, 25, 1398, 1993.

29. Effros, R. B., Svoboda, K., and Walford, R. L., Influence of age and caloric restriction on macrophage IL-6 and TNF production, *Lymphokine Cytokine Res.*, 10, 347, 1991.

30. Effros, R. B., Walford, R. L., Weindruch, R., and Mitcheltree, C., Influences of dietary restriction on immunity to influenza in aged mice, *J. Gerontol.*, 46, B142, 1991.

31. Evans, W. J., Meredith, C. N., Cannon, J. G., Dinerello, C. A., Frontera, W. R., Hughes, B. A., Jones, B. H., and Knuttgen, H. G., Metabolic changes following eccentric exercise in trained and untrained men, *J. Appl. Physiol.*, 61, 1864, 1986.

32. Fasol, R., Schindler, M., Schumacher, B., Schlaudraff, K., Hannes, W., Seitelberger, R., and Schlosser, V., The influence of obesity on perioperative morbidity: retrospective study of 502 aortocoronary bypass operations, *Thorac. Cardiovasc. Surgeon*, 40, 126, 1992.

33. Ferguson, A. V., Veale, W. L., and Cooper, K. E., Age-related differences in the febrile response of the New Zealand White rabbit to endotoxin, *Can. J. Physiol. Pharmacol.*, 59, 613, 1981.
34. Fernandes, G. and Talal, N., SLE: homones and diet, *Clin. Exp. Rheumatol.*, 4, 183, 1986.
35. Field, C. J., Gougeon, R., and Marliss, E. B., Changes in circulating leukocytes and mitogen responses during very-low-energy all-protein reducing diets, *Am. J. Clin. Nutr.*, 54, 123, 1991.
36. Fietta, A., Merlini, C., Dos Santos, C., Rovida, S., and Grassi, C., Influence of aging on some specific and nonspecific mechanisms of the host defense system in 146 healthy subjects, *Gerontology*, 40, 237, 1994.
37. Filteau, S. M., Menzies, R. A., Kaido, T. J., O'Grady, M. P., Gelderd, J. B., and Hall, N. R. S., Effects of exercise on immune functions of undernourished mice, *Life Sci.*, 51, 565, 1992.
38. Fitzgerald, L., Overtraining increases the susceptibility to infection., *Int. J. Sports Med.*, 12, S5, 1991.
39. Foster, K. D., Conn, C. A., and Kluger, M. J., Fever, tumor necrosis factor and interleukin-6 in young, mature, and aged Fischer 344 rats, *Am. J. Physiol.*, 262, R211, 1992.
40. Freischlag, J., Weight loss, body composition, and health of high school wrestlers, *Physician Sports Med.*, 12, 121, 1984.
41. Gershwin, N. E., Beach, R. S., and Hurley, L. S., *Nutrition and Immunity*, Academic Press, Orlando, 1985, 82, 90.
42. Gladstone, J. L. and Recco, R., Host factors and infectious diseases in the elderly, *Med. Clin. N. Am.*, 60, 1225, 1976.
43. Golla, J. A., Larson, L. A., Anderson, C. F., Lucas, A. R., Wilson, W. R., and Tomasi, T. B., An immunological assessment of patients with anorexia nervosa, *Am. J. Clin. Nutr.*, 34, 2756, 1981.
44. Good, R. A. and Lorenz, E., Influence of energy levels and trace metals on health and life span, *JPEN*, 14, 230S, 1990.
45. Good, R. A., Jose, D. G., and Cooper, W. C., The relation between nutritional deprivation and immunity, in *Microenvironmental Aspects of Immunity, Advances in Experimental Medicine and Biology*, Jankovic, B. D. and Isakovic, K., Eds., Plenum Press, New York, 29, 321, 1973.
46. Good, R. A., Fernandes, G., Yunis, E. J., Cooper, W. C., Jose, D. C., Kramer, T. R., and Hansen, M. A., Nutritional deficiency, immunologic function, and disease, *Am. J. Pathol.*, 84, 599, 1976.
47. Goodrick, C. L., Effects of long-term voluntary wheel exercise on male and female Wistar rats, *Gerontology*, 26, 22, 1980.
48. Goodrick, C. L., Ingram, D. K., Reynolds, M. A., Freeman, J. R., and Cider, N. L., Differential effects of intermittent feeding and voluntary exercise on body weight and lifespan in adult rats, *J. Gerontol.*, 38, 36, 1983.
49. Gortmaker, S. L., Dietz, W. H., and Cheung, L. W. Y., Inactivity, diet, and the fattening of America, *J. Am. Diet. Assoc.*, 90, 1247, 1990.
50. Gotch, F. M., Spry, C. J. F., Mowat, A. G., Beeson, P. B., and Maclennan, I. C. M., Reversible granulocyte killing defect in anorexia nervosa, *Clin. Exp. Immunol.*, 21, 244, 1975.
51. Grimble, R. F., Dietary manipulation of the inflammatory response, *Proc. Nutr. Soc.*, 51, 285, 1992.
52. Gross, R. L. and Newberne, P. M., Role of nutrition in immunologic function, *Physiol. Rev.*, 60, 188, 1980.
53. Grossman, C. J., Interactions between the gonadal steroids and the immune system, *Science*, 227, 257, 1985.
54. Halberg, F., Some aspects of the chronobiology of nutrition: more work is needed on "when to eat," *J. Nutr.*, 119, 333, 1989.
55. Halberg, F., Johnson, E. A., Brown, B. W., and Bitner, H. H., Susceptibility rhythm to *E. coli* endotoxin and bioassay, *Proc. Soc. Exp. Biol.*, 103, 142, 1960.

56. Hart, B. L., Biological basis of the behavior of sick animals, *Neurosci. Biobehav. Rev.*, 12, 123, 1988.

57. Hegsted, D. M., Exercise, calories, and fat: future challenges, *Adv. Exp. Med. Biol.*, 322, 1, 1992.

58. Hicks, J. E., Exercise in patients with inflammatory arthritis and connective tissue disease, *Rheum. Dis. Clin. N. Am.*, 16, 845, 1990.

59. Hirokawa, K., Understanding the mechanism of the age-related decline in immune function, *Nutr. Rev.*, 50, 361, 1992.

60. Hoffman-Goetz, L., Exercise, natural immunity, and tumor metastasis, *Med. Sci. Sports Exerc.*, 26, 157, 1994.

61. Hoffman-Goetz, L. and Pedersen, B. K., Exercise and the immune system: a model of the stress response?, *Immunol. Today*, 15, 382, 1994.

62. Hoffman-Goetz, L. and Kluger, M. J., Protein-deprivation: its effects on fever and plasma iron during bacterial infection in rabbits, *J. Physiol. (London)*, 295, 419, 1979.

63. Holloszy, J. O. and Schechtman, K. B., Interaction between exercise and food restriction: effects on longevity of male rats, *J. Appl. Physiol.*, 70, 1529, 1991.

64. Holloszy, J. O., Smith, E. K., Vining, M., and Adams, S., Effect of voluntary exercise on longevity of rats, *J. Appl. Physiol.*, 59, 826, 1985.

65. Horswill, C. A., Applied physiology of amateur wrestling, *Sports Med.*, 14(1), 14, 1992.

66. Ingram, D. K. and Reynolds, M. A., The relationship of body weight to longevity within laboratory rodent species, in *Evolution of Longevity in Animals: a Comparative Approach*, Woodhead, A. D. and Thompson, K. H., Eds., Plenum Press, New York, 1986, 247.

67. Irwin, M., Daniels, M., Bloom, E. T., Smith, T. L., and Weiner, H., Life events, depressive symptoms, and immune function, *Am. J. Psychol.*, 144, 437, 1987.

68. Janssen, G. M. E., Graef, C. J. J., and Saris, W. H. M., Food intake and body composition in novice athletes during a training period to run a marathon, *Int. J. Sports Med.*, 10, S17, 1989.

69. Jennings, G. and Elia, E., Independent effects of protein and energy deficiency on acute-phase protein response in rats, *Nutrition*, 7, 430, 1991.

70. Kanis, J. A., Brown, P., Fitzpatrick, K., Hibbert, D. J., Horn, D. B., Nairn, I. M., Shirling, D., Strong, J. A., and Walton, H. J., Anorexia nervosa: a clinical, psychiatric, and laboratory study, *Q. J. Med.*, 170, 321, 1974.

71. Kauffman, C. A., Jones, P. G., and Kluger, M. J., Fever and malnutrition: endogenous pyrogen/interleukin-1 in malnourished patients, *Am. J. Clin. Nutr.*, 44, 449, 1986.

72. Kaufman, J. C., Harris, T. J., Higgins, J., and Maisel, A. S., Exercise-induced enhancement of immune function in the rat, *Circulation*, 90, 525, 1994.

73. Kaye, W. H., Gwirtsman, H. E., George, D. T., Ebert, M. H., and Peterson, R., Caloric consumption and activity levels after weight recovery in anorexia nervosa: a prolonged delay in normalization, *Int. J. Eating Disorders*, 5, 489, 1986.

74. Kaye, W. H., Gwirtsman, H. E., Obarzanek, E., and George, D. T., Relative importance of calorie intake needed to gain weight and level of physical activity in anorexia nervosa, *Am. J. Clin. Nutr.*, 47, 989, 1988.

75. Keusch, G. T., Nutrition and infection, in *Modern Nutrition in Health and Disease*, Shils, M. E., Olson, H. A., and Shike, M., Eds., Lea & Febiger, Philadelphia, 1994, 1241.

76. Keys, A., Brozek, J., Henschel, A., Mickelsen, O., and Taylor, H. L., *The Biology of Human Starvation*, The University of Minnesota Press, Minneapolis, 1950.

77. Khansari, D. N., Murgo, A. J., and Faith, R. E., Effects of stress on the immune system, *Immunol. Today*, 11, 170, 1990.

78. Kono, I., Kitao, H., Matsuda, M., Haga, S., Fukushima, H., and Kashiwagi, H., Weight reduction in athletes may adversely affect the phagocytic function of monocytes, *Physician Sports Med.*, 16, 56, 1988.

79. Kozak, W., Conn, C. A., and Kluger, M. J., Lipopolysaccharide induces fever and depresses locomotor activity in unrestrained mice, *Am. J. Physiol.*, 266, R125, 1994.

80. Kritchevsky, D., Influence of caloric restriction and exercise on tumorigenesis in rats, *PSEBM*, 193, 35, 1990.
81. Kritchevsky, D., Undernutrition and chronic disease: cancer, *Proc. Nutr. Soc.*, 52, 39, 1993.
82. Kuczmarski, R. J., Flegal, K. M., Campbell, S. M., and Johnson, C. L., Increasing prevalence of overweight among U.S. adults, the National Health and Nutrition Examination Surveys, 1960 to 1991, *J. Am. Med. Assoc.*, 272, 205, 1994.
83. Lew, E. A. and Garfinkel, L., Variations in mortality by weight among 750,000 men and women, *J. Chron. Dis.*, 32, 563, 1979.
84. Lewicki, R., Tchorzewski, H., Denys, A., Kowalska, M., and Golinska, A., Effect of physical exercise on some parameters of immunity in conditioned sportsmen, *Int. J. Sports Med.*, 8, 309, 1987.
85. Lieberman, M. D., Reynolds, J., Redmond, H. P., Leon, P., Shou, J., and Daly, J. M., Comparison of acute and chronic protein-energy malnutrition on host antitumor immune mechanisms, *JPEN*, 15, 15, 1991.
86. Liu, Y. G. and Wang, S. Y., The enhancing effect of exercise on the production of antibody to *Salmonella typhi* in mice, *Immunol. Lett.*, 14, 117, 1987.
87. Lusk, G., The physiological effect of undernutrition, *Physiol. Rev.*, 1, 523, 1921.
88. MacKinnon, L. T., *Exercise and Immunology,* Human Kinetics Books, Champaign, 1992, 4.
89. MacNeil, B. and Hoffman-Goetz, L., Chronic exercise enhances in vivo and in vitro cytotoxic mechanisms of natural immunity in mice, *J. Appl. Physiol.*, 74, 388, 1993.
90. Martinez-Lopez, L. E., Moore, R. H., Friedl, K. E., and Kramer, T. R., A longitudinal study of infections and injuries of Ranger students, *Military Med.*, 158, 433, 1993.
91. Masoro, E. J., Dietary restriction and aging, *J. Am. Geriatric Soc.*, 41, 994, 1993.
92. Maughan, R. J., Nutritional aspects of endurance exercise in humans, *Proc. Nutr. Soc.*, 53, 181, 1994.
93. McArdle, W. D., Katch, F. I., and Katch, V. L., *Exercise Physiology*, Lea & Febiger, Philadelphia, 1981, 393.
94. McCarthy, D. O., Ouimet, M. E., and Dunn, J. M., The effects of noise stress on leukocyte function in rats, *Res. Nurs. Health*, 15, 131, 1992.
95. McCay, C. M., Maynard, L. A., Sperling, G., and Osgood, H. S., Nutritional requirements during the latter half of life, *J. Nutr.*, 21, 45, 1941.
96. McMurray, R. W., Bradsher, R. W., Steele, R. W., and Pilkington, N. S., Effect of prolonged modified fasting in obese persons on in vitro markers of immunity: lymphocyte function and serum effects on normal neutrophils, *Am. J. Med. Sci.*, 299, 379, 1990.
97. Miller, R. A., Aging and the immune response, in *Handbook of the Biology of Aging*, Schneider, E. L., Ed., Academic Press, San Diego, 1990, 157.
98. Murray, J. and Murray, A., Toward a nutritional concept of host resistance to malignancy and intracellular infection, *Persp. Biol. Med.*, 24, 290, 1981.
99. Murray, M. J. and Murray, A. B., Starvation suppression and refeeding activation of infection, *Lancet*, 1, 123, 1977.
100. Myrvik, Q. N., Immunology and nutrition, in *Modern Nutrition in Health and Disease*, Shils, M. E., Olson, H. A., and Shike, M., Eds., Lea & Febiger, Philadelphia, 1994, 623.
101. Nelson, W. and Halberg, F., Meal-timing, circadian rhythms and life span of mice, *J. Nutr.*, 116, 2244, 1986.
102. Nicholas, P. and Dwyer, J., Diets for weight reduction: nutritional considerations, in *Handbook of Eating Disorders*, Brownell, K. D., Ed., Basic Books, New York, 1986, 123.
103. Nieman, D. C., Exercise, infection, and immunity, *Int. J. Sports Med.*, 15, s131, 1994.
104. Nieman, D. C., Exercise, upper respiratory tract infection, and the immune system, *Med. Sci. Sports Exerc.*, 26, 128, 1994.
105. Nieman, D. C., The effects of moderate exercise training on natural killer cells and acute upper respiratory tract infections, *Int. J. Sports Med.*, 11, 467, 1990.

106. Nieman, D. C., Miller, A. R., Henson, D. A., Warren, B. J., Gusewitch, G., Johnson, R. L., Davis, J. M., Butterworth, D. E., and Nehlsen-Cannarella, S. L., Effects of high- vs moderate-intensity exercise on natural killer cell activity, *Med. Sci. Sports Exerc.*, 25, 1126, 1993.
107. Nieman, D. C. and Henson, D. A., Role of endurance exercise in immune senescence, *Med. Sci. Sports Exerc.*, 26, 172, 1994.
108. Nieman, D. C., Henson, D. A., Gusewitch, G., Warren, B. J., Dotson, R. C., Butterworth, D. E., and Nehlsen-Cannarella, S. L., Physical activity and immune function in elderly women, *Med. Sci. Sports Exerc.*, 25, 823, 1993.
109. Norman, D. C., Yamamura, R. H., and Yoshikawa, T. T., Fever response in old and young mice after injection of interleukin 1, *J. Gerontol.*, 43, M80, 1988.
110. Northoff, H. and Berg, A., Immunologic mediators as parameters of the reaction to strenuous exercise, *Int. J. Sports Med.*, 12, s9, 1991.
111. Ortega, E., Physiology and biochemistry: influence of exercise on phagocytosis, *Int. J. Sports Med.*, 15, S172, 1994.
112. Ortega, E., Barriga, C., and de la Fuente, M., Study of the phagocytic process in neutrophils from elite sportswomen, *Eur. J. Appl. Physiol.*, 66, 37, 1993.
113. Paffenbarger, R. S., Jr., Kampert, J. B., Lee, I.-M., Hyde, R. T., Leung, R. W., and Wing, A. L., Changes in physical activity and other lifeway patterns influencing longevity, *Med. Sci. Sports Exerc.*, 26, 857, 1994.
114. Palmblad, J., Hafstrom, I., and Ringertz, B., Antirheumatic effects of fasting, *Rheum. Dis. Clin. N. Am.*, 17, 351, 1991.
115. Palmblad, J., Fohlin, L., and Lundstrum, M., Anorexia nervosa and polymorphonuclear (PMN) granulocyte reactions, *Scand. J. Haematol.*, 19, 334, 1977.
116. Pederson, B. K. and Ullum, H., NK cell response to physical activity: possible mechanisms of action, *Med. Sci. Sports Exerc.*, 26, 140, 1994.
117. Pertschuk, M.J., Crosby, L. O., Barot, L., and Mullen, J. L., Immunocompetency in anorexia nervosa, *Am. J. Clin. Nutr.*, 35, 968, 1982.
118. Pieri, C., Recchioni, R., Moroni, F., Marcheselli, F., and Marra, M., Food restriction in female Wistar rats. VII. Mitochondrial parameters in resting and proliferating splenic lymphocytes, *Arch. Gerontol. Geriatr.*, 19, 31, 1994.
119. Post, D. J., Carter, K. C., and Papaconstantinou, J., The effect of aging on constitutive mRNA levels and lipopolysaccharide inducibility of acute phase genes, *Ann. N. Y. Acad. Sci.*, 621, 66, 1991.
120. Refinetti, R., Ma, H., and Satinoff, E., Body temperature rhythms, cold tolerance, and fever in young and old rats of both genders, *Exp. Gerontol.*, 25, 533, 1990.
121. Reiger, W., Brady, J. P., and Weisberg, E., Hematologic changes in anorexia nervosa, *Am. J. Psychiatry*, 135, 984, 1978.
122. Reynolds, J., Shou, J., Sigel, R., Ziegler, M., and Daly, J. M., The influence of protein malnutrition on T cell, natural killer cell, and lymphokine-activated killer cell function, and on biological responsiveness to high-dose interleukin-2, *Cell. Immunol.*, 128, 569, 1990.
123. Russell, G. F. M., The nutritional disorder in anorexia nervosa, *J. Psychosom. Res.*, 11, 141, 1967.
124. Salimonu, L. S., Natural killer cell activity in protein-calorie malnutrition, in *Nutrient Modulation of the Immune Response*, Cunningham-Rundles, S., Ed., Marcel Dekker, New York, 1993, 359.
125. Sevier, T. L., Infectious disease in athletes, *Med. Clin. N. Am.*, 78, 389, 1994.
126. Short, S. H., Surveys of dietary intake and nutrition knowledge of athletes and their coaches, in *Nutrition in Exercise and Sport*, Wolinsky, I. and Hickson, J. F., Jr., Eds., CRC Press, Boca Raton, FL, 1994, 367.
127. Simon, H. B., Exercise and human immune function, in *Psychoneuroimmunology*, Ader, R., Felten, D. L., and Cohen, N., Eds. Academic Press, New York, 1991, 869.

128. Simpson, J. R. and Hoffman-Goetz, L., Nutritional deficiencies and immunoregulatory cytokines, in *Nutrient Modulation of the Immune Response*, Cunningham-Rundles, S., Ed., Marcel Dekker, New York, 1993, 31.

129. Sletvold, O., Circadian rhythms of peripheral blood leukocytes in aging mice, *Mech. Aging Dev.*, 39, 251, 1987.

130. Smith, J. A., Telford, R. D., Baker, M. S., Hapel, A. J., and Weidemann, M. J., Cytokine immunoreactivity in plasma does not change after moderate endurance exercise, *J. Appl. Physiol.*, 73, 1396, 1992.

131. Sommer, A., Vitamin A status, resistance to infection, and childhood mortality, *Ann. N.Y. Acad. Sci.*, 587, 17, 1990.

132. Spinedi, E., Suescun, M. O., Hadid, R., Daneva, T., and Gaillard, R. C., Effects of gonadectomy and sex hormone therapy on the endotoxin-stimulated hypothalamo-pituitary-adrenal axis: evidence for a neruoendocrine-immunological sexual dimorphism, *Endocrinology*, 131, 2430, 1992.

133. Sprenger, H., Jacobs, C., Nain, M., Gressner, A. M., Prinz, H., Wesemann, W., and Gemsa, D., Enhanced release of cytokines, interleukin-2 receptors, and neopterin after long-distance running, *Clini. Immunol. Immunopathol.*, 63, 188, 1992.

134. Stallone, D. D., The influence of obesity and its treatment on the immune system, *Nutr. Rev.*, 52, 37, 50, 1994.

135. Steen, S. N. and Brownell, K. D., Patterns of weight loss and regain in wrestlers: has the tradition changed?, *Med. Sci. Sports Exerc.*, 22, 762, 1990.

136. Sternberg, E. M., Hill, J. M., Chouras, G. P., Kamilaris, T., Listwak, S. H., Gold, P. W., and Wilder, R. L., Inflammatory mediator-induced hypothalamic-pituitary-adrenal axis activation is defective in streptococcal cell wall arthritis-susceptible Lewis rats, *Proc. Natl. Acad. Sci.*, 8, 2374, 1989.

137. Strauss, R. H., Lanese, R. R., and Leizman, D. J., Illness and absence among wrestlers, swimmers, and gymnasts at a large university, *Am. J. Sports Med.*, 16, 653, 1988.

138. Stuchlikova, E., Juricova-Horakova, M., and Deyl, Z., New aspects of the dietary effect of life prolongation in rodents. What is the role of obesity in aging?, *Exp. Geront.*, 10, 141, 1975.

139. Subcommittee on the Tenth Edition of the RDAs Food and Nutrition Board, Commission on Life Sciences, National Research Council, *Recommended Dietary Allowances*, 10th ed., National Academy Press, Washington, D. C., 1989.

140. Tchervenkov, J. I. and Meakins, J. L., Altered host defense mechanisms in septic patients, in *Surgical Infections,* Fry, D. E., Ed., Little, Brown, Boston, 1994, 19.

141. The Office of Disease Prevention and Health Promotion, U.S. Public Health Service, U. S. Department of Health and Human Services, *Disease Prevention/Health Promotion: The Facts*. Bull Publishing, Palo Alto, 1988, 99.

142. Thibault, L. and Roberge, A. G., The nutritional status of subjects with anorexia nervosa, *Int. J. Vitam. Res.*, 57, 447, 1987.

143. Torun, B. and Chew, F., Protein-energy malnutrition, in *Modern Nutrition in Health and Disease*, Shils, M. E., Olson, H. A., and Shike, M., Eds. Lea & Febiger, Philadelphia, 1994, 950.

144. Tvede, N., Pedersen, B. K., Hansen, F. R., Bendix, T., Christensen, L. D., Galbo, H., and Halkjer-Kristensen, J., Effect of physical exercise on blood mononuclear cell subpopulations and in vitro proliferative responses, *Scand. J. Immunol.*, 29, 383, 1989.

145. Vaisman, N., Hahn, T., Dayan, Y., and Schattner, A., The effect of different nutritional states on cell-mediated cytotoxicity, *Immunol. Lett.*, 24, 37, 1990.

146. Van der Meer, J. W. M., Vogels, M. T. E., and Kullberg, B.-J., Interleukin-1 and related pro-inflammatory cytokines in the treatment of bacterial infections in neutropenic and non-neutropenic animals, *Biotherapy*, 7, 161, 1994.

147. Vande Wiele, R. I., Anorexia nervosa and the hypothalamus, *Hosp. Pract.*, 12, 45, 1977.

148. Wada, M., Morimoto, A., Watanabe, T., Sakata, Y., and Murakami, N., Effects of physical training on febrile and acute-phase responses induced in rats by bacterial endotoxin or interleukin-1, *J. Physiol. (London)*, 430, 595, 1990.

149. Weber, D. J., Rutala, W. A., Samsa, G. P., Santimaw, J. E., and Lemon, S. M., Obesity as a predictor of poor antibody response to Hepatitis B plasma vaccine, *J. Am. Med. Assoc.*, 22, 3187, 1985.

150. Weimer, H. E., Roberts, D. M., and Comb, J. C., The α-macrofetoprotein response to an inflammatory stimulus in fasted rats, *J. Nutr.*, 102, 873, 1972.

151. Weindruch, R. and Walford, R. L., *The Retardation of Aging and Disease by Dietary Restriction*, Charles C. Thomas, Springfield, 1988, 31, 186.

152. Weindruch, R., Albanes, D., and Kritchevsky, D., The role of calories and caloric restriction in carcinogenesis, *Hematol./Oncol. Clin. N. Am.*, 5, 79, 1991.

153. Weindruch, R., Walford, R. L., Fligiel, S., and Guthrie, D., The retardation of aging in mice by dietary restriction: longevity, cancer, immunity and lifetime energy intake, *J. Nutr.*, 116, 642, 1986.

154. Wing, E. J., Stanko, R. T., Winkelstein, A., and Adibi, S. A., Fasting-enhanced immune effector mechanisms in obese subjects, *Am. J. Med.*, 75, 91, 1983.

155. Wing, R. R. and Greeno, C. G., Behavioural and psychosocial aspects of obesity and its treatment, *Baillere's Clin. Endocrinol. Metab.*, 8, 689, 1994.

156. Xusheng, S., Yugi, X., Yongguang, Z., and Li, S., Effect of ballet on immunity in young people, *J. Sports Med. Phys. Fitness*, 30, 392, 1990.

157. Yoshikawa, T. T., Geriatric infectious diseases, *J. Am. Geriatr. Soc.*, 31, 34, 1983.